Sixth Edition

HEALTH PROMOTION IN NURSING PRACTICE

Sixth Edition

HEALTH PROMOTION IN NURSING PRACTICE

Nola J. Pender, PhD, RN, FAAN
Professor Emerita
University of Michigan
School of Nursing
Ann Arbor, Michigan

Carolyn L. Murdaugh, PhD, RN, FAAN
Professor and Associate Dean for Research
University of Arizona
College of Nursing
Tucson, Arizona

Mary Ann Parsons, PhD, RN, FAAN
Professor Emerita and Dean Emerita
University of South Carolina
College of Nursing
Columbia, South Carolina

Pearson

Boston   Columbus   Indianapolis   New York   San Francisco   Upper Saddle River
Amsterdam   Cape Town   Dubai   London   Madrid   Milan   Munich   Paris   Montréal   Toronto
Delhi   Mexico City   São Paulo   Sydney   Hong Kong   Seoul   Singapore   Taipei   Tokyo

Library of Congress Cataloging-in-Publication Data

Pender, Nola J., (Date)
  Health promotion in nursing practice/Nola J. Pender, Carolyn L. Murdaugh,
Mary Ann Parsons.—6th ed.
    p. cm.
  Includes bibliographical references and index.
  ISBN-13: 978-0-13-509721-2
  ISBN-10: 0-13-509721-5
  1. Health promotion.   2. Preventive health services.   3. Nursing.   I. Murdaugh, Carolyn L.
II. Parsons, Mary Ann.   III. Title.
  [DNLM: 1. Health Promotion—Nurses' Instruction.   2. Nursing Care—Nurses' Instruction.
3. Health Behavior—Nurses' Instruction.   4. Health Policy—Nurses' Instruction. WY 100 P397h 2011]
RT67.P56 2011
610.73—dc22

                                                                                    2009046239

Notice: Care has been taken to confirm the accuracy of information presented in this book. The authors, editors, and the publisher, however, cannot accept any responsibility for errors or omissions or for consequences from application of the information in this book and make no warranty, express or implied, with respect to its contents.

The authors and publisher have exerted every effort to ensure that drug selections and dosages set forth in this text are in accord with current recommendations and practice at time of publication. However, in view of ongoing research, changes in government regulations, and the constant flow of information relating to drug therapy and reactions, the reader is urged to check the package inserts of all drugs for any change in indications or dosage and for added warning and precautions. This is particularly important when the recommended agent is a new and/or infrequently employed drug.

Publisher: Julie Levin Alexander
Assistant to Publisher: Regina Bruno
Editor-in-Chief: Maura Connor
Assistant to the Editor-in-Chief: Deirdre MacKnight
Executive Acquisitions Editor: Kim Mortimer
Editorial Assistant: Marion Gottlieb
Assistant Editor: Sarah Wrocklage
Media Product Manager: Travis Moses-Westphal
Director of Marketing: David Gesell
Marketing Coordinator: Michael Sirinides
Managing Editor, Production: Patrick Walsh

Production Editor: Elm Street Publishing Services
Production Liaison: Anne Garcia
Permissions Researcher: Mary Dalton-Hoffman
Media Project Manager: Rachel Collett
Manufacturing Manager: Ilene Sanford
Design Coordinator: Kristine Carney
Cover Designer: Laura Ierardi
Composition: Integra Software Services Pvt. Ltd.
Printer/Binder: R.R. Donnelley
Cover Printer: R.R. Donnelley

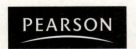

www.pearsonhighered.com

ISBN-13: 978-0-13-509721-2
ISBN-10:   0-13-509721-5

To all nurses who teach and role model health promotion.

—C. Murdaugh

To my five grandsons, Blake, Andrew, Sterling, Campbell, and Graham, for whom I wish a happy and healthy life.

—M. A. Parsons

CONTENTS

Part 2   Planning for Health Promotion and Prevention   87

FOREWORD

I am delighted to write the foreword for the sixth edition of *Health Promotion in Nursing Practice*. The value added to health care by health promotion can no longer be debated. Impressive data support the critical role of health promotion in decreasing health care costs and adding quality years to the life span of each individual. Nurses must accept the challenge of designing and providing high-quality health promotion services in every health care setting. As I travel to countries on every continent, I hear about exciting plans to integrate health promotion into the fabric of national health plans. There is worldwide recognition that priorities in health care must change to make health promotion the key global strategy for improving health and decreasing health disparities. In the United States, health care reform is a major issue that Americans must address. This is the time to create a health care system in which health promotion is the leading edge of health care.

Healthy individuals have the right to live in healthy communities that are supported by healthy public policies. This is an unbeatable combination for quality existence. Every nursing school should have a comprehensive plan for integrating health promotion knowledge and skills in all levels of the curriculum. Students should develop expertise in behavioral counseling to deliver health promotion services in primary, acute care, and chronic care settings. Further, students need skills to work with communities to inspire and empower citizens as well as educate community leaders to build healthy neighborhoods in which they can live and prosper. Nurses also have exciting roles in the development of positive local and national health policies through advocacy and political action. Experiential learning in health promotion in clinics, schools, work sites, acute care facilities, and policy-making agencies is an essential part of nursing education. This text is intended to support quality classroom and clinical experiences in health promotion and prevention for undergraduate and graduate students.

Aspects of this new edition that are particularly noteworthy include the enhanced discussion of the role of the environment in health promotion, new information about use of technology for prevention and health promotion, and additional valuable Web resources. The reader is also introduced to Healthy People 2020, the national health goals for the next decade. You will find that each chapter offers thought-provoking information that challenges you as a nurse to expand your role in delivering health promotion services and conducting health promotion research.

Dr. Carolyn Murdaugh and Dr. Mary Ann Parsons are ideal authors for this text. Their rich experience in teaching health promotion to nursing students as well as their research in health promotion for vulnerable populations enable them to offer exceptional insights into strategies for health promotion as an integral part of nursing in the 21st century.

Designing health promotion services as an essential component of all health care systems is an exciting adventure with professional satisfaction derived from making an important difference in the lives of individuals and families. I hope as a nurse you will accept the challenge to participate in this adventure.

Nola J. Pender, PhD, RN, FAAN
Professor Emerita
School of Nursing
University of Michigan
Distinguished Professor
Marcella Niehoff School of Nursing
Loyola University, Chicago

PREFACE

Major changes are occurring to promote health and health care reform as we complete the sixth edition of this book. Health care disparities exist and continue to increase as the uninsured and underinsured populations in this country intensify. Obesity, a preventable health problem, is an epidemic in our children and adults and annually consumes almost $150 billion in direct health care costs and lost productivity. The American society has become obesogenic, one characterized by an environment that promotes a greater caloric intake, unhealthy foods, and an inactive lifestyle. Now, more than ever, healthy lifestyles must be promoted and established, beginning in early childhood.

The purpose of the book has not changed and continues to be threefold: (1) to present an overview of the major individual and community models and theories that guide health promotion interventions; (2) to offer evidence-based strategies that can be used in practice settings to implement health promotion programs to promote healthy life styles for diverse populations; and (3) to foster critical thinking about future opportunities for health promotion research and the most effective interventions for practice. We believe information in the book is the foundation on which to build the science and practice of health promotion.

The content of the book is organized into six sections. In Part 1, "The Human Quest for Health," *health* and *health promotion* are defined, and individual and community models to promote health are described. Part 2, "Planning for Health Promotion and Prevention," strategies are described to effectively assess health, health beliefs, and health behaviors and develop a health promotion plan. "Interventions for Health Promotion and Prevention" are addressed in Part 3, focusing on physical activity, nutrition, stress management, and social support. In Part 4, strategies for "Evaluating the Effectiveness of Health Promotion" interventions are addressed. Part 5, "Health Promotion in Diverse Populations," includes strategies for self-care and approaches to promote health in vulnerable populations. In Part 6, "Approaches for Promoting a Healthier Society," community partnerships for health promotion are described as well as policies and programs to promote social and environmental changes. The content in all chapters has been expanded and updated based on published research evidence. The Healthy People 2020 overarching goals are introduced, and an ecological approach to health promotion has been woven throughout the book, as research has substantiated the need to move beyond the individual to promote healthy lifestyles. In addition, the role of technology in health promotion is described, as well as the role of the electronic health record in health promotion. The term *client* is used rather than *patient* throughout the book to refer to individuals, families, and communities who are active participants in health promotion. *Health* and *wellness* are used interchangeably. Last, *health protection* and *prevention* are also used interchangeably throughout the book.

Sincere appreciation is extended to Pearson Education's Kim Mortimer and Sarah Wrocklage, who have worked with us in the preparation of the book. We are also indebted to Melinda Fletcher, Administrative Associate in the College of Nursing, University of Arizona, who performed the typing, formatting, preparation of tables and figures, and editing of chapters.

Carolyn Murdaugh
Mary Ann Parsons

Reviewers

Carolyn L. Blue, PhD, RN, CHES
*The University of North Carolina
at Greensboro
Greensboro, North Carolina*

Darrice E. Kelley, RN, MS
*Excelsior College
Albany, New York*

Margaret Lunney, PhD, RN
*College of Staten Island, City University
of New York
Staten Island, New York*

Holly Evans Madison, PhD (c), RN
*Excelsior College
Albany, New York*

Margaret McAllister PhD, FNP-C,
FAANP
*University of Massachusetts—Boston
Boston, Massachusetts*

Vanessa Miller, DrPH, MSN
*California State University—Fullerton
Fullerton, California*

Jeanne Morrison, PhD, MSN
Kaplan University

Global Health Promotion: Challenges of the 21st Century

The establishment of health promotion as an integral aspect of health care and society continues to present challenges for all nations. Accumulating evidence indicates that health promotion holds promise for maintaining vigor, vitality, and productivity into the eighth and ninth decades of life for an increasing proportion of the world population. Governments of many countries are developing national health promotion plans to shape the future direction of health care, as the link between a healthy and productive population and national welfare and economic prosperity is now recognized. Overall goals are to help people of all ages stay healthy, to optimize health in the presence of chronic disease or disability, and to create healthy environments in which to live.

The Commission on Social Determinants of Health, formed by the World Health Organization (WHO) in 2005, examined the evidence on equity in implementing health promotion strategies and how to foster a worldwide approach to achieve equity. The commission's final report, *Closing the Gap in a Generation* (WHO, 2008a), expressed the commission's aspirations for actions that involve government, civil society, local communities, businesses, global and international organizations, and research institutions. Resulting health-oriented public policy can facilitate positive changes in health behavior norms as well as provide health-promoting and health-enhancing environments on a national and international scale (Laxminarayan et al., 2006). Health is the responsibility of all, not just the health care sector. Individual, community, and political will and resources all working together are necessary to achieve health for all (WHO, 2008a).

GLOBAL PROGRESS TOWARD HEALTH PROMOTION

All people of the world are part of a global community or health mega system. In today's world, what affects one country affects other countries as well. The *Bangkok Charter for Health Promotion in a Globalized World* identifies actions and commitments needed to address the determinants of health in a globalized world through health promotion (WHO, 2005). The charter builds on the values and strategies for health promotion established by the Ottawa Charter for Health Promotion, which defines health promotion as a process enabling people to increase control over and improve their health (WHO, 1986). Both charters emphasize the necessity of including individuals as well as communities, societies, governments at all levels, and international organizations to achieve health.

This broader approach to health promotion is well illustrated by the Healthy Cities Projects, which WHO initiated more than 25 years ago in Europe. The ongoing project engages local governments in health development through extensive community participation and institutional changes to implement comprehensive city plans for health promotion. The target endpoints are evaluated on not only morbidity and mortality but also prevalence of health-promoting behaviors, quality of the physical and social environment, and extent of community empowerment and action. Each five-year plan focuses on core priority themes. The Phase V (2009–2013) overarching goal focuses on health equity through caring and supportive environments, healthy living, and healthy urban design. Building healthy cities is an ecological approach that has yet to reach its full potential for improving the health of people. An improvement in well-being throughout the life span, especially for vulnerable populations, will enable cities and nations to benefit from greater economic prosperity and improved national welfare (WHO, 2008b).

The health-promoting features of social policies, organizations, and environments are highlighted in a report published 30 years after the defining international primary health care conference in 1978 at Alma-Ata, Kazakhstan. The 2008 report, *Primary Health Care: Now More Than Ever* (WHO, 2008c), was dedicated to reemphasizing primary health care and offers an assessment of global health with a focus on primary care. The report emphasizes primary care as a way to help meet the challenge of considerable and increasing health inequities and the effects of globalization on the burden of chronic and communicable as well as noncommunicable diseases.

Reforms identified in the report reflect a convergence among the values of primary care, the performance of the health system, and the expectation of citizens. They include:

- Universal coverage to ensure equity, social justice, and the end of exclusion
- Service delivery organized around people's needs and expectations
- Public policy that secures healthier communities through integration of public health and primary care
- Leadership that is reflective of inclusion, participation, and negotiation (WHO, 2008c)

A major challenge worldwide is to develop credible, widely recognized, high-quality standards to evaluate the effectiveness of multicultural health promotion interventions. This task presents a formidable challenge given the complexity of health promotion interventions ranging from changing individual and group behaviors to changing policies that set norms for behavior. Use of behavioral surveillance systems is critical to assessing progress toward health promotion objectives, as are time-sensitive strategies to analyze and use data to make strategic decisions about "what works." Meeting these challenges is essential to further the global agenda for health promotion (Abbott & Coenen, 2008).

INFLUENCE OF TECHNOLOGICAL ADVANCES ON GLOBAL HEALTH PROMOTION

In an age of rapid advances in technology, innovations in communication technology offer unprecedented opportunities to provide health-related information worldwide. Innovative use of interactive computer technology and interactive television through worldwide networks is enabling health professionals and consumers to collaborate as never before in tailoring health communications to the special needs of individuals and families from diverse cultures and sociocultural backgrounds (Smeets, Brug, & de Vries, 2008; McDaniel, Schutte, & Keller, 2008).

The accelerated technological revolution has multiplied the potential for improving health globally. Health systems are increasing their capabilities to literally "reach around the world" to provide open access to the latest health knowledge and create a national and international resource for informed health care decision making by both providers and consumers. Improving vulnerable populations' accessibility to and competence in using computerized information systems must be a top priority.

NATIONAL PROGRESS TOWARD HEALTH PROMOTION

Unhealthy lifestyles and environments are responsible for a high percentage of the morbidity and mortality in the United States. Unless the health care system is significantly changed to influence lifestyles and environments, the nation's health profile will continue to deteriorate (Brahan & Bauchner, 2005). Demographic changes toward an older population and a more ethnically and culturally diverse population create new demands for health promotion and prevention services in primary care and public health (U.S. Department of Health and Human Services, 2006).

Public support continues to grow for coverage of health promotion and illness prevention services by third-party payers. There is also an increased interest in health promotion and preventive services that have been shown to be effective in promoting positive behavior change and decreasing health care costs. The federal government and private insurers have a mandate to continue to evaluate the impact of providing an array of health promotion services to individuals and families, including the millions of citizens in the United States who are currently uninsured or underinsured.

Healthy People: The U.S. Surgeon General's Report on Health Promotion and Disease Prevention is an initiative to set science-based objectives for promoting health and preventing disease, and to monitor the outcomes of these national health objectives. The objectives address a broad range of health needs, encourage informed decision making, promote collaboration, and measure the effect of the outcomes on individuals, groups, families and communities. *Healthy People* provides users with up-to-date information on health status, public health priority setting, and significant statistical analyses on health promotion and disease prevention. Initiated in 1979, the process involves governmental officials, businesses, professional groups, researchers and academic institutions in setting the vision, mission, goals and objectives every 10 years.

Midway through each decade the U.S. Department of Health and Human Services conducts a midcourse review of the national objectives and assesses progress toward meeting them. In 2006 the midcourse review of the 2010 objectives showed that only 10% met the set target of 281 objectives with baseline data available. Less than half (49%) moved toward the target, and 14% demonstrated mixed progress. Moreover, 6% showed no change, and 20% moved away from the target. The assessment of the quality and years of healthy life showed that while overall life expectancy continues to improve, the white population continues to have a longer life expectancy than the black population; all women have a longer life expectancy than men with greater expected years in good or better health and free of limitations and chronic diseases; a slight increase was noted for men in expected years in good or better health.

The assessment of the second goal of Healthy People 2010—to eliminate health disparities—concluded that substantial disparities continue between all minority populations and the white non-Hispanic population. There was no change in disparities among all racial populations for 81% of the objectives. Disparity based on education level, gender, income level, geographic location, and disability status had mixed outcomes, but overall minimal improvement was noted at the midcourse review (U.S. Department of Health and Human Services, 2006).

The process for developing *Healthy People 2020* was initiated in 2009 with a vision of "a society in which all people live long and healthy lives" (www.healthypeople.gov/HP2020). Addressing a long-standing criticism, the *Healthy People 2020* process moves from setting aspirational goals (i.e., increase quality and years of life, and eliminate health disparities), to setting realistic and achievable goals:

- Achieve health equity, eliminate disparities, and improve health for all groups
- Eliminate preventable disease, disability, injury, and premature death
- Create social and physical environments that promote good health for all and
- Promote healthy development and healthy behaviors across every stage of life

The development and implementation of *Healthy People 2020* can be viewed at www.healthypeople.gov/HP2020.

Achieving Healthy People objectives is a continuing challenge. The process of developing the plan has been very successful, but the resources required and commitment needed from individuals, families, schools, and communities to implement the plans have resulted in meeting or exceeding only a minimal number of objective targets. Increased attention to the social determinants of health means that local, state and national policy changes and resources are necessary to improve the health and well-being of persons of all ages and increase the prevalence of healthy lifestyles in the population.

The National Health Interview Survey (NHIS) provides another view of our national progress toward health. The Centers for Disease Control and Prevention's National Center for Health Statistics (2007) sponsor the annual NHIS household survey conducted by the U.S. Census Bureau. The result of the 2006 survey of 24,275 civilian, noninstitutionalized adults was based on a response rate of 71%. Of adults over 18 years of age, 61% reported excellent or very good health, yet 62% reported they never participated in vigorous leisure-time physical activity, One-fifth (21%) were smokers. Based on body mass index estimates, 35% were overweight and 26% were obese (Pleis & Lethbridge-Cejku, 2007). Females were more likely to report fair or poor health.

The Youth Risk Behavioral Surveillance System (YRBSS) is administered annually to monitor priority health risk behaviors that contribute to the leading causes of death, disability, and social problems among youth in America (Eaton et al., 2008). A 2007 midyear report showed that motor vehicle crashes, other unintentional injuries, homicide, and suicide accounted for 72% of all deaths among persons aged 10–24 years.

Age-adjusted and non-age-adjusted health statistics for U.S. children are available from the 2006 NHIS on selected health measures for noninstitutionalized population of children under 18 years of age. In this survey, 82% of children had excellent or very good health. Only 5% of children had no usual place of health care and 10% had no health insurance. Poverty status was associated with the health of the respondent. Four out of ten children in poor families reported excellent health while six out of ten children in families that were not poor reported excellent health (Bloom & Cohen, 2007).

A national children's prospective, multiyear, epidemiologic study of 100,000 American children, funded by the U.S. Congress through the Children's Act of 2000, began in 2007. Children will be followed from conception to 21 years of age. Environmental exposures are assessed in the children's homes, schools, and communities. Genetic material is also collected to permit study of gene–environment interactions. The results of this study will guide future development of a comprehensive blueprint for health promotion and disease prevention in children (Landrigan et al., 2006).

Much progress has been made to prevent and control disease processes. The priority health problems among America's children, youth, and adults stem from risky behaviors and lifestyle choices. More effective individual, family, and community interventions are needed to reduce risk and improve health outcomes to move the nation toward a more healthy society.

HEALTH PROMOTION AND DISEASE PREVENTION: IS THERE A DIFFERENCE?

The most important difference between health promotion and disease or illness prevention is in the underlying motivation for the behavior on the part of individuals and aggregates. *Health promotion* is behavior motivated by the desire to increase well-being and actualize human health potential. *Disease prevention*, also called *health protection*, is behavior motivated by a desire to actively avoid illness, detect it early, or maintain functioning within the constraints of illness. The *actualizing tendency* underlying health promotion increases states of positive tension in order to promote change and growth, which is often experienced as a challenge and facilitates behaviors expressive of human potential. The *stabilizing tendency* underlying disease prevention is evident in the functioning of homeokinetic mechanisms and is directed toward maintaining balance and equilibrium. The stabilizing tendency is responsible for protective maneuvers, primarily maintaining the internal and external environments within a range compatible with continuing existence.

The purest form of motivation for health promotion exists in childhood through young adulthood when energy, vitality, and vigor are important to attain but the threat of chronic illness seems remote. Youth may engage in health behaviors for the pleasure of doing so or for the improvement of physical appearance and attractiveness to others. In the adult years, when human vulnerabilities become more apparent, both motivations for health behavior usually coexist. For example, an older adult may be motivated to jog in order to improve stamina and energy (health promotion) but also to avoid cardiovascular disease (disease prevention). Regulatory measures for clean air may be passed to prevent exposure to asbestos as a cancer risk factor (disease prevention) but also to improve the overall quality of the environment (health promotion). Three important theoretical differences exist between health promotion and disease prevention:

1. Health promotion is not illness or disease specific; prevention is.
2. Health promotion is "approach" motivated, whereas prevention is "avoidance" motivated.
3. Health promotion seeks to expand positive potential for health, whereas prevention seeks to thwart the occurrence of insults to health and well-being.

In reality, health promotion and disease prevention are complementary processes. Both processes are critical to the quality of life at all developmental stages. Although attention is given to prevention throughout the book, a much greater emphasis is placed on health promotion.

THE MULTIDIMENSIONAL NATURE OF HEALTH PROMOTION

Community, socioeconomic level, culture, and environment affect the health of individuals and families markedly. The context either sustains and expands health potential or inhibits the emergence of health and well-being. Health promotion is a process that enables individuals, groups, families and communities to exhibit control over the determinants of their health behaviors and to take action.

It is important for health care providers to appreciate and consider the complexity of health promotion, as it focuses on six dimensions.

- Individual
- Family
- Community
- Socioeconomic
- Cultural
- Environmental

Individual Dimension

Individuals play a critical role in determining their own health status, because self-care represents the dominant mode of health care in our society. Many personal decisions are made daily that shape lifestyle and the social and physical environments. Health promotion at the individual level improves personal decision making and health practices.

Throughout this book, the frame of reference for individual prevention and health promotion activities is the total life span from childhood to the older adult years. Every developmental stage must be considered in formulating national health policy and programs if the quality of life for people of all ages is to be significantly enhanced through health promotion efforts.

Family Dimension

The family plays a critical role in the development of health beliefs and health behaviors. Almost all individuals identify with a family group in which members influence one another's ideas and actions. Each family has a characteristic value, role, and power structure as well as unique communication patterns. In addition, families fulfill affective, socialization, health care, and coping functions in varying ways. Parenting styles and family environments encourage healthy and/or unhealthy behaviors that may persist throughout the life span. The health of children is linked to family stress and health-promoting or health-damaging behaviors of parents. Much more attention must be given to the development of strategies to promote family wellness to initiate healthy behaviors early in childhood.

Community Dimension

Community wellness is achieved by multiple actions that improve the conditions of family and community life. Benefits of community-based health promotion programs are as follows:

1. Enhanced opportunities for information exchange and social support among members of the target population
2. Reduced unit cost of programming because large groups, rather than individuals, receive health promotion services
3. Availability of networks that facilitate and coordinate health promotion efforts
4. Potential for widespread change in social norms about health and health behavior
5. Coordinated approach to promote the health of large populations
6. Access to a broad array of media/technology to disseminate health information
7. Availability of aggregate indices to track the health status of the population
8. Inclusion of the talents and resources of community residents resulting in a sense of commitment to health promotion programs

Community programs for prevention and health promotion enhance the dissemination of health information and encourage changes in cultural norms relevant to health and health behavior.

Socioeconomic Dimension

The social conditions in which people live have a dramatic influence on their health. Poverty, insufficient food, inadequate housing, poor sanitation, and limited education are major factors that must be addressed to improve the health of individuals. New health promotion strategies are needed to address these factors through social, institutional, and political change, as traditional individual approaches have not been effective.

Cultural Dimension

The role of culture underlies the effectiveness of health promotion efforts and must be emphasized to achieve individual, family, community, and societal goals (Armer & Radina, 2006). The complexity of culture includes race and ethnicity, socioeconomic status, gender, age, sexual orientation, disability, and geographic setting. Culture is the learned and shared experiences that create a person's worldview. Hereditary factors, customs, language, clothing, ideas, music, art, religion, food habits, and other components contribute to the cultural identity of an individual, a family, a community, or a group. Although groups may share core values, not all members of the group have identical experiences; therefore, diversity is seen in every group or community in every society. Culture says who we are but not what we can be. Cultural stereotyping assumes that all individuals share the same characteristics as others in their cultural group. Members of a group may have different experiences that result in different approaches to decision making and health behaviors. Without understanding the role of culture and linguistic competence in health promotion programs, these programs will not be successful. Everyone must be treated as an individual within a cultural framework and health promotion activities tailored accordingly. The challenge of the 21st century is to create a future in which people's chances for a healthy life are possible by coherent action on a global strategy and where cultural differences, economics, and social standing are not the determinants of who benefits from societal resources (Fields et al., 2006).

Environmental Dimension

The level of environmental wellness affects the extent to which individuals, families, and communities achieve their optimum potential. *Environment* is a comprehensive term meaning the physical, interpersonal, and economic circumstances in which we live. The quality of the environment is dependent on the absence of toxic substances, availability of aesthetic or restorative experiences, and accessibility of human and economic resources needed for healthful and productive living. Socioeconomic conditions such as unemployment, poverty, crime, prejudice, and isolation have adverse effects on the health of adults as well as children and youth. Environmental wellness is manifest in harmony and balance between human beings and their surroundings.

THE CONTRIBUTION OF NURSES TO THE HEALTH PROMOTION TEAM

Health professionals have been slow to promulgate curricula to ensure development of knowledge and expertise in delivering evidenced-based health promotion (Genuis, 2008; Whitehead, 2007). Greater expediency is needed to move scientific breakthroughs into evidence-based practice in order for the public to benefit in a timely manner from new knowledge.

Breakthroughs in understanding the human genome will shift the balance from diagnosis and disease to prediction and health enhancement. Molecular prevention is fast becoming such a reality that soon disease will be managed prior to symptoms. Nurses are pivotal in helping clients combine knowledge about personal genetic makeup, genetic prevention techniques, and behavior change strategies to prevent illnesses for which they are at high risk. Nursing research agendas must pioneer and test innovative biopsychosocial nursing care strategies.

Nurses, because of their biopsychosocial expertise and frequent, continuing contact with clients, have the unique opportunity of providing global leadership to health professionals in the promotion of better health for the global community. Nurses should be at the forefront in developing interactive health education counseling programs and behavioral interventions that capitalize on emerging information technology breakthroughs. A "one size fits all" approach to health promotion programming has become outdated. Technology offers nurses new tools to further develop individualized health care, to which they have long been committed. Nurses must serve as role models of health-promoting lifestyles and as leaders to activate communities for health promotion. Nurses, as the largest single group of health care providers, continue to play a vital role in making health promotion and illness prevention services available to all populations, including the underserved and vulnerable. Payers are increasingly willing to reimburse for health promotion and prevention services that add value to health care (Aldana, Merrill, Price, Hardy, & Hager, 2005; Parks & Steelman, 2008). Nurses can provide leadership in bringing these resources together to improve the health of individuals, families, and communities.

Primary care and community care delivery systems must continue to eliminate barriers to delivering high-quality health promotion services. Nurses must continue to work toward the redistribution of health care resources so that high-quality health promotion and illness prevention services are available to all. In an environment of economic constraints, this requires that resources spent on health care are balanced with other resource demands (Borghi & Jan, 2008). A continuing challenge of the 21st century is to provide access to knowledge and services that promote health for all segments of an increasing culturally diverse global population.

In summary, globalization has resulted in challenges to health promotion that are beyond the dominion of individuals, communities, and nations (Mittelmark, 2007). Population growth, urbanization, and consumerism are challenging global resources and damaging the environment. In addition, the spread of communicable diseases and increases in chronic disease are affecting all societies. More importantly, the origins of chronic diseases can be found in childhood, pointing to the critical need to focus health-promoting approaches on young children as well as adults. These new challenges warrant new approaches. Health promotion must be linked to empowering individuals and communities, and evidence that supports the effectiveness of health promotion must be used to develop policy and guide practice. A new agenda for health promotion will play a critical role in shaping the health for all.

Selected Web Sites

World Health Organization (WHO)
www.who.int/about/en/
WHO is the directing and coordinating authority for health within the United Nations system. It is responsible for providing leadership on global health matters, shaping the health research agenda, setting norms and standards, articulating evidence-based policy, providing technology support to countries, and monitoring and assessing health trends.

Healthy People 2010 Summary of Progress
http://www.healthypeople.gov/data/midcourse/html/execsummary/progress.htm
Healthy People 2010 is a comprehensive, national health promotion and disease prevention program. It is a road map for improving the health of all the people in the United States during the 21st century. The midcourse review provides an assessment of the progress made during the first half of the decade.

Healthy People 2020 Vision, Mission, and Overarching Goals
http://www.healthypeople.gov/HP2020/Comments/SubjectFocus
The process for defining the vision, mission, and goals for 2020 involves government officials, professional organizations, researchers, businesses, and academic institutions.

Summary Health Statistics for U.S. Adults: National Health Interview Survey, 2007
http://www.cdc.gov/nchs/about/major/nhis/released 200806.htm
This early release report presents health statistics from the NHIS for the noninstitutionalized adult population, classified by sex, age, race and ethnicity, education, family income, poverty status, health insurance coverage, marital status, and place and region of residence.

Summary Statistics for U.S. Children: National Health Interview Survey: 2006
www.childstats.gov/americaschildren07/surveys.asp
This report represents both age-adjusted and un-adjusted statistics from the 2006 NHIS on selected health measures for children under 18 years of age, classified by sex, age, race, Hispanic origin, family structure, parent education, family income, poverty status, health insurance coverage, place of residence, region, and current health status.

Forum on Child and Family Statistics
www.childstats.gov/americaschildren07
America's Children: Key National Indicators of Well-Being, 2007 is a compendium of indicators—drawn from the most reliable official statistics—illustrative of both the promises and the difficulties confronting young Americans. The report presents

38 key indicators on important aspects of children's lives. These indicators are easily understood by broad audiences, objectively based on substantial research, balanced so that no single area of children's lives dominates the report, measured regularly so that they can be updated to show trends over time, and representative of large segments of the population rather than one particular group.

Youth Risk Behavior Surveillance System (YRBSS)
http://www.cdc.gov/HealthyYouth/yrbs
The YRBSS monitors priority health risk behaviors of 9th to 12th grade students. The YRBSS includes national, state, and local school-based surveys conducted every two years.

References

Abbott, P., & Coenen, A. (2008). Globalization and advances in information and communication technologies: The impact on nursing and health. *Nursing Outlook, 56*(5), 238–246.

Aldana, S. G., Merrill, R. M., Price, K., Hardy, A., & Hager, R. (2005, February). Financial impact of a comprehensive multisite workplace health promotion program. *Preventive Medicine, 40*(2), 131–137.

Armer, J. M., & Radina, M. E. (2006). Definition of health and health promotion behaviors among Midwestern old order Amish families. *Journal of Multicultural Nursing & Health, 12*(3), 44–53.

Bloom, B., & Cohen, R. A. (2007). Summary health statistics for U.S. children: National health interview survey, 2006. *Vital Health Statistics, 10*(234), 1–79.

Borghi, J., & Jan, S. (2008). Measuring the benefits of health promotion programmes: Application of the contingent valuation method. *Health Policy, 87*(2), 235–248.

Brahan, D., & Bauchner, H. (2005). Current child health challenges and opportunities in the United States. *Current Paediatrics, 15*(3), 239–245.

Centers for Disease Control and Prevention's National Center for Health Statistics. (2007). *National Health Interview Survey (NHIS)— Celebrating the first 50 years: 1957–2007.* Retrieved from http://www.cdc.gov/nchs/about/major/nhis/about200806.htm

Eaton, D. K., Kann, L., Kinchen, S., Shanklin, S., Ross, J., Hawkins, J., et al. (2008). Youth risk behavior surveillance—United States, 2007. *Morbidity and Mortality Weekly Report.* Retrieved from http://www.cdc.gov/mmwr/preview/mmwrhtml/ss5704a1.htm

Fields, N., Pongsiri, M., Wetzel, D., Reynolds, J., Miller, P., Waghiyi, V., et al. (2006). Promoting tribal science and wellness: Linking subsistence culture to differential exposures. *Abstracts of the U.S. Environmental Protection Agency Science Forum.* Washington, DC, May 16–18, 2006.

Genuis, S. J. (2008). Medical practice and community health care in the 21st Century: A time of change. *Public Health, 12*(7), 671–680.

Landrigan, P. J., Trasande, L., Thorpe, L. E., Gwynn, C., Lioy, P. J., D'Alton, M. E., et al. (2006). Special article: The national children's study: A 21-year prospective study of 100,000 American children. *Pediatrics, 118*(5), 2173–2186.

Laxminarayan, R., Jamison, D. T., Mills, A., Breman, J., Measham, A., Alleyne, G., et al. (2006). Advancement of global health: Key messages from the disease control priorities project. *The Lancet, 367*(9517), 1193–1208.

McDaniel, A., Schutte, D., & Keller, L. (2008). Consumer health informatics: From genomics to population health. *Nursing Outlook, 56*(5), 216–223.

Mittelmark, M. (2007). Shaping the future of health promotion: priorities for action. *Health Promotion International, 23*, 98–102.

Parks, K. M., & Steelman, L. A. (2008). Organizational wellness programs: A meta-analysis. *Journal of Occupational Health Psychology, 13*(1), 58–68.

Pleis, J. R., & Lethbridge-Cejku, M. (2007). Summary health statistics for U.S. adults: National Health Interview Survey, 2006. *Vital and Health Statistics, 10*(235), 1–153.

Smeets, T., Brug, J., & de Vries, H. (2008, June). Effects of tailoring health messages on physical activity. *Health Education Research,* 23(3): 402–413.

U.S. Department of Health and Human Services. (2006). *Midcourse review of Healthy People 2010.* Retrieved from http://www .healthypeople.gov/data/midcourse/default .htm

Whitehead, D. (2007). Reviewing health promotion in nursing education. *Nurse Education Today,* 27(3), 225–237.

World Health Organization. (1986). *Ottawa charter for health promotion.* Geneva, Switzerland: WHO.

———— (2005). *Bangkok charter for health promotion in a globalized world.* Retrieved from http://www.who.int/healthpromotion/ conferences/6gchp/bangkok_charter/en/ index.html

———— (2008a). *Closing the gap in a generation: Health equity through action on the social determinants of health.* Commission on Social Determinants of Health, Final Report, Executive Summary. Geneva, Switzerland: WHO.

———— (2008b). *Healthy cities and urban governance.* Geneva: WHO. Retrieved from http:/ /www.euro.who.int/healthy-cities

———— (2008c). *The world health report 2008: Primary health care: Now more than ever.* Geneva, Switzerland: WHO.

PART 1

The Human Quest for Health

CHAPTER 1

Toward a Definition of Health

OBJECTIVES

This chapter will enable the reader to:

1. Compare traditional and holistic definitions of health.
2. Contrast conceptions of individual health as stability and health as actualization.
3. Describe conceptions of health by nurse theorists.
4. Discuss family and community definitions of health.
5. Describe the social determinants of health.
6. Discuss the emergence and significance of global health.
7. Describe the changing conceptions of health promotion.

Outline

- Health as an Evolving Concept
- Health and Illness: Distinct Entities or Opposite Ends of a Continuum?
- Definitions of Health that Focus on Individuals
  - A. Health as Stability
  - B. Health as Actualization
  - C. Health as Actualization and Stability
  - D. An Integrated View of Health
- Definitions of Health That Focus on the Family
- Definitions of Health That Focus on the Community
- Social Determinants of Health
- Social Determinants and Global Health
- Conceptions of Health Promotion
- Measurement of Health

- **Opportunities for Research on Health**
- **Considerations for Practice in the Context of Holistic Health**
- **Summary**
- **Learning Activities**
- **Selected Web Sites**
- **References**

Health, person, environment, and nursing constitute the commonly accepted metaparadigm of the discipline of nursing (American Nurses Association, 2003; Fawcett, 2005). Although health is the frequently articulated goal of nursing, different conceptions about the meaning of health are common. These differences result from the increasingly diverse social values and norms that shape conceptualizations of health in societies with many distinct ethnic, religious, or cultural groups. What many health professionals once assumed was a universally accepted definition of health—the absence of diagnosable disease—is actually only one of many views of health held today. All people who are free of disease are not equally healthy. Furthermore, health can exist without illness, but illness never exists without health as its context (Pender, 1990).

The emergence of health promotion as the central strategy for improving health has shifted the paradigm from defining health in traditional medical terms (the curative model within a biologic perspective) to a multidimensional definition of health with social, economic, cultural, and environmental dimensions. In a multidimensional model of health, benefits can potentially be achieved from positive changes in any one of the health dimensions (Benson, 1996). This expanded perspective of health opens up multiple options for improving health and no longer places the responsibility for poor health entirely on the individual.

During the course of human development, the definition of health changes over the life span. As children mature and move into adolescence, their definition of health becomes more inclusive and more abstract (Millstein, 1994). Health definitions of adolescents show a trend toward greater thematic diversity (physical, mental, social, and emotional health) and less emphasis on the absence of illness with increasing age (Millstein & Irwin, 1987). Older adults hold a definition of health that integrates the physical, mental, spiritual, and social aspects of health, reflecting how health is embedded in everyday experiences (Arcury, Quandt, & Bell, 2001). In addition, gender differences in health have been put forth because perceived determinants of health differ between men and women (Denton, Prus, & Walters, 2004). Possible explanations for these differences include genetic and biologic factors as well as social and behavioral factors (Erikssen, Delive, Eklof, & Hagberg, 2007). The social structural context of men and women has been documented to be a major determinant of gender differences, as the power balance between men and women plays a major role in women's health (Belhadj & Toure', 2008). The promotion of gender equality and empowerment interventions is crucial to improving women's health. Nursing can have a significant role in provision of education and knowledge sharing to promote empowerment to increase the health and well-being of women.

In a positive model of health, emphasis is placed on strengths, resiliencies, resources, potentials, and capabilities rather than on existing pathology. Despite a philosophic and conceptual shift in thinking about health, the nature of health as a positive life process is less understood empirically, as attention continues to focus on forces that undermine health and lead to disease, rather than factors that lead to health. Morbidity (prevalence of illness) and mortality (death) are still commonly used to define the health of a population. These indicators are problematic, as they more accurately reflect disease burden and the need for health care, not health (Congdon, 2001). A focus on disease morbidity and mortality frames health within a biologic definition: the body without disease. However, evidence indicates that complex interwoven forces embedded in the social context of people's lives determine health. Health cannot be separated from one's life conditions, as neighborhood, social relationships, food, work, and leisure, which lie outside the realm of health practice, positively or negatively influence health long before morbid states are evident (McMullin, 2005).

HEALTH AS AN EVOLVING CONCEPT

A brief review of the historical development of the concept of health provides the background for examining definitions of health found in the professional literature. The word *health* as it is commonly used did not appear in writing until approximately AD 1000. It is derived from the Old English word *health,* meaning being safe or sound and whole of body (Sorochan, 1970). Historically, physical wholeness was of major importance for acceptance in social groups. Persons suffering from disfiguring diseases, like leprosy, or congenital malformations were ostracized from society. Not only was there fear of contagion of physically obvious disease, there was also repulsion at the grotesque appearance. Being healthy was construed as natural or in harmony with nature, whereas being unhealthy was thought of as unnatural or contrary to nature (Dolfman, 1973).

With the advent of the scientific era and the resultant increase in medical discoveries, illness came to be regarded with less disgust, and society became concerned about helping individuals escape its catastrophic effects. *Health* in this context was defined as "freedom from disease." Because disease could be traced to a specific cause, often microbial, it could be diagnosed. The notion of health as a disease-free state was extremely popular into the first half of the 20th century and was recognized by many as *the* definition of health (Wylie, 1970). Health and illness were viewed as extremes on a continuum; the absence of one indicated the presence of the other. This gave rise to "ruling out disease" to assess health, an approach still prevalent in the medical community today. The underlying erroneous assumption is that a disease-free population is a healthy population.

The concept of mental health as we now know it did not exist until the latter part of the 19th century. Individuals who exhibited unpredictable or hostile behavior were labeled "lunatics" and ostracized in much the same way as those with disfiguring physical ailments. Being put away with little if any human care was considered their "just due," because mental illness was often ascribed to evil spirits or satanic powers. The visibility of the ill only served as a reminder of personal vulnerability and mortality, aspects of human existence that society wished to ignore.

For several decades, the importance of mental health became obscured in the rapid barrage of medical discoveries for treatment of physical disorders. However, the psychologic trauma resulting from the high-stress situations of combat during World War II expanded the scope of health as a concept to include consideration of the mental status of the individual. Mental health was manifest in the ability of an individual to withstand stresses imposed by the environment. When individuals succumbed to the rigors of life around them and could no longer carry out the functions of daily living, they were declared to be mentally ill. Despite efforts to develop a more holistic definition of health, the dichotomy between individuals suffering from physical illness and those suffering from mental illness persisted for many years (Congdon, 2001; Sorochan, 1970).

In 1974, the World Health Organization (WHO) proposed a definition of health that emphasized "wholeness" and the positive qualities of health: "Health is a state of complete physical, mental, and social well-being and not merely the absence of disease and infirmity" (WHO, 1974, 1986, 1996). The definition was revolutionary in that it (1) reflected concern for the individual as a total person, (2) placed health in the context of the social environment, and (3) equated health with productive and creative living. The breadth of this historical definition mandated a comprehensive approach to health promotion, and intrinsically, created an imperative for health equity (Marmot, Friel, Bell, Houweling, & Taylor, 2008).

The WHO definition has been criticized by many who think the definition is utopian, too broad, inflexible, and not subject to scientific application (Awofeso, 2009). Despite these criticisms, the WHO definition of health continues to be the most popular and comprehensive definition of health worldwide and has been expanded to focus on both the individual and the environment.

It is now accepted that individual health cannot be separated from the health of society and that individuals are interdependent with the totality of the world. Moreover, the relationship of human health to the health of the earth's ecosystem is also recognized as an important dimension. In other words, one cannot be healthy in an unhealthy society or world. Within these dimensions health has been defined as the ability to adapt to one's environment. Health is not a fixed state, as it varies depending on an individual's life state. This conception, originally proposed by Conguilhem in 1943, enables the changing context to be taken into consideration to understand the meaning of health ("What Is Health?" 2009).

In the following sections, definitions of health are discussed that focus on the individual, the family, and the community. In the past, defining health for individuals received more attention than defining health for families and communities. However, it has become clear that individual health is almost inseparable from the health of the larger community, and the health of every community determines the overall health status of the nation (U.S. Department of Health and Human Services, 2000).

HEALTH AND ILLNESS: DISTINCT ENTITIES OR OPPOSITE ENDS OF A CONTINUUM?

Theorists who present health and illness as a continuum usually identify possible reference points such as (1) optimum health, (2) suboptimal health or incipient illness, (3) overt illness and disability, and (4) very serious illness or approaching death (Dunn, 1959). These descriptors have only one point representing health, whereas multiple points on the scale represent varying states of illness. Dunn's model of wellness maintains that health and illness are separate concepts and continua must allow the differentiation of varying levels of health as well as varying levels of illness (Dunn, 1975).

When health and illness are assumed to represent a single continuum, it is difficult to discuss healthy aspects of the ill individual. The presence of illness ascribes the "sick

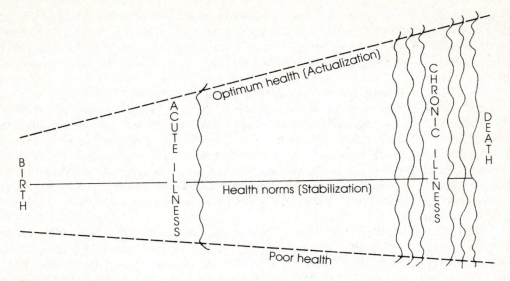

FIGURE 1–1   The Health Continuum Throughout the Life Span

role," and the individual is expected to direct all energies toward finding the cause of the illness and engaging in behaviors that will result in a return to health as soon as possible.

Health can be manifested in the presence of illness, so a case can be made for separate but parallel continua for health and illness. Poor health can exist even if disease is not present and good health can be present in spite of disease (Tamm, 1993). Oelbaum (1974) stresses the interrelationship of health and illness, even though she considers the concepts to be separate entities rather than opposite ends of a continuum. She states that apathy toward the work of wellness is the precursor of disease. The particular health behaviors or functions that are poorly performed will influence the type of disease, disorder, or damage that will follow.

The authors of this book believe health and illness are qualitatively different, interrelated concepts that may coexist (Sullivan, 2003). In Figure 1–1, multiple levels of health are depicted in interaction with episodes of illness. Illness, which may have a short (acute) or long (chronic) duration, is represented as discrete events within the life span. Health can still be an aspiration to those with a chronic illness, and health can be achieved despite being diagnosed with a disease (Hwu, Coates, & Boore, 2001). Illness experiences can either hinder or facilitate one's continuing quest for health. Thus, good health or poor health may exist with or without overt illness (Neuman & Fawcett, 2002).

DEFINITIONS OF HEALTH THAT FOCUS ON INDIVIDUALS

Health as Stability

For individuals, stability-based definitions of health derive primarily from the physiologic concepts of homeostasis and adaptation. Dubos (1965), an early advocate of the stability position, defines health as a state or condition that enables the individual to adapt to the environment. The degree of health experienced is dependent on one's ability to adjust to the various internal and external tensions that one faces. Dubos considers optimum health to be a mirage because in the real world individuals must face the physical and social forces that are forever changing, frequently unpredictable, and often dangerous. According to Dubos, the closest approach to optimum or high-level health is a physical and mental state free of discomfort and pain that permits one to function effectively within the environment.

Definitions of health based on normality can be described as stability-oriented. Statistical norms for a variety of human functions are already well defined. A significant problem with normative definitions of health is that they predict "what could be" based on "what is," leaving little room for incorporating growth, maturation, and evolutionary emergence into a definition of health. In addition, norms represent average or middle-range effectiveness rather than excellence or exceptional effectiveness in human functioning.

Environmentally focused models of health can also be described as stability oriented, as the essence of these models is adaptation of individuals to their environment. Health is related to the ability of individuals to maintain a balance with the environment, with relative freedom from pain, disability, or limitations, including social limitations. Health exists when one is able to adapt to the environment successfully and is able to grow, function, and thrive. In contrast, lack of adaptation is seen as a gap between one's ability and the demands of the environment (Verbrugge & Jette, 1994).

Parson's conceptualization of health is compatible with an environmental model. More than 50 years ago he defined health in terms of social norms rather than physiologic norms, describing health as individuals' effective performance of roles and tasks for which they have been socialized (Parsons, 1958). This definition is relevant today.

Similar to Parsons' sociologic model of health, Patrick, Bush, and Chenn (1973) and Feeny et al. (2002) define health in terms of functional norms. Their conception of health is the ability to perform socially valued activities usual for a person's age and social roles with a minimum probability of change to less valued functional levels. The desirability of the immediate functional level, as well as the probability that the current condition or state will change to a higher or lower preference functional level, must be considered in assessing current health status.

A number of nurse-theorists have proposed definitions of health emphasizing stability. Levine defines health as a state in which there is balance between input and output of energy and in which structural, personal, and social integrity exists (Schaefer & Pond, 1991). Johnson, in her behavioral system model, does not explicitly define health. However, a conception of health that focuses on stability can be inferred from her conceptualization of internal homeostasis. Health or wellness is balance and stability among the following behavioral systems: attachment or affiliative, dependency, ingestive, eliminative, sexual, aggressive, and achievement. Behavioral system stability is demonstrated by efficient and effective behavior that is purposeful, goal directed, orderly, and predictable (Loveland-Cherry & Wilkerson, 1989). Newman has defined health or wellness as a condition in which all subsystems—physiologic, psychologic, and sociocultural—are in balance and in harmony with the whole of humankind. Health is a state of saturation, of inertness, free of disruptive needs. Disrupting forces or noxious stressors with which individuals cannot cope create disharmony, reducing the level of wellness. In a wellness state, total needs are met and more energy is generated and stored than expended. A strong, flexible line of defense is maintained, providing the individual with considerable resistance to disequilibrium (Newman, 1991).

Roy also subscribes to a stability definition of health. The central concept in Roy's model is adaptation. Health is a state and process of successful adaptation that promotes being and becoming an integrated whole person. The four adaptive modes through which coping energies are expressed are physiologic, self-concept, role performance, and interdependence modes. Adaptation promotes integrity, which implies soundness or an unimpaired condition that can lead to completeness and unity. The person in an adapted state is freed from ineffective coping attempts that deplete energy. Available energy can be used to enhance health (Roy & Andrews, 2008).

Tripp-Reimer (1984) also proposes a model for health that is stability oriented. The conceptualization of health is based on a two-dimensional perspective: an *etic* dimension (disease–nondisease), which reflects a quantitative, objective interpretation of health by a health care professional; and an *emic* dimension (wellness–illness), which represents the subjective perception and experiences of health by an individual. The etic–emic approach has been further described by Arcury et al. (2001), who state that the etic dimension focuses on a medical model of normality or homeostasis, whereas the emic approach, which focuses on the lay perspective, is well suited to social scientists, who understand the interactions concerning health. The two approaches shed light on reasons for differing conceptions of health between medical personnel and clients of differing ethnic backgrounds.

Health as Actualization

When individual health is defined more broadly as actualization of human potential, it has been called *wellness*. Wellness is considered an expanded term, not as restricted as the concept of health. Despite these differences, *health* and *wellness* tend to be used interchangeably in the health promotion literature and is used interchangeably in this text.

Halbert Dunn was an early advocate for emphasizing actualization in definitions of health. Dunn coined the term *high-level wellness,* which he described as integrated human functioning that is oriented toward maximizing an individual's potential. This requires that individuals maintain balance and purpose within the environment where they are functioning (Dunn, 1980). Although the definition identifies balance as a dimension of health, emphasis is on the realization of human potential through purposeful activity. There is a single optimum level of wellness, as individuals move toward their personal optimum level based on their capabilities and potential.

Dunn states that high-level wellness, or an ideal state of optimum health, involves three components: (1) progress in a forward and upward direction toward a higher potential of functioning, (2) an open-ended and ever-expanding challenge to live at a fuller potential, and (3) progressive maturation of the individual at increasingly higher levels throughout the life cycle (Oelbaum, 1974; Tamm, 1993). Dunn proposes that high-level wellness can only emerge in a favorable environment. Health, according to Dunn, is not simply a passive state of freedom from illness; it is an emergent process characteristic of the entire life span (Dunn, 1980).

Orem uses *health* and *well-being* to refer to two different but related human states in her self-care theory (Orem, Taylor, & Renpenny, 2003). She defines *health* as a state characterized by soundness or wholeness of human structures and bodily and mental functions. *Well-being* is defined as an ideal state characterized by experiences of contentment, pleasure, and happiness; by spiritual experiences; by movement toward fulfillment of one's self-ideal; and by continuing personalization. Personalization is movement toward maturation and achievement of human potential. Engaging in responsible self-care and continuing development of self-care competency are facets of the process of personalization. Individuals can experience well-being even under conditions of adversity, including disorders of human structure and function (Orem et al., 2003).

Parse, in describing her man-living-health theory of nursing, presents five assumptions about health that define the term from her perspective (Parse, 1981):

1. Health is an open process of becoming, experienced by individuals.
2. Health is a rhythmically co-constituting process of the individual–environment relationship.
3. Health is an individual's patterns of relating value priorities.
4. Health is an intersubjective process of transcending with the possible.
5. Health is an individual's negentropic (toward increasing order, complexity, and heterogeneity) unfolding.

Newman, building on the work of Martha Rogers, defines health as the totality of the life process, which is evolving toward expanded consciousness (Newman, 1991). This definition emphasizes the actualizing properties of individuals throughout the life span. Four dimensions of health as a concept are identified:

1. Health is a fusion of disease and nondisease.
2. Health is the manifestation of an individual's unique pattern.
3. Health is expansion of consciousness. Time is a measure of consciousness, and movement is a reflection of consciousness.
4. Health encompasses the entire life process, which evolves toward higher and greater frequency of energy exchange.

Key life process phenomena include consciousness, movement, space, and time. Newman's model of health addresses holistic characteristics of human beings. However, there is no intent to create measures for many of the terms within the model, limiting potential testing and empirical applicability of the model.

Both Newman and Parse build on Martha Rogers' theory of a unitary person. Both represent early attempts to define health in terms of holism as opposed to defining health in terms of component parts. The emergent nature or actualization potential of the healthy individual and the capacity for open energy exchange with the environment are characteristics of both Newman's and Parse's definitions of health.

Actualization or wellness models have been criticized because of the difficulties in measuring subjective perceptions. In addition, perceptions of health and wellness vary according to age and cultural context. Another criticism is that the expanded definitions of health in these models do not distinguish health from happiness, quality of life, and other global concepts (Saracci, 1997). In spite of these criticisms, the wellness models provide a focus on the whole person and promote the positive aspects of health. Also, persons who accept the wellness model of health are more likely to seek alternative sources of therapy, not because of dissatisfaction with conventional medicine but because of their different beliefs and values about life and health. They are also more likely to view themselves as healthy in the presence of illness.

Health as Actualization and Stability

Models of individual health also incorporate both stability and actualization. For example, Wu has described health as a feeling of well-being, a capacity to perform to the best of one's ability, and the flexibility to adapt and adjust to varying situations created by the systems in which one exists (Wu, 1973). Wu proposes that wellness and illness represent distinct entities, with a repertory of behaviors for each. Within this frame of reference, both wellness and illness can exist simultaneously, so an evaluation of both wellness and illness are critical to a comprehensive health assessment.

King proposes a definition of health that emphasizes both stabilizing and actualizing tendencies. She defines *health* as a dynamic state in the life cycle of a person that implies adjustment to stressors in the environment through optimum use of resources to achieve maximum potential for daily living (King, 1983). In King's model, a holistic health perspective relates to the way individuals handle stressors while functioning within the culture to which they were born and attempt to conform (King, 1990). King views health as a functional state in the life cycle, with illness defined as interference in the life cycle.

Smith (1983) proposes a model of health encompassing four dimensions: Three focus on stability and one on actualization. Each health dimension is defined by the extremes on the health–illness continuum identified by the dimension.

- *Clinical dimension*: Health extreme: Absence of signs or symptoms of disease or disability; Illness extreme: Presence of signs or symptoms or obvious disability.
- *Role-performance dimension*: Health extreme: Performance of social roles with maximum expected output; Illness extreme: Failure to perform one's social roles.
- *Adaptive dimension*: Health extreme: Flexible adaptation to the environment; Illness extreme: Alienation of the person from environment.
- *Eudaimonistic dimension*: Health extreme: Exuberant well-being; Illness extreme: Devitalized, increasing debility.

Each dimension requires a distinct approach and a different mode of intervention, depending on which dimension is used as the guiding framework.

A definition of health must be applicable to everyone—to the well, to those with a treatable disease or illness, and to those with chronic disease or disability (Institute of the Future, 2000). The authors of this text believe a definition of health should incorporate both actualizing and stabilizing tendencies and define *health* as the realization of human potential through goal-directed behavior, competent self-care, and satisfying relationships with others, while adapting to maintain structural integrity and harmony with the social and physical environments. This broad conceptual definition has led to a classification system that describes affective and behavioral expressions of health by individuals (Table 1–1). The major culture-free dimensions of health expression include affect, attitudes, activity, aspirations, and accomplishments. The physical, mental, social, and spiritual components of health that are now cited in expanded definitions of health, including the WHO definition, are encompassed in this classification. The dimensions are further divided into 15 subcategories that may be culture specific. The

TABLE 1–1   Classification System for Affective and Behavioral Expressions of Health

Affect

Serenity	Harmony	Vitality	Sensitivity
Calm	Spiritual	Energetic	Aware
Relaxed	Contemplative	Vigorous	Connected
Peaceful	At one with the universe	Zestful	Intimate
Content		Alert	Loving
Comfortable			Warm

Attitudes

Optimism	Relevancy	Competency
Hopeful	Useful	Purposive
Enthusiastic	Contributing	Initiating
Open	Valued	Self-motivating
Reverent	Committed	Self-affirming
Resilient	Involved	Innovative

Activity

Positive Life Patterns	Meaningful Work	Invigorating Play
Healthy eating	Realistic goals	Meaningful hobbies
Regular exercise	Varied activities	Satisfying leisure
Stress management	Challenging tasks	activities
Adequate rest	Collaboration	Energizing diversions
Positive relationships		
Health monitoring		
Constructive coping		

Aspirations

Self-Actualization	Social Contribution
Growth	Global harmony and
Personal mastery	interdependence
	enhancement
	Environmental preservation

Accomplishments

Enjoyment	Creativity	Transcendence
Pleasure from daily	Maximum use of capacities	Freedom, harmony
living	Innovative contribution	Purpose in life
Sense of achievement		

system is based on the assumptions that health is a manifestation of person and environment interactional patterns that become increasingly complex throughout the life span. The classification system provides a framework for a comprehensive assessment of health that is consistent with a positive, unitary, humanistic view.

An Integrated View of Health

Health is a holistic experience and only becomes fragmented in the minds of health professionals. Although the biological model provides technological excellence and sophisticated medical care, it has led to a narrow focus on disease. An expansive view of health goes beyond disease prevention and risk reduction. An expansive view emphasizes personal and social resources as well as physical capacities and can be integrated with traditional biomedical models (disease) and public health models (mortality, morbidity, risks) of health to provide a holistic biopsychosocial view (Engel, 1997; Hanson & Boyd, 1996). The biopsychosocial view eliminates the need to reject one view of health at the cost of another and enables clinicians and researchers to work with health and disease together rather than separating the concepts (Loveland-Cherry, 2000). Last, the social context is now recognized as a powerful determinant of health (Dunn, 1959; Engel, 1997). Therefore, understanding the relevance of a broad definition of health to individuals in their everyday experiences in different social contexts is critical to improving their health.

DEFINITIONS OF HEALTH THAT FOCUS ON THE FAMILY

The complexity of the family and the diversity of family life in different ethnic, cultural, and geographic settings pose a challenge for defining and promoting family health. The traditional definition of family as two or more persons living together who are related by marriage, blood, or adoption is no longer adequate in American society. A broad definition of *family* now accepted is two or more persons who depend on one another for emotional, physical, or financial support (Klein & White, 1996). In this definition family members are self-defined and may include any individuals who make a significant commitment to each other outside of marriage. It is critical that variation in family structure be taken into consideration in defining and measuring family health.

Conceptual frameworks of family health have evolved with the changing definition of family. There is no single conceptual framework, as family nursing conceptual models and theories are found in the family social science disciplines, family therapy, and nursing (Loveland-Cherry, 2000). Four major social science theories that have provided direction for development of nursing knowledge in family health include developmental theory, systems theory, structural functional theory, and interactional theory.

Loveland-Cherry observes that family health is a concept often referred to as a goal of nursing but seldom defined. She defines family health as possessing the abilities and resources to accomplish the development tasks of the family. Adapting Smith's model of health to families, she proposes the following dimensions of family health (McCubbin, 1999):

- *Clinical model*: Lack of evidence of physical, mental, or social disease; deterioration or dysfunction of family system.
- *Role-performance model*: Ability of family system to carry out family functions effectively to achieve family developmental tasks.

- *Adaptive model*: Family patterns of interaction with the physical and social environment, characterized by flexible, effective adaptation or ability to change and grow.
- *Eudaimonistic model*: Ongoing provision of resources, guidance, and support to realize the family's maximum well-being and potential throughout the life span.

This framework specifies the critical dimensions of family health conceptually to enable the nurse to assess each of the dimensions.

Other approaches to family nursing have been proposed to promote health (Baranowski, Perry, & Parcel, 2008). These include the family as context, client, system, and a component of society. A model of family reciprocal determinism takes into account the complexity of the family environment in promoting health (Fisher et al., 1998). Within this model, behavior is a function of the shared environment with other family members and their behavior and personal characteristics. The family plays an important role in the promotion of health because health information is shared and behaviors are learned, practiced, and reinforced in the daily routine, which are facilitated or hindered by family values and beliefs. All of the perspectives move the basic unit of analysis from the individual to the family system, as the interaction of the individual with other members of the family or other units in society is emphasized.

A biopsychosocial definition of *family health* describes family health as a dynamic changing state of well-being, including biologic, psychologic, sociologic, spiritual, and cultural factors of the family system (Engel, 1997). In this definition an individual's health affects the functioning of the family, and in turn, family functioning affects the health of the individual. Thus, both the family system and the individual members must be part of the health assessment.

Characteristics of healthy families have been described. These characteristics include affirmation and support for one another, shared sense of responsibility, shared leisure time, shared religious core, respect, trust, and family rituals and traditions. These qualities address stability of family functioning and balance in interaction among family members. Family typologies have also been developed to identify a common profile that may be linked to health in families. For example, four family types (balanced, traditional, disconnected, and emotionally strained) have differentiated health in two community-based samples (Fisher et al., 1998). These typologies also suggest that health promotion interventions must be implemented in ways that are compatible with family values, beliefs, and orientations. Additional research is needed to evaluate the effects of health-related interventions based on family type.

Many factors influence how family health is defined. Social, cultural, environmental and religious factors play a central role in determining how families view their health. Families' strengths, resources, and competencies are also an integral part of a positive conceptualization of health. Family health processes are being given increased attention by scientists in nursing and other disciplines. Development and testing of theoretical models to describe family health will help health professionals identify determinants of family well-being to promote the health of families.

DEFINITIONS OF HEALTH THAT FOCUS ON THE COMMUNITY

Communities are usually defined within one of two frameworks: geographical area or relational. Geographical definitions are based on legal or geopolitical areas such as cities, towns, or census tracts. Relational definitions are based on how people interact to achieve common goals. The WHO defines community as a social group determined by both geographical area and common values, with members who know each other and interact within a social structure (WHO, 1974). Members of the community create norms, values, and social institution for its members. The WHO definition focuses on the spatial, personal, and functional dimensions of a community.

Social ecological theories of community health emphasize the interaction and interdependence of the individual with the family, community, social structure, and physical environment (Green, 1999). A social ecology model described in the *Ottawa Charter for Health Promotion*, a landmark policy statement, outlines the essential dimensions of community health (WHO, 1986). Fundamental to community health are peace, shelter, education, food, income, a stable ecosystem, sustainable resources, social justice, and equity. The Healthy Cities projects in the United States, Europe, and Australia are based on a social ecological view that the roots of ill health lie in social and economic factors, and support the premise that the responsibility for health is widely shared in the community with collaborative decision making about health issues (Baum, Jolley, Hicks, Saint, & Parker, 2006). Informed political action and public policies are essential to a healthy community.

Three major dimensions have been identified in an effort to develop a broad understanding of community health. These dimensions, which can be assessed by multiple measures, provide information that is complementary for developing a clear picture of the health of the community (Shuster & Goeppinger, 2003):

1. *Status dimension*: Biological, emotional and social components, measured by morbidity, mortality, life expectancy, risk factors, consumer satisfaction, mental health, crime rates, functional levels, worker absenteeism, and infant mortality.
2. *Structural dimension*: Community health services and resources measured by utilization patterns, treatment data, and provider/population ratios; social indicators measured by socioeconomic and racial distributions and median education level.
3. *Process dimension*: Effective community functioning or problem solving that results in community competence as evidenced by commitment, self–other awareness, effective communication, conflict containment and accommodation, participation, management of relations with larger society, and mechanisms to facilitate interaction and decision making.

Based on these dimensions, *community health* can be defined as meeting the collective needs of its members through identifying problem and managing interactions within the community and between the community and the larger society (Hemstrom, 1995).

Community health is more than the sum of the health of its individual members; it encompasses the characteristics of the community as a whole. Individual, family, and community health are intimately related. The health of the community depends on individual health as well as whether the social, physical, and political aspects that enable individuals to live healthy lives exist. Research indicates that characteristics of communities have an important influence on health and individual risk behaviors (DiClemente, Crosby, Sionean, & Holtgrave, 2004). Studies have also documented the relationship between social and economic conditions and the health of individuals in a community. Social capital has also been described as a major determinant of health in communities. This term, which includes trust, reciprocity, and cooperation among families, neighborhoods, and entire communities, is discussed in more detail in Chapter 3. Healthy communities support healthy lifestyles. Likewise the collective attitudes, beliefs, and behaviors of individuals who live in the community influence community health (Dunn, 1959). An overarching goal of *Healthy People 2020* is to create social and physical environments that promote good health of all. All components of the social and physical environments that interact with individuals must be assessed prior to developing strategies to create healthier communities.

The traditional focus on an individual, curative model, while successful in the care of chronic diseases, unintentionally relegates individual and community health to a position of secondary importance. However, the focus now goes beyond the individual to include community-level factors. A body of evidence supports an expanded view of individual health that is inseparable from the community and larger society. Effective health promotion interventions are beginning to be based on the assessment of a community's social environment as well as societal and physical environmental level factors, as recommended in the *Healthy People 2020* document (http://www.healthypeople.gov/HP2020/).

SOCIAL DETERMINANTS OF HEALTH

More than 100 years ago, European physicians understood that social and economic conditions, as well as physical defects, were major contributors to health and disease (Levin & Browner, 2005). The social determinants of health are the conditions in which people are born, live, work, and age, including the health care system (Marmot et al., 2008). The social determinants of health are responsible for inequities in health, or the differences in health seen within and between communities and countries. The social conditions under which people live indeed have a dramatic impact on their health, including poverty with its accompanying inadequate housing, poor sanitation, suboptimal food; lack of education, and social discrimination. Differences in health can be attributed to socioeconomic, political, cultural, and geographic dimensions; the influence of these factors is evident when comparing the health of those at the top with those at the bottom of the social ladder.

In the first phase of *Healthy People 2020*, the national health agenda, one of the four major goals is to create social and physical environments that promote health (U.S. Department of Health and Human Services, 2009). The *Healthy People 2020* agenda documents the multiple determinants of health and health behaviors, including personal, social, and physical environments and the interrelationships that exist among these different levels of health determinants. The need to address multilevel interventions is emphasized to promote health and well-being.

Some people have criticized use of the term *social determinant*, as they believe that the expanded focus results in a loss of individual identity. Still others believe that the term *social* should not be used. Rather, determinants of health should be the focus to avoid the politicized view of health. Regardless of the terms used, it is now understood that a broader view of health is necessary to improve the health of all. An understanding of the social determinants is important for nurses and other health care professionals to effectively intervene in neighborhoods, communities, and organizations to improve individual health (Marmot, 2005). This is discussed in more detail in Chapter 15.

SOCIAL DETERMINANTS AND GLOBAL HEALTH

Global health has been defined as the transnational impact of globalization (interconnectedness) on the determinants of health and health problems, which are beyond the control of institutions or individual countries (Smith, Tang, & Nutbeam, 2006). Global health issues include the vulnerability of refugee populations, the marketing of harmful products, the erosion of social and environmental conditions, the exacerbation of income differences, and global climate change. Although the major drivers in global health are government and nongovernment agencies, health care providers must be aware of the increasing importance of addressing community and population health, as international borders are increasingly becoming invisible (see Chapter 15).

CONCEPTIONS OF HEALTH PROMOTION

The changing, expanding definitions of health have led to changing views of health promotion. Early health promotion efforts focused on individual responsibility for health and emphasized behavioral determinants and educational approaches. However, evidence has shown that health promotion programs must also address social and physical environments, as these are also sources of poor health. This view was expressed in the *Ottawa Charter for Health Promotion*, the first document to focus on health promotion as a process to enable people to overcome challenges and increase control over their environments to improve their health (WHO, 1986). This document laid the foundation for the theory and practice of health promotion and emphasized the role of social and personal resources as well as physical capabilities and the need to achieve equity in health. The *Ottawa Charter* also documented the responsibility of nongovernment and government agencies in creating supportive environments and health public policy.

The *Bangkok Charter for Health Promotion* updated the Ottawa Charter to make health promotion central to the global development agenda and a core responsibility of all governments (Porter, 2006; WHO, 2005). The Bangkok Charter addressed the changing context of health promotion that had occurred since the adoption of the Ottawa Charter. The document has been described as moving health promotion from a socioecological approach to a regulative and legislative approach to manage the challenges of global health. In the document the many challenges are recognized due to the multiple determinants of health in a globalized world, and health promotion is considered a core responsibility for all governments.

Health promotion and *health education* are often used interchangeably. Although the terms are closely linked, they are not the same. Health education focuses on learning activities and experiences for individuals and groups. It is considered a component of health promotion, which is a much broader concept. Health promotion has three components: health education, prevention, and health protection. Tannahill defines health protection as legal or fiscal controls and other regulations to enhance health and prevent disease (Tannahill, 2009). His expanded definition of health promotion includes health fostering and ill health prevention policies; strategies and activities to address social, economic, and physical environments; cultural factors; equity and diversity; education and learning; services, amenities, and products; and community-led and community-based activities.

Health promotion has moved from being considered a goal or desired end point to a process or tool to facilitate accomplishment of goals. It is both the art and science of helping people make lifestyle changes and is considered a combination of educational and ecological supports for actions and conditions of living conducive to health (Green & Kreuter, 1999). A combination of supports or strategies are needed to address the multiple determinants of health with multiple health promotion interventions. Ecological supports include the social, economic, and physical environments that influence health.

MEASUREMENT OF HEALTH

In general, few health measures incorporate the holistic and expansive views of health, as most health status measures are derived from an illness or curative model (Hinshaw, 1999). Many commonly used measures of health status continue to focus primarily on mortality- or on morbidity-related indices such as dysfunction, disability, or impairment. Such "measures of health" are really "measures of illness." Measures of health need to encompass the complexity of health. They should (1) characterize health by conditions that define its presence rather than its absence, (2) identify a spectrum of health states, and (3) reflect a life-span developmental perspective. In addition, measures of the social determinants of the health of individuals and communities must be taken into consideration when measuring health.

On the basis of the WHO definition, Ware (1987) proposes five distinct dimensions as a minimum standard for a comprehensive health measure: physical health (functional and structural integrity), mental health (emotional and intellectual functioning), social functioning, role functioning, and general perceptions of well-being. These dimensions are now widely accepted measures of health status. Another classification includes subjective health status, or individuals' global assessment of their health; chronic health problems, or illnesses diagnosed by a physician that are expected to last six months or more; functional health, or characteristics of the individuals' health in eight domains (vision, hearing, speech, mobility, cognition, emotion, pain/discomfort, and distress or an unpleasant subjective state) (Denton et al., 2004). As can be seen in both classifications, there is a greater focus on limitations in performance or functioning and/or disease, reflecting the illness model of health.

Two views of self-rated health assessments have been proposed: spontaneous assessment and enduring self-concept. In the spontaneous assessment view, self-rated assessments of health are considered responsive to observable indicators of illness and have been shown to take a wide range of factors into consideration, including functional ability, lifestyle and health practices, sociocultural constructions of health, and physical symptoms (Ballis, Segall, & Chipperfield, 2004). Individual ratings of health may be transitory, with respect to multiple dimensions of one's health status. The enduring self-concept view characterizes self-rated health as a reflection of one's established beliefs about one's health. In this view, self-rated health is stable over time and is based on one's self concept. Therefore, self-rated health may not reflect the objective indicators of health, as it is independent of one's physical status. This view is more congruent with an expansive definition of health, as an individual's self-evaluation of global health is more related to an overall sense of well-being. However, if one takes the view that health depends on one's circumstances, then the individual's social and physical context must be taken into consideration in assessing one's view of health.

The multilevel nature of health and its determinants points to the need for measurable personal, social, and physical environmental indicators. Standardized measures are needed to evaluate the effectiveness of multilevel health promotion interventions across individuals, families, and communities. In addition, both individual and aggregate measures are needed to assess and monitor health at the individual, family, and community levels. Measurement of health and its multiple determinants is complex; it becomes even more so when all perspectives are taken into account. This challenge poses multiple research opportunities.

OPPORTUNITIES FOR RESEARCH ON HEALTH

The fundamental purpose of nursing research is to build knowledge to improve health. Nursing research has been on the forefront in knowledge development to improve the health of all. However, many questions remain unanswered. How is human health expressed both biologically and behaviorally? What are the gender, culture, and racial differences in the expressions of health? How does health differ at varying points of life-span development? What interactive conditions between persons and their environment enhance or deplete health? Which health determinants are critical to assess the health of families? Which health determinants are key to improving the health of communities? How do issues related to globalization affect the health of individuals and communities? Generating knowledge relevant to these questions will advance nursing science and provide an empirical base to guide effective health-promoting interventions and begin policy discussions for change.

Models of health that incorporate ethnic, cultural, social, environmental, political, and global factors are needed to examine the diversity of health conceptions. Attention should be given to developing more rigorous, consistent definitions of family health and community health. Furthermore, longitudinal studies are needed to determine the developmental variations in health perceptions across the life span. Multidisciplinary research teams are suggested to develop and test multilevel interventions to address the social determinants of health. Measures to assess the expanded conceptualizations of health should be constructed that will provide information needed to guide interventions to improve individual, family, community, and global health.

CONSIDERATIONS FOR PRACTICE IN THE CONTEXT OF HOLISTIC HEALTH

The definition of *health* has evolved from traditional usage in a medical, curative model to a multidimensional phenomenon with biopsychosocial, spiritual, environmental, and cultural dimensions. Nurses and other health care professionals must understand and assess all dimensions in their health assessments. The assessment information can then be used to develop interventions. For example, the traditional biomedical assessment may be useful in guiding genetic counseling or screening interventions. Information gleaned from a spiritual and cultural assessment can provide valuable knowledge in developing health promotion interventions for diverse populations. An assessment of the social and physical environment will provide useful information about aspects of the environment that may be positively or negatively affecting the health of the individual or community. In a holistic view of health, an assessment is not complete unless it involves the individual and the family and community in which the individual functions. Nurses work in partnership with clients to provide the knowledge and skills needed to empower them to achieve their health goals or adapt to their circumstances to move toward their health goals. Last, health must be viewed from a positive perspective when conducting an assessment or designing health promotion strategies. This means that the focus should be on available resources, potentials, and capabilities. When health is viewed in a positive model, strategies can be developed that concentrate on strengthening resources as well as decreasing negative risks.

Summary

Varying definitions of *health* have been presented that provide the foundation on which health promotion programs for individuals, families, and communities can be based. To address the promotion of health, one must know how health, the desired outcome, is defined and how achievement of health can be measured at individual, family, and community levels. Evidence has shown that individual health cannot be separated from the health of the family, community, nation, and world. A shift to this broader perspective of health will facilitate development of proactive policy to improve the health of all. However, the complexity of factors known to determine the health of individuals also raises many challenges, as no one dimension or determinant can be ignored.

Learning Activities

1. Write your own definition of *health* and state the rationale for the factors you considered in developing the definition.
2. Interview three persons at varying points in the life span to obtain their perspective of their health, health promotion strategies they perform to stay healthy, and personal, social, and environmental barriers to promoting a healthy lifestyle.
3. Categorize your interviewees' conceptions of health based on the information obtained as stability, actualization, or traditional.
4. Develop a plan to conduct an assessment to determine the health of a community, using the social determinants of health.

Selected Web Sites

Healthy People 2020
http://www.healthypeople.gov/HP2020/

The Bangkok Charter for Health Promotion
http://www.who.int/healthpromotion/conferences/6gchp/bangkok_charter/en/

References

American Nurses Association. (2003). *Nursing's social policy statement: Second edition.* Pub # 03NSPS. Silver Spring, MN: ANA.

Arcury, T. A., Quandt, S. A., & Bell, R. A. (2001). Staying healthy: The salience and meaning of health maintenance behaviors among rural older adults in North Carolina. *Social Science and Medicine, 53*, 1541–1556.

Awofeso, N. (2009). Re-defining health. *Bulletin of the World Health Organization.* Retrieved June 2009 from http://www.who.int/bulletin/bulletin_board/83/ustun11051/en/

Ballis, D. S., Segall, A., & Chipperfield, J. G. (2004). Two views of self-rated general health status. *Social Science and Medicine, 56*(2), 203–217.

Baranowski, T., Perry, C. L., & Parcel, G. S. (2008). How individuals, environments and health behavior interact: Social cognitive theory. In K. Glanz, B. K. Rimer, & R. Viswanath (Eds.), *Health behavior and health education* (3rd ed., pp. 153–178). San Francisco: Jossey-Bass.

Baum, F., Jolley, G., Hicks, R., Saint, K., & Parker, S. (2006). What makes for sustainable Healthy Cities initiatives? A review of the evidence from Noarlunga, Australia after 18 years. *Health Promotion International, 21,* 259–265.

Belhadj, H., & Touré, A. (2008). Gender equality and the right to health. *The Lancet, 372*(9655), 2008–2009.

Benson, H. (1996). *Timeless healing: The power and biology of belief.* New York: Scribner.

Congdon, P. (2001). Health status and healthy life measures for population health need assessment: Modeling variability and uncertainty. *Health & Place, 7,* 13–25.

Denton, M., Prus, S., & Walters, V. (2004). Gender differences in health: A Canadian study of the psychosocial, structural and behavioral determinants of health. *Social Science and Medicine, 58*(12), 2585–2600.

DiClemente, R. J., Crosby, R. A., Sionean, C., & Holtgrave, D. (2004). Community intervention trials: Theoretical and methodological considerations. In D. S. Blumenthal & R. J. DiClemente (Eds.), *Community-based health research* (pp. 171–178). New York: Springer.

Dolfman, M. L. (1973). The concept of health: An historic and analytic examination. *Journal of School Health, 43,* 493.

Dubos, R. (1965). *Man adapting* (p. 349). New Haven, CT: Yale University Press.

Dunn, H. L. (1959, November). What high-level wellness means. *Canadian Journal of Public Health, 50*(11), 447–457.

———— (1975). Points of attack for raising the level of wellness. *Journal of National Medical Association, 49,* 223–235.

———— (1980). *High-level wellness.* Thorofare, NJ: Charles B Slack Inc.

Engel, G. (1997). From biomedical to biopsychosocial: Being scientific in the human domain. *Psychosomatics, 38*(6), 521–526.

Erikssen, J., Delive, L., Eklof, M., & Hagberg, M. (2007). Early inequities in excellent health and performance among young adult women and men in Sweden. *Gender Medicine, 4*(2), 170–182.

Fawcett, J. (2005). *Contemporary nursing knowledge: Analysis and evaluation of nursing models and theories* (2nd ed.). Philadelphia: FA Davis Co.

Feeny, D., Furlong, W., Torrance, G. W., Goldsmith, C. H., Zhu, Z., DePauw, S., et al. (2002). Multiattribution and single attribute utility functions for the health utilities index mark 3 system. *Medical Care, 40,* 113–128.

Fisher, L., Paradis, G., Soubhi, H., Mansai, O., Gauvin, L., & Potvin, L. (1998). Family process in health research: Extending a family typology to a new cultural context. *Health Psychology, 17*(4), 358–366.

Green, L. (1999). Health education's contribution to public health in the twentieth century: A glimpse through health promotion's rearview mirror. *Annual Review of Public Health, 20,* 67–88.

Green, L. W., & Kreuter, M. W. (1999). Health promotion and a framework for planning. In *Health promotion planning* (3rd ed., pp. 1–44). Boston: McGraw Hill.

Hanson, S. M., & Boyd, S. T. (1996). *Family healthcare nursing: Theory, practice and research.* Philadelphia: FA Davis.

Hemstrom, M. M. (1995). Application as scholarship: A community client experience. *Public Health Nursing, 12*(30), 279–283.

Hinshaw, A. S. (1999). Evolving nursing research traditions: Influencing factors. In A. S. Hinshaw, S. L. Feetham, & J. Shaver (Eds.), *Handbook of clinical nursing research* (pp. 19–38). Thousand Oaks, CA: Sage Publications.

Hwu, Y., Coates, V., & Boore, J. (2001). The evolving concept of health in nursing research: 1988–1998. *Patient Education and Counseling, 42,* 105–114.

Institute of the Future. (2000). *Health and healthcare 2010.* San Francisco: Jossey-Bass.

King, I. M. (1983). *A theory for nursing: Systems, concepts, processes* (p. 31). New York: Teachers College Press.

———— (1990). Health as the goal for nursing. *Nursing Science Quarterly, 3*(3), 123–128.

Klein, D. M., & White, J. M. (1996). *Family theories: An introduction.* Thousand Oaks, CA: Sage Publications.

Levin, B. W., & Browner, C. H. (2005). The social production of health: Critical contributions from evolutionary, biological and cultural anthropology. *Social Science and Medicine, 61,* 745–750.

Loveland-Cherry, C., & Wilkerson, S. A. (1989). Dorothy Johnson's behavioral system model. In J. Fitzpatrick & A. Whall (Eds.), *Conceptual models of nursing: Analysis and application* (2nd ed.). Norwalk, CT: Appleton & Lange.

Loveland-Cherry, C. J. (2000). Family health risks. In M. Stanhope & J. Lancaster (Eds.), *Community & public health nursing* (5th ed., pp. 506–525). St Louis, MO: Mosby.

Marmot, M. (2005). Social determinants of health inequalities. *The Lancet, 365,* 1999–1201.

Marmot, M., Friel, S., Bell, R., Houweling, T. A., & Taylor, S. (2008). Closing the gap in a generation: Health equity through action on the social determinants of health. *The Lancet, 372,* 1661–1669.

McCubbin, M. M. (1999). Normative family transitions and health outcomes. In A. Hinshaw, S. Feetham, & J. Shaver (Eds.), *Handbook of clinical nursing research* (pp. 201–230). Thousand Oaks, CA: Sage Publications.

McMullin, J. (2005). The call to life: Revitalizing a healthy Hawaiian identity. *Social Science and Medicine, 61,* 809–820.

Millstein, S. G. (1994). A view of health from the adolescent's perspective. In S. G. Millstein, A. C. Petersen, & E. O. Nightingale (Eds.), *Promoting the health of adolescents: New directions for the twenty-first century* (pp. 97–118). New York: Oxford University Press, Inc.

Millstein, S. G., & Irwin, C. E. (1987). Concepts of health and illness: Different constructs or variation in a theme. *Health Psychology, 6,* 515–524.

Neuman, B., & Fawcett, J. (Eds.). (2002). *The Neuman systems model* (4th ed.). Upper Saddle River, NJ: Prentice Hall.

Newman, M. A. (1991). Health conceptualization. In J. Fitzpatrick, R. L. Taunton, & A. K. Jacox (Eds.), *Annual review of research* (pp. 221–243), New York: Springer Publishing Co.

Oelbaum, C. H. (1974). Hallmarks of adult wellness. *American Journal Nursing, 74,* 1623.

Orem, D. E., Taylor, S. G., & Renpenny, K. N. (2003). *Self care theory in nursing.* New York: McGraw-Hill Inc.

Parse, R. R. (1981). *Man-living-health: A theory of nursing* (pp. 25–36). New York: John Wiley & Sons.

Parsons, T. (1958). Definitions of health and illness in the light of American values and social structure. In E. G. Jaco (Ed.), *Patients, physicians and illness* (p. 176). New York: The Free Press.

Patrick, D. L., Bush, J. W., & Chenn, M. M. (1973). Toward an operational definition of health. *Journal of Health and Social Behavior, 14,* 6.

Pender, N. J. (1990). Expressing health through lifestyle patterns. *Nursing Science Quarterly, 3*(3), 115–122.

Porter, C. (2006). Ottawa to Bangkok: Changing health promotion discourse. *Health Promotion International, 23,* 72–79.

Roy, C., & Andrews, H. A. (2008). *The Roy adaptation model* (3rd ed.). Norwalk, CT: Appleton & Lange.

Saracci, R. (1997). The World Health Organization needs to reconsider its definition of health. *British Medical Journal, 314,* 1409–1410.

Schaefer, K. M., & Pond, J. B. (1991). *Levine's conservation model: A framework for nursing practice* (p. 17). Philadelphia: FA Davis Co.

Shuster, G. F., & Goeppinger, J. (2003). Community as client: Using the nursing process to promote health. In M. Stanhope & J. Lancaster (Eds.), *Community & public health nursing* (6th ed., pp. 306–329). St. Louis, MO: Mosby.

Smith, B. J., Tang, K. C., & Nutbeam, D. (2006). WHO health promotion glossary: New terms. *Health Promotion International, 21,* 340–345.

Smith, J. (1983). *The idea of health: Implications for the nursing profession* (p. 31). New York: Teachers College Press.

Sorochan, W. (1970). Health concepts as a basis for orthobiosis. In E. Hart & W. Sechrist (Eds.), *The dynamics of wellness.* Belmont, CA: Wadsworth, Inc.

Sullivan, M. (2003). The new subjective medicine: Taking the patient's point of view on health care and health. *Social Science and Medicine, 56,* 1595–1604.

Tamm, M. E. (1993). Models of health and disease. *British Journal of Medical Psychology, 66,* 213–228.

Tannahill, A. (2009). Health promotion: The Tannahill model revisited. *Public Health, 123,* 396–399.

Tripp-Reimer, T. (1984). Reconceptualizing the concept of health: Integrating emic and etic perspectives. *Research in Nursing & Health, 7,* 101–109.

U.S. Department of Health and Human Services. (2000). *Healthy People 2010: Understanding and improving health.* Washington, DC: U.S. Government Printing Office.

—— (2009). *Phase 1 report: Recommendations for the framework and format for Healthy People 2020.* Retrieved from http://www.healthypeople .gov/HP2020/

Verbrugge, L., & Jette, A. (1994). The disablement process. *Social Science & Medicine, 38,* 1–14.

Ware, J. E. (1987). Standards for validating health measures: Definition and content. *Journal of Chronic Diseases, 40,* 473–480.

What is health? The ability to adapt. [Editorial] (2009, March 7). *The Lancet, 373*(9666), 781.

World Health Organization. (1974). Community health nursing: Report of a WHO expert committee. *Technical Report Series No. 558.* Geneva, Switzerland: WHO.

—— (1986). Ottawa charter for health promotion. *Health Promotion, 1*(4), ii–v.

—— (1996). *Basic document* (36th ed.). Geneva, Switzerland: WHO.

—— (2005). *The Bangkok Charter for health promotion in a globalized world.* Retrieved August 11, 2005 from http://who.int/healthpromotion /conference/6gchp/ bangkok _charter/en

Wu, R. (1973). *Behavior and illness.* Englewood Cliffs, NJ: Prentice-Hall, Inc.

Wylie, C. M. (1970, February). The definition and measurement of health and disease. *Public Health Report, 85,* 100–104.

CHAPTER 2

Individual Models to Promote Health Behavior

OBJECTIVES

1. Discuss the rationale for using behavior change theory to structure interventions.
2. Describe commonalities and differences in the social cognitive models.
3. Apply the stages of change model to health behavior.
4. Discuss the revised health promotion model and its usefulness in nursing practice.
5. Describe theory-based strategies for behavior change.
6. Discuss the concept and application of tailoring behavior strategies to promote healthy behavior outcomes.

Outline

- Human Potential for Change
- Use of Theories and Models for Behavior Change
- Social Cognition Theories and Models
  A. The Health Belief Model
  B. Theory of Reasoned Action and Theory of Planned Behavior
  C. Self-Efficacy and Social Cognitive Theory
  D. The Health Promotion Model
- Theoretical Basis for the Health Promotion Model
- The Health Promotion Model (Revised)
  A. Individual Characteristics and Experiences
  B. Behavior-Specific Cognitions and Affect
  C. Commitment to a Plan of Action
  D. Immediate Competing Demands and Preferences
  E. Behavioral Outcome
- Stage Models of Behavior Change
  A. Transtheoretical Model

- **Interventions for Health Behavior Change**
  - A. Raising Consciousness
  - B. Reevaluating the Self
  - C. Promoting Self-Efficacy
  - D. Enhancing the Benefits of Change
  - E. Modifying the Environment
  - F. Managing Barriers to Change
- **Tailoring Behavior Change Interventions**
- **Maintaining Behavior Change**
- **Ethics of Behavior Change**
- **Opportunities for Research with Health Behavior Theories and Models**
- **Considerations for Practice in Motivating Health Behavior**
- **Summary**
- **Learning Activities**
- **Selected Web Sites**
- **References**

Health promotion services provided by health professionals in the United States are directed toward assisting individuals, families, and communities to achieve their full health potential by adopting healthy behaviors. Although early detection of disease, referred to as secondary prevention, is extremely important, it has produced limited health, quality-of-life, and economic benefits. Secondary prevention is based on a disease model of health care. Health promotion (action to contribute to health) and primary prevention (action to avoid or forestall the development of illness/disease) have been shown to have substantial benefits in improving quality of life and longevity. In contrast to secondary prevention, health promotion and primary prevention are based on behavioral or sociopolitical models of health care that recognize the effects of multiple systems on health outcomes. The goal of improving the health of the population is best served by emphasizing health promotion and primary prevention throughout the life span. Progress toward this goal requires an understanding of the motivational dynamics of actions that enhance health. This chapter focuses on models and theories useful in explaining and predicting individual health behaviors—those actions motivated by the desire to prevent disease or promote health. Examples of interventions that have been tested using the theories and models are described to provide examples of successful strategies for changing behavior.

Health behavior may be motivated by a desire to protect one's health by avoiding illness or a desire to increase one's level of health in either the presence or absence of illness. *Health promotion* is directed toward increasing the level of well-being and self-actualization of a given individual or group (see Chapter 1). Health promotion focuses on efforts to approach or move toward a positive state of high-level wellness and well-being. In reality, for many health behaviors, both "approaching a positive state" and "avoiding a negative state" serve as sources of motivation for behavior. Health behaviors of adults middle age and older can be explained by approach and avoidance. In contrast, children are more likely to be motivated toward positive healthy behaviors because negative states (illness) are more likely to occur in the future; therefore, avoidance lacks relevance.

HUMAN POTENTIAL FOR CHANGE

Individuals have tremendous potential for self-directed change due to their capacity for self-knowledge, self-regulation, decision making, and creative problem solving. *Self-change* is defined as new behaviors that clients willingly undertake to achieve self-selected goals or desired outcomes. Clients have the power and skill to change health behaviors or modify health-related lifestyles. The nurse's role is to promote a positive climate for change, serve as a catalyst for change, assist with various steps of the change process, and increase the individual's capacity to maintain change.

USE OF THEORIES AND MODELS FOR BEHAVIOR CHANGE

Theories and models of health behavior are attempts to explain why individuals do or do not engage in health behaviors and how individuals change negative behaviors (Noar, Chabot, & Zimmerman, 2008). They specify the concepts that influence the desired health behavior and the relationship among these concepts, indicate how to intervene to promote change, and predict the expected outcomes. Understanding the mechanisms for behavior change and sustainability of these changes is necessary to develop and evaluate health promotion and prevention interventions. To understand the possible mechanisms of change, the mediators—or intervening variables that describe the process responsible for the effect of the intervention on the health behavior—must be examined. Mediators describe why the change occurs. The mediators or mechanisms of behavior change enable health care providers to develop and deliver effective theoretically driven interventions based on the most powerful predictors of health behavior.

To date, no one theory or model completely predicts behavior or behavior change, so multiple theories are presented. The models and theories presented in this chapter focus primarily on individual, intrapersonal, and interpersonal influences to promote health. These models have their origins in educational and social psychology and expectancy-value, social cognitive, and decision-making theories. Key concepts in these theories include cognition, motivation, behavior, and environment. Cognitive processing of information is important in all of the models because individuals' perceptions and interpretations of what they experience directly affect their behaviors. Further, the potential of individuals to respond to alter their environment is recognized. Knowledge of the elements and mechanisms of behavior-change theories that have been shown to influence health behavior enables nurses and other health care professionals to optimize their counseling effectiveness and success in structuring behavioral interventions for clients.

SOCIAL COGNITION THEORIES AND MODELS

Social cognition models are those that incorporate cognitive and affective factors as proximal determinants of behavior (Conner & Norman, 1998; Sutton, 2004). They have been called social cognition models because of the focus on cognitive variables as the major determinant of individual health. Although other factors influence behavior, social cognition models assume that the effects of these factors are mediated by the proximal factors specified in the model. The proximal determinants are amenable to change and can be used as the basis for health promotion interventions. Two types of social cognition models have been applied to explain health related behaviors: The first, attribution models, focuses on an individual's understanding of the causes of the health related events, and the second attempts to predict future health-related behaviors and outcomes. These include the health belief model, the theory of reasoned action and planned behavior, social cognitive and self-efficacy theory, the wellness motivation model, and the health promotion model. Each of these models provides an understanding of the determinants of health behaviors and behavior change.

The Health Belief Model

The health belief model (HBM) was developed in the 1950s to describe why some people who are free of illness will take actions to prevent illness, whereas others fail to do so (Champion & Skinner, 2008; Rosenstock, 1960). The model was developed at a time when there were public health concerns about the widespread reluctance to accept screening for tuberculosis, screening for detection of cervical cancer, immunizations, and other preventive measures that were often free or provided at nominal charge. The model was viewed as potentially useful to predict individuals who would or would not use preventive measures and to suggest interventions that might increase the willingness of resistant individuals to engage in preventive behaviors.

The HBM is derived from social psychology and Lewin's value-expectancy theory (Lewin, Dembo, Festinger, & Sears, 1944). Lewin, a cognitive theorist, conceptualized the life space in which an individual exists as composed of regions, some regions having negative valence, some having positive valence, and others being relatively neutral. Illnesses are conceived to be regions of negative valence exerting a force moving the person away from the regions of positive valence. Preventive behaviors are strategies for avoiding the negatively valenced regions of illness. The model, as modified by Becker, is presented in Figure 2–1.

Evidence has shown that individuals will take action if two conditions are present: (1) a perceived threat to personal health and (2) the conviction that the benefits of taking action to protect health outweigh the barriers that will be encountered. Beliefs about personal susceptibility and the seriousness of a specific illness combine to produce the degree of threat or negative valence of that illness. Perceived susceptibility reflects an individual's feelings of personal vulnerability or risk for a specific health problem. Perceived seriousness of a given health problem may be judged either by the degree of emotional arousal created by the thought of having the disease, or by the medical, clinical, or social difficulties (family and work life) that individuals believe a given health condition would create for them. Perceived benefits are beliefs about the effectiveness of recommended actions in preventing the health threat. Perceived barriers are perceptions regarding the potential negative aspects of taking action such as expense, danger, unpleasantness, inconvenience, and time required. Cues to action are events, internal or external, that trigger action, such as a bodily or environmental event. Modifying factors such as demographic, social, psychological, and structural variables, as well as cues to action, affect action tendencies indirectly through their relationship with perception of threat. However, little research has been conducted on the significance of cues to taking action.

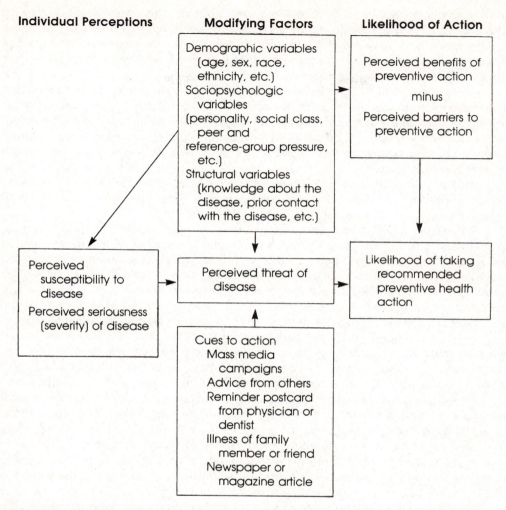

FIGURE 2–1   The Health Belief Model   *Source:* From M. H. Becker, D. P. Haefner, and S. V. Kasl, et al., 1997, "Selected Psychosocial Models and Correlates of Individual Health-Related Behaviors," *Medical Care*, May 1977, Vol. XV, No. 5, Supplement, 27–46. Used with permission.

The HBM continues to be used to explain preventive and health promotion behaviors as well as sick role behaviors, including breast self-examination (Norman & Brain, 2005), condom use (Hounton, Carabin, & Henderson, 2005), screening (Wai et al., 2005), and intent to reduce stroke risk (Sullivan et al., 2008). Prior reviews have shown perceived barriers to be the most powerful HBM dimension in explaining or predicting various preventive behaviors followed by perceived susceptibility (Champion & Skinner, 2008). In general, these two factors are the best predictors of preventive behaviors, and perceived severity and barriers are the best predictors for persons with a diagnosed illness (Armitage & Conner, 2000). The HBM was partially tested in an intervention study in which perceived susceptibility was targeted in smokers, regardless of their interest in quitting smoking (McClure, Ludman, Grothaus, Pabiniak, & Richards, 2009). The group who received brief, personally tailored counseling using biologically based feedback was not more likely to quit than the control group. One possible explanation is that the control group also received an intervention that focused on their health, so the two groups were not substantially different.

Rosenstock, Stretcher, and Becker (1988) proposed expansion of the perceived barriers component to consider feelings of confidence in one's ability to perform a behavior (self-efficacy) as an explanatory variable and suggest that it be incorporated in interventions based on the model. When the HBM was first developed, it was intended for application to one-time behaviors such as immunization. However, application of the model to more complex behavioral risks such as smoking and unsafe sexual practices necessitates attending to individual perceptions of competence, or self-efficacy. to repeatedly engage in preventive behaviors over a long period of time. The absence of this social cognitive concept has been a criticism of the model.

An extended HBM that includes self-efficacy has begun to undergo testing. Norman and Brain (2005) used the extended model to predict breast self-examination and found that women who performed breast self-examinations infrequently reported perceived lower self-efficacy, greater emotional barriers, and fewer benefits. In another study using the extended HBM model, perceived benefits to undertaking exercise and self-efficacy were the two most important determinants of exercise for stroke prevention (Sullivan et al., 2008). Willingness to select healthy bread was studied across four countries with the extended health promotion model (Vassallo et al., 2009). The perceived benefit (health) was the major significant predictor across all four countries, followed by perceived barriers. Self-efficacy was a predictor in three countries, although not significant in two. Results of these studies substantiate the addition of self-efficacy to the HBM.

Protection motivation theory builds on the concepts of the HBM; it is an attempt to explain health behavior motivation based on a disease prevention perspective. In the model health threat appraisal and coping appraisal are theorized to form one's prevention (protection) motivation (Rogers, 1983). Threat appraisal encompasses perceived severity and perceived vulnerability or susceptibility to contracting the disease. Coping appraisal encompasses response efficacy and self-efficacy, a concept in the extended HBM (Plotnikoff, Trinh, Courneya, Karunamunit, & Sigal, 2009). Further work is needed to test which model is more effective in explaining preventive behaviors.

Theory of Reasoned Action and Theory of Planned Behavior

In the theory of reasoned action (TRA), a person's intention to perform a behavior is the most immediate determinant and best predictor of that behavior. Attitudes and subjective norms, intrapersonal factors, constitute the fundamental building blocks of the theory (Fishbein & Ajzen, 1975). Attitudes and subjective norms influence behavioral intention. The first determinant of intention, attitude toward a behavior, is an overall evaluation of the consequences (outcomes) of performing the behavior as either positive or negative. When the evaluation of the behavior outcome is primarily desirable, the result is a positive attitude, whereas a negative attitude results when the evaluation is primarily undesirable. The second determinant of intention, subjective norms, is individuals' beliefs about whether significant others expect them to engage in the behavior—that is, would they approve or disapprove?—and the motivation of the individual to comply with others' expectations. The relative importance of attitudes and subjective norms in predicting any given behavior varies, depending on the target behavior, the context, and the population being studied (Montano, Kasprzyk, & Taplin, 2002).

The TRA is based on the assumption that both attitudes and subjective norms are amenable to change. Interventions by health care professionals may target attitudes by addressing beliefs about outcomes and values related to the outcomes, or subjective norms by focusing on perceptions regarding normative expectations of others and motivation to comply with what others expect. Research has tested the applicability of the TRA to various health behaviors. A review of research indicates that for the most part, intentions moderately to highly correlate with behavior, attitudes are moderately correlated with behavior, and subjective norms are only modestly correlated with behavior. Research has shown that components of the TRA influence a range of health behaviors.

The TRA assumes that behavior is under volitional control; that is, that there are no barriers to performance of the intended behavior. Ajzen, in a critique of the TRA, commented that behavior is not completely under the control of the individual. Thus, he added a third variable, perceived behavioral control, to the original Fishbein and Ajzen concepts of attitude and subjective norms. He labeled the extended theory the theory of planned behavior (TPB) (Ajzen, 1991). Perceived behavioral control is an individual's expectancy that performance of the behavior is within his or her control and is measured by beliefs about the opportunities to engage in the behavior as well as the power of various factors to inhibit or facilitate the behavior. An example of a control belief is "How likely is it that I can get a ride to the gym tomorrow with my friend?" An inhibiting factor is illustrated by "If I cannot get a ride to the gym tomorrow, how likely am I to walk in my neighborhood?"

The TPB has been widely applied in research related to physical activity. In a study of young people 16–19 years, physical activity behavior was explained by both intention and perceived behavioral control (Everson, Daley, & Ussher, 2007). Intention was explained by attitude, subjective norms, and perceived behavioral control, indicating the potential usefulness of the model for guiding physical activity interventions. In an intervention targeting exercise behavior in sedentary college students, the treatment group received email messages targeting attitude with positive framed messages about the health benefits of physical activity (Parrott, Tennant, Olejnik, & Poudevigne, 2008). The group receiving positive framed messages reported higher intention levels, higher levels of affective attitude, and higher exercise behavior levels at follow-up. These findings support the use of the TPB in guiding health promotion interventions for physical activity. The role of ethnicity and gender was examined when using the TPM in a study to understand fruit and vegetable consumption (Blanchard et al., 2009). Both affective attitude and behavioral control predicted intention to meet "5-A-Day" recommendations for blacks, white, males, and females. However, subjective norms were significantly stronger for black males and females than whites.

Despite the strengths of the TPB, there have been suggestions to include additional variables to further increase understanding of behavior. Some behavioral scientist have extended the TPB to include habit strength, which relates to behavioral factors, such as unawareness in performing the behavior (automatic), difficulty in controlling the behavior, and mental efficiency in performing the behavior (de Bruijin, Kroeze, Oenema, & Brug, 2008). Although the interaction of habits with intention has been in the literature for more than 30 years, the role of habit has received little attention due to measurement issues. However, reliable and valid measures are now available, and the relationship has been tested in several studies in which both habit strength and TPB concepts have been measured (Verplanken & Melkevik, 2008). Findings indicate that habit strength interacts with intentions in explaining behavior. When habit strength is strong, intentions are weakly correlated with behavior (de Bruijin, Kremers, Singh, van den Putte, & van Mechelen, 2009; de Bruijin & van den Putte, 2009). When habit strength is weak, intention is a stronger predictor of behavior. These findings have important implications for practitioners as they provide a beginning explanation for the limited success in breaking strong unhealthy habits. Traditional programs using the TPB are aimed at changing attitudes. However, because habits are triggered by situational and environmental cues, change interventions should focus on these things to modify unhealthy behaviors (Honkanen, Olsen, & Verplanken, 2005).

Habit strength is a potentially important determinant of behavior in the TPM and other health behavior models. The few studies that have been reported offer exciting avenues for further research.

Self-Efficacy and Social Cognitive Theory

In social cognitive theory, environmental events, personal factors, and behavior act as reciprocal determinants of each other. The core determinants include knowledge of health risks and benefits of reducing risks; perceived self-efficacy, or the belief that one has the ability to change one's health habits; both positive and negative outcome expectations about changing behavior; personal health goals and strategies for achieving them; and perceived facilitators and structural impediments to achieving them (Bandura, 1997, 2004).

Self-efficacy plays a central role in personal change and is the foundation of human motivation and action. Knowledge is a precondition for change. However, individuals must believe they have control to change the behavior in order to take action. Health behaviors are also influenced by outcome expectancies and goals set by the individual, as they serve as incentives for change. Both facilitators and impediments are determinants of behavior and must be taken into account when assessing self-efficacy (Bandura, 2004). Bandura also recognizes the role of impediments outside one's personal control. The model presented in Figure 2–2 shows the central relationship of self-efficacy with behavior (Bandura, 2004).

According to social cognitive theory, self-beliefs formed through self-observation and self-reflective thought greatly influence human functioning. Self-efficacy expectations develop through mastery experiences (accomplishments), vicarious learning (models), verbal persuasion, and somatic responses to particular situations to build competencies and confidence. The greater the perceived efficacy, the more vigorous and persistent individuals will engage in a behavior, even in the face of obstacles and aversive experiences (Bandura, 1997, 2004). Individuals with high levels of self-efficacy expectations are more likely to set higher goal challenges, expect that their efforts will produce favorable change, and believe that obstacles to their goals are surmountable.

Self-efficacy beliefs are measured in terms of three parameters: magnitude, strength, and generality (Conner & Norman, 2001). *Magnitude* refers to the level of difficulty of the behavior and is an assessment of individuals' perceived capability of

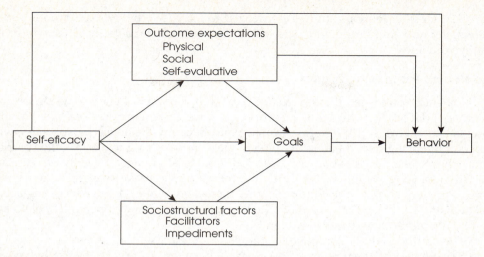

FIGURE 2–2   Sociocognitive Model (showing influence of self-efficacy)   *Source:* From E. Bandura (2004). *Health Education and Behavior: The Official Publication of the Society for Public Health Education, 31*, p. 143. Used with permission.

their level of performance. Individuals with low self-efficacy expectations feel capable of only performing very simple behaviors. *Strength* refers to the individual's confidence in performing the behavior. *Generality* refers to the generalizability of expectations across situations. There is a massive amount of research using the self-efficacy concept; therefore, measures for almost all health behaviors are available in the literature.

The self-efficacy construct has been found to be one of the most important predictors of behavior, and research continues to support social cognitive theory in health behavior change. The theory has been used to predict smoking relapse in adolescents who smoke (Van Zundert, Nijhof, & Engels, 2009). Low self-efficacy to quit was a major predictor for relapse. However, its effects were accounted for by the intensity of smoking. In a longitudinal study of the role of self-efficacy on the relationship between perception of workplace environment and physical activity, self-efficacy partially mediated the relationship of perceptions and physical activity (Plotnikoff, Pickering, Flaman, & Spence, 2009). Self-efficacy has also been shown to be a predictor of physical activity in African-American women (Martin et al., 2008). Lower health literacy has been shown to be associated with less knowledge seeking and lower self-efficacy (von Wagner, Semmler, Good, & Wardle, 2009). This finding reinforces the need to also address health literacy when developing health promotion materials for vulnerable populations.

Interventions to increase self-efficacy have also been conducted. For example, the "Smart Bodies" school wellness program was a clinical trial to increase knowledge and preference for a diet rich in fruits and vegetables in fourth and fifth graders (Tuuri et al., 2009). Children who participated in the 12-week program had greater nutrition knowledge and expressed confidence (self-efficacy) that they could choose fruits instead of less healthy alternatives. A pilot online nutrition course for public librarians to help patrons reduce saturated fat was also shown to increase knowledge and self-efficacy (Turner-McGrievy & Campbell, 2009).

Further interventions studies are needed to increase efficacy expectations and to understand how the concept interacts with other motivational determinants to improve health behaviors.

The Health Promotion Model

In 1990 Pender published the first test of the initial version of Pender's health promotion model (HPM) (Pender, Walker, Sechrist, & Frank-Stromborg, 1990). The HPM proposes a framework for integrating nursing and behavioral science perspectives with factors influencing health behaviors. The model offers a guide to explore the complex biopsychosocial processes that motivate individuals to engage in behaviors directed toward enhancing health. In the 1980s the term *health behavior* was being used with increasing frequency in the literature, and there was renewed interest in high-level wellness and behavior that was motivated by a desire to promote personal health and well-being, rather than disease avoidance.

The initial HPM stimulated studies to describe the potential of seven cognitive–perceptual factors and five modifying factors to predict health behaviors. The cognitive–perceptual factors are importance of health, perceived control of health, definition of health, perceived health status, perceived self-efficacy, perceived benefits, and perceived barriers. The modifying factors are demographic and biologic characteristics, interpersonal influences, situational influences, and behavioral factors. Assumptions and theoretical propositions, a summary of empirical support for constructs in the HPM, and studies using the HPM can be reviewed in earlier editions of this book (Pender, Murdaugh, & Parsons, 2002).

The HPM is a competence- or approach-oriented model. Unlike prevention models, such as the HBM, the HPM does not include "fear" or "threat" as a source of motivation for health behavior. Although immediate threats to health have been shown to motivate action, threats in the distant future lack the same motivational strength. Thus, avoidance-oriented models of health behavior are of limited usefulness in motivating overall healthy lifestyles, particularly in children, youths, and young adults, who often perceive themselves to be invulnerable to illness. The HPM is applicable to any health behavior in which threat is not proposed as a major source of motivation for the behavior. The initial model has since been replaced by the HPM (revised).

THEORETICAL BASIS FOR THE HEALTH PROMOTION MODEL

The HPM is an attempt to depict the multidimensional nature of persons interacting with their interpersonal and physical environments as they pursue health. The HPM integrates constructs from expectancy-value theory and social cognitive theory, within a nursing perspective of holistic human functioning (Bandura, 1986; Feather, 1982).

THE HEALTH PROMOTION MODEL (REVISED)

The revised HPM that first appeared in the third edition of *Health Promotion in Nursing Practice* (Pender, 1996) is shown in Figure 2–3. The variables in the revised HPM and their interrelationships are described in the next section. Three new variables in the revised model are activity-related affect, commitment to a plan of action, and immediate competing demands and preferences.

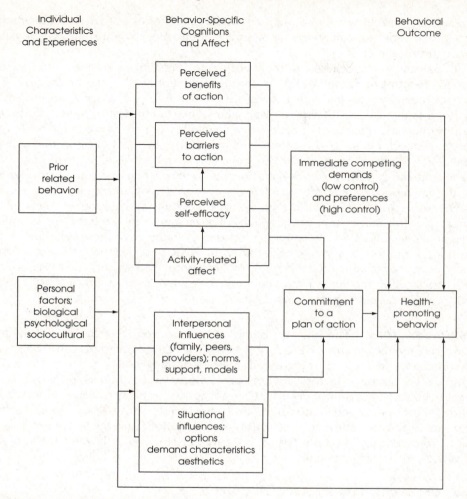

FIGURE 2–3   Health Promotion Model (revised)

Individual Characteristics and Experiences

Each person has unique personal characteristics and experiences that affect subsequent actions. The importance of their effect depends on the target behavior being considered. Individual characteristics and experiences include prior related behavior and personal factors.

PRIOR RELATED BEHAVIOR.   Behavioral factors have been retained in the HPM as "prior related behavior." Research indicates that often the best predictor of behavior is the frequency of the same or a similar behavior in the past. Prior behavior is proposed to have both direct and indirect effects on the likelihood of engaging in health-promoting behaviors. The direct effect of past behavior on current health-promoting behavior may be due to habit formation, predisposing one to engage in the behavior automatically with little attention to the specific details of its execution. Habit strength accrues each time the behavior occurs and is augmented by concentrated, repetitive practice of the behavior.

Consistent with social cognitive theory, prior behavior is proposed to indirectly influence health-promoting behavior through perceptions of self-efficacy, benefits, barriers, and activity-related affect. According to Bandura (1985), actual enactment of a behavior and its associated feedback is a major source of efficacy or "skill" information. Bandura refers to anticipated or experienced benefits from engaging in the behavior as "outcome expectations." If short-term benefits are experienced early in the course of the behavior, the behavior is more likely to be repeated. Barriers to a given behavior are experienced and stored in memory as "hurdles" that must be overcome to engage successfully in the behavior. Every behavior is also accompanied by emotions or affect. Positive or negative affect before, during, or following the behavior is encoded into memory as information that is retrieved when engaging in the behavior is contemplated at a later time. Prior behavior is proposed to shape all of these behavior-specific cognitions and affect. The nurse helps individuals shape a positive behavioral history for the future by focusing on the benefits of a behavior, teaching how to overcome hurdles to performing the behavior, and engendering high levels of efficacy and positive affect through successful performance experience and positive feedback.

PERSONAL FACTORS.   The relevant personal factors predictive of a given behavior are shaped by the nature of the target behavior being considered. In the revised HPM, personal factors are categorized as biologic, psychologic, and sociocultural. Examples of biologic factors include age, body mass index, pubertal status, menopausal status, aerobic capacity, strength, agility, or balance. Psychologic factors include self-esteem, self-motivation, and perceived health status. Sociocultural factors include race, ethnicity, acculturation, education, and socioeconomic status. Personal factors should be limited to those that are theoretically relevant to explain or predict a given target behavior.

Behavior-Specific Cognitions and Affect

Behavior-specific variables within the HPM are considered to have major motivational significance. These variables constitute a critical "core" for intervention, because they can be modified through interventions. These variables include perceived benefits, perceived barriers, perceived self-efficacy, activity-related affect, interpersonal influences, and situational influences. Measuring these variables is essential to assess whether change actually results from the intervention.

PERCEIVED BENEFITS OF ACTION.   Perceived benefits of action are mental representations of the positive or reinforcing consequences of a behavior. An individual's expectations to engage in a particular behavior hinge on the anticipated benefits. In the HPM, perceived benefits are proposed to directly and indirectly motivate behavior through determining the extent of commitment to a plan of action to engage in the behaviors. According to expectancy-value theory, the motivational importance of anticipated benefits is based on personal outcomes from prior direct experience with the behavior or vicarious experience through observing others engaging in the behavior. Individuals tend to invest time and resources in activities that have a high likelihood of positive outcomes. Benefits may be intrinsic or extrinsic. Intrinsic benefits include increased alertness and energy and increased perceived attractiveness. Extrinsic benefits include monetary rewards or social interactions possible as a result of engaging in the behavior. Initially, extrinsic benefits of health behaviors may be highly significant, whereas intrinsic benefits may be more powerful in motivating sustainability of health behaviors. Beliefs in positive outcome expectations have generally been shown to be a necessary although not sufficient condition to engage in a specific health behavior.

PERCEIVED BARRIERS TO ACTION.   Barriers consist of perceptions about the unavailability, inconvenience, expense, difficulty, or time-consuming nature of a particular action. Barriers are often viewed as mental blocks, hurdles, and personal costs of undertaking a given behavior. Barriers usually arouse motives of avoidance in relation to a given behavior. Anticipated barriers have been repeatedly found to affect intentions to engage in a particular behavior . Loss of satisfaction from giving up health-damaging behaviors such as smoking or eating high-fat foods to adopt a healthier lifestyle may also constitute a barrier.

When readiness to act is low and barriers are high, action is unlikely to occur. Perceived barriers to action in the revised HPM affect health-promoting behavior directly by serving as blocks to action as well as indirectly through decreasing commitment to a plan of action.

PERCEIVED SELF-EFFICACY.   Self-efficacy is the judgment of personal capability to organize and carry out a particular course of action. Self-efficacy does not involve skill but judgments of what one can do with whatever skills one possesses. Judgments of personal efficacy are distinguished from outcome expectations. Perceived self-efficacy is a judgment of one's abilities to accomplish a certain level of performance, whereas an outcome expectation is a judgment of the likely consequences (benefits, costs) the behavior will produce (Siela & Wieseke, 2000). Perceptions of skill and competence in a particular domain motivate individuals to engage in behaviors in which they excel. Feeling efficacious and skilled is likely to encourage one to engage in the target behavior more frequently than is feeling inept and unskilled.

The HPM proposes that perceived self-efficacy is influenced by activity-related affect. The more positive the affect, the greater the perceptions of efficacy. However, in reality this relationship is reciprocal: Greater perceptions of efficacy, in turn, increase positive affect. Self-efficacy influences perceived barriers to action, with higher efficacy resulting in lowered perception of barriers. Self-efficacy motivates health-promoting behavior directly by efficacy expectations and indirectly by affecting perceived barriers and level of commitment or persistence in pursuing a plan of action.

ACTIVITY-RELATED AFFECT.   Activity-related affect consists of three components: emotional arousal to the act itself (act related), the self acting (self related), and the environment in which the action takes place (context related). The resultant feeling state is likely to affect whether an individual will repeat the behavior again or maintain the behavior long term. Subjective feeling states occur prior to, during, and following an activity, based on the stimulus properties associated with the behavioral event. These affective responses may be mild, moderate, or strong and are cognitively labeled, stored in memory, and associated with subsequent thoughts of the behavior. The affect associated with the behavior reflects a direct emotional reaction or gut-level response to the behavior, which can be positive or negative—is it fun, delightful, enjoyable, disgusting, or unpleasant? Behaviors associated with positive affect are likely to be repeated, whereas those associated with negative affect are likely to be avoided. Both positive and negative feeling states are induced for some behaviors. Thus, the relative balance between positive and negative affect prior to, during, and following the behavior is important to ascertain. Activity-related affect is different from the evaluative dimension of attitude proposed by Fishbein and Ajzen (1975). The evaluative dimension of attitude reflects affective evaluation of the specific outcomes of a behavior rather than the response to the stimulus properties of the behavioral event itself.

For any given behavior, the full range of negative and positive feelings states in relation to the act, self as actor, and context for action should be measured. In many instruments proposed to measure affect, negative feelings are elaborated more extensively than positive feelings. This is not surprising because anxiety, fear, and depression have been studied much more than have joy, elation, and calm. Emotional responses and their induced physiologic states during a behavior serve as sources of efficacy information (Bandura, 1985). Thus, activity-related affect is proposed to influence health behavior directly as well as indirectly through self-efficacy and commitment to a plan of action.

INTERPERSONAL INFLUENCES. Interpersonal influences are cognitions involving the behaviors, beliefs, or attitudes of others. These cognitions may or may not correspond with reality. Primary sources of interpersonal influence on health-promoting behaviors are family, peers, and health care providers. Interpersonal influences include norms (expectations of significant others), social support (instrumental and emotional encouragement), and modeling (vicarious learning through observing others engaged in a particular behavior). These three interpersonal influences determine individuals' predisposition to engage in health-promoting behaviors.

Social norms set standards for performance that individuals may adopt or reject. Social support for a behavior taps the sustaining resources offered by others. Modeling portrays the sequential components of a health behavior and is an important strategy for behavior change in social cognitive theory. The HPM proposes that interpersonal influences affect health-promoting behavior directly as well as indirectly through social pressures or encouragement to commit to a plan of action. Individuals vary in the extent to which they are sensitive to the wishes, examples, and praise of others. However, given sufficient motivation, individuals are likely to undertake behaviors that will be socially reinforced. Susceptibility to the influence of others may vary developmentally and be particularly evident in adolescence. Some cultures place more emphasis on interpersonal influences than others. For example, *familismo* among Hispanic populations may encourage individuals to engage in a particular behavior for the good of the family rather than for personal gain.

SITUATIONAL INFLUENCES. Personal perceptions and cognitions of any situation or context facilitate or impede behavior. Situational influences on health-promoting behavior include perceptions of options available, demand characteristics, and aesthetic features of the environment in which a given behavior is proposed to take place. Individuals are drawn to and perform more competently in situations or environmental contexts in which they feel compatible, related, and safe and reassured. Environments that are fascinating and interesting are also desirable contexts for performing health behaviors.

In the revised HPM, situational influences have been reconceptualized to directly and indirectly influence health behavior. Situations may directly affect behaviors by presenting an environment "loaded" with cues that trigger action. For example, a "no smoking" environment creates demand characteristics for nonsmoking behavior. Company regulations for hearing protection to be worn create demand characteristics that employees comply with regulations. Both situations enforce commitment to health actions.

Situational influences have received moderate support as determinants of health behavior and may be an important key to develop new and more effective strategies to facilitate the acquisition and maintenance of health-promoting behaviors in diverse populations.

Commitment to a Plan of Action

Commitment to a plan of action initiates a behavioral event. Commitment propels the individual into action unless there is a competing demand that cannot be avoided or a competing preference that is not resisted. Individuals generally engage in organized rather than disorganized behavior. In the revised HPM, *commitment to a plan of action* implies the following underlying cognitive processes: (1) commitment to carry out a specific action at a given time and place and with specified persons or alone, irrespective of competing preferences (implementation intention), and (2) identification of definitive strategies for eliciting, carrying out, and reinforcing the behavior. Identification of specific strategies to be used at different points in the behavioral sequence goes beyond intentionality to further the likelihood that the plan of action will be successfully implemented. For example, the strategy of contracting consists of a mutually agreed-upon set of actions to which one party commits with the understanding that the other party will provide some tangible reward or reinforcement if the commitment is sustained. Strategies are selected to energize and reinforce health behaviors according to individual preferences and stage of change. Commitment alone without associated strategies often results in "good intentions" but failure to perform the health behavior. Commitment to a plan is similar to the concept of implementation intentions in which strong commitment is supplemented with when, where and how the commitment will be realized (Rise, Thompson, & Verplanken, 2003).

Immediate Competing Demands and Preferences

Immediate competing demands or preferences refer to alternative behaviors that intrude into consciousness as possible courses of action immediately prior to the intended occurrence of a planned health-promoting behavior. Competing demands are alternative behaviors over which individuals have a relatively low level of control because of environmental contingencies such as work or family care responsibilities. Failure to respond to a competing demand may have untoward effects for the self or for significant others. Competing preferences have powerful reinforcing properties over which individuals exert a relatively high level of control. The extent to which an individual resists competing preferences depends on the ability to be self-regulating. Examples of "giving in" to competing preferences are selecting a food high in fat rather than low in fat because of taste or flavor preferences; driving past the recreation center where one usually exercises to stop at the mall based on a preference for shopping rather than physical activity. Both competing demands and preferences can derail a plan of action. Competing preferences are differentiated from barriers such as lack of time, because competing preferences are last-minute urges based on one's preference hierarchy that derail a plan for positive health action.

Individuals vary in their ability to sustain attention and avoid disruption of health behaviors. Some individuals may be predisposed developmentally or biologically to be more easily swayed from a course of action. Inhibiting competing preferences requires the exercise of self-regulation and control capabilities. Strong commitment to a plan of action may sustain dedication to complete a behavior in light of competing demands or preferences. In the HPM, immediate competing demands and preferences are proposed to directly affect the probability of occurrence of health behavior as well as moderate the effects of commitment.

Behavioral Outcome

HEALTH-PROMOTING BEHAVIOR. Health-promoting behavior is the end point or action outcome in the HPM. However, health-promoting behavior is ultimately directed toward *attaining positive health outcomes* for the client. Health-promoting behaviors, particularly when integrated into a healthy lifestyle, results in improved health, enhanced functional ability, and better quality of life at all stages of development.

Studies continue to be conducted to support the HPM model constructs. Most of the studies reported in the past 10 years have focused on testing the predictability of the model rather than as a theoretical basis for developing and testing interventions to study the mechanisms of change proposed in the model. The model has been applied to predict health-promoting behaviors of homeless women in shelters (Wilson, 2005); women with female-specific cancers (Eschiti, 2008); adolescent cancer survivors (Smith & Bashore, 2006); pre-university students (Morowatisbarifabad & Karimzadeh, 2007); married couples (Padula & Sullivan, 2006); and construction workers (Ronis, Hong, & Lusk, 2006). Health-promoting behaviors have included physical activity, nutrition, oral health, and hearing. An issue that continues is the incomplete testing of the entire HPM model in many studies. Instead, only a few of the model concepts are tested for their predictive ability on health-promoting lifestyles. Several studies report only measuring health behavior using Pender's Health-Promoting Lifestyle Measure (HPLII) as a test of the model. A possible reason may be the complexity of the model and the large number of concepts that need to be measured to test the full model. In spite of the limitation, self-efficacy, perceived barriers, and social support are consistent predictors of health behaviors. In addition, when many of the model concepts are included in structural equation model testing, the amount of explained variance in modified models has ranged as high as 73% (Shin, Kang, Park, Cho, & Heitkemper, 2008). Research to date points to the need to carefully examine the model to eliminate nonsignificant concepts and add new concepts while maintaining parsimony. The

HPM remains a widely used model in nursing and other health care disciplines to predict health promoting behaviors. The behavior-specific cognitions (perceived benefits, barriers, self-efficacy, and affect), as well as other model components amenable to change, must be used to develop and test theoretically driven interventions to further test the model.

STAGE MODELS OF BEHAVIOR CHANGE

The fundamental assumption underlying a stage model of change is that differences exist in people in their likelihood of action, and different explanations are necessary for different stages of change. Stage models, also known as continuum models, have four major principles (Weinstein, Rothman, & Sutton, 1998):

1. A category system to define the stages
2. An ordering of the stages
3. Common barriers to change people face in the same stage
4. Different barriers to change facing people in different stages

The best-known stage model is the transtheoretical model of change, which is discussed in the next section. The precaution adoption process model is another stage model of change (Weinstein, Sandman, & Blalock, 2008). The seven-stage adoption process model focuses on risk and changing behavior to reduce risks (prevention). Further information on this model is available in the literature.

Transtheoretical Model

The transtheoretical model, which is derived from psychotherapy and theories of behavior change, is an integrative framework to describe how individuals progress toward adopting and maintaining behavior change (Prochaska, Johnson, & Lee, 2009). The premise of the model is that health-related behavior change progresses through five stages, regardless of whether the client is trying to quit a health-threatening behavior or adopt a healthy behavior (Prochaska & DiClemente, 1983). These stages are as follows:

- *Precontemplation*: An individual is not thinking about quitting or adopting a particular behavior, at least not *within the next six months* (no intention to take action).
- *Contemplation*: An individual is seriously thinking about quitting or adopting a particular behavior *in the next six months* (intends to change).
- *Planning or Preparation*: An individual is seriously thinking about engaging in the contemplated change *within the next month* and has taken some steps in this direction (making small or sporadic changes).
- *Action*: The individual has made the behavior change and it has persisted *for less than six months* (actively engaged in behavior change).
- *Maintenance:* The change has been in place for at least six months and is continuing (sustaining the change over time).

An attempt has been made to integrate various core concepts from other models of behavior change into the transtheoretical model. The concept of *decisional balance* from

Janis and Mann's decision-making model (Janis & Mann, 1977) is integral to the model. The Janis and Mann conflict model assumes sound decision making involves comparison of all potential gains and losses. Behavior should occur when the potential gains of engaging in the behavior outweigh the losses.

Self-efficacy is also considered a core concept in the model. Self-efficacy shifts in a predictable way across the stages of behavior change, with clients progressively becoming more efficacious. The concept was integrated from Bandura's social cognitive theory.

The third core concept is temptation, or the intensity of urges to engage in a specific behavior in the midst of a difficult situation (Prochaska et al., 2009). Emotional distress, positive social situations, and cravings account for the most common temptations.

Prochaska proposes that different processes of change are appropriate at different stages of behavior change. The 10 processes of change are presented in Table 2–1. They are categorized as either experiential or behavioral processes or strategies.

Experiential processes are more important than behavioral processes in the early stages of change for understanding and predicting progress. Experiential processes are to a large extent internally focused on behavior-linked emotions, values, and cognitions. Behavioral processes are more important for understanding and predicting transition

TABLE 2–1   Processes of Change

Process	Definition
Experiential Processes	
Consciousness raising	Efforts by the individual to seek new information and to gain understanding and feedback about the problem
Dramatic relief	Affective aspects of change, often involving intense emotional experiences related to the problem behavior
Environmental reevaluation	Consideration and assessment by the individual of how the problem affects the physical and social environments
Self-reevaluation	Emotional and cognitive reappraisal of values by the individual with respect to the problem behavior
Social Liberation	Awareness, availability, and acceptance by the individual of alternative lifestyles in society
Behavioral Processes	
Counterconditioning	Substitution of alternative behaviors for the problem behavior
Helping relationships	Trusting, accepting, and utilizing the support of caring others during attempts to change the problem behavior
Reinforcement management	Changing the contingencies that control or maintain the problem behavior
Self-liberation	The individual's choice and commitment to change the problem behavior, including the belief that one *can* change
Stimulus Control	Control of situations and other causes that trigger the problem behavior

Source: From Marcus, B. H., Rossi, J. S., Selby, V. C., et al. (1992). The stages and processes of exercise adoption and maintenance in a worksite example. *Health Psychology, 11*, 387. American Psychological Association. Reprinted with permission.

from preparation to action and from action to maintenance. Behavioral processes focus directly on behavioral change. When an individual's stage has been assessed, appropriate processes are implemented to help the client progress from stage to stage.

Many intervention studies have been conducted using the transtheoretical model. The largest number has focused on smoking, followed by physical activity. Other topics have included stress management, bullying prevention, condom use, and obesity (see Prochaska et al. (2009), for a review). Behavior change is most successful when all of the core concepts are integrated, not just the stages of change. Evidence also supports that those who are ready to change respond more to stage-based interventions than those who are not ready (Aveyard, Massey, Parsons, Maneski, & Griffin, 2009). In a dietary intervention program for youth using the transtheoretical model concepts, stages of changes and processes were consistent mediators of program effects, providing some evidence for the mechanisms producing the intervention effects (Di Noia & Prochaska, 2009).

Despite the success of the model in helping explain health behavior, additional concepts should be considered. This is a major challenge for all of the behavior change models.

INTERVENTIONS FOR HEALTH BEHAVIOR CHANGE

Increasing healthy behaviors and decreasing risky or health-damaging behaviors are the major challenges facing health professionals. Thus, a core question is this: What are the critical interventions, based on health promotion and prevention models and theories, that will enable nurses to assist clients to make desired changes in health-related behaviors? Behavior-change strategies based on the theories presented here are used to illustrate evidence-based counseling and behavioral interventions.

Raising Consciousness

The transtheoretical model emphasizes the importance of raising consciousness at the point when the client is either not considering behavior change or just beginning to consider a change. Awareness of the benefits of adopting a healthy behavior or discontinuing a risky behavior is enhanced through seeking and processing information, observing others, and interpreting information in light of one's personal situation. Materials should be provided about health-related issues relevant to the target behavior, including the short- and long-term consequences for the individual. "Headliners" from national newspapers and magazines that focus on the benefits of change or the negative consequences of not changing may be particularly effective in raising consciousness due to the "eye-catching" format in which the information is presented. The client should be given a list of information resources and encouraged to become an active participant in information gathering. The materials used for raising consciousness must address health literacy issues and be culturally specific to optimize impact.

Reevaluating the Self

Self-reevaluation, a process identified in social cognitive theory, is based on the premise that change results from the arousal of an affective state of dissatisfaction within oneself as a result of recognition of disturbing inconsistencies between self-standards (values, beliefs) and behaviors. The client may ask questions such as these: Will I like myself better if I am thinner, more physically active, or no longer smoke? A contradiction between personal values and current behavior is most directly resolved by engaging in behavior change. Further, the more individuals perceive that they are the type of person who engages in a particular behavior; the more likely they are to perform the behavior. Adherence to personal behavior standards will enhance self-concept through feelings of pride and self-satisfaction, whereas violation of self-standards for behavior results in negative feelings of guilt and self-censure. Strong intentions to meet personal standards will likely increase performance of the behavior and eventually lead to sustained behavior change.

Self-reevaluation may involve mental contrasting, in which individuals name their most important wish related to changing a behavior (physical inactivity), name and imagine the most positive outcome of successfully changing the behavior (better physical shape), and name and imagine the most critical obstacle standing in the way of accomplishing the wish (family responsibilities) (Oettingen, Pak, & Schnetter, 2001). If clients expect they can achieve the goal and overcome the obstacles, they are more likely to strongly commit to their goals.

Promoting Self-Efficacy

The most powerful input to self-efficacy is successful performance of a behavior. Whenever possible, the nurse facilitates the client to perform the target behavior and provides positive feedback on aspects of the behavior that were performed appropriately. For example, having the client select low-fat foods from an array of pictures or food models and providing immediate feedback on correct choices enhances task self-efficacy. Praise and positive feedback along with persuasion and reassurance are concrete ways to build self-efficacy relevant to a particular behavior. The nurse builds regulatory self-efficacy by providing clients with strategies to overcome barriers to performing the target behavior as well as enhancing confidence that the client can successfully overcome the barriers. Learning from the experiences of others or directly observing others' behaviors increases clients' perceptions of self-efficacy and lowers perceived barriers to successful behavior change.

Observation of others engaging in the desired behavior is important during the action phase to refine one's performance capabilities and enhance self-efficacy. Modeling of behavior by others is especially helpful when clients have articulated specific health goals but are uncertain about the exact behaviors that should be developed to move toward the goals. The following considerations are important to effectively use modeling to facilitate self-efficacy and resultant behavior change:

- Clients must share characteristics with the model, such as gender, age, ethnicity, race, language.
- Clients must have an opportunity to observe the desired behavior.
- Clients must have the requisite knowledge and skills to engage in the behavior.
- Clients must perceive benefits from engaging in the target behavior.
- Clients must have the opportunity to practice the target behavior.

Enhancing the Benefits of Change

Behavioral beliefs in the TPB as well as outcome expectations in social cognitive theory are considered necessary conditions for behavior change. Planning for reward or reinforcement is a unique way to expand the benefits or positive outcomes derived from behavior change. The importance of reinforcement is based on the premise that all behaviors are determined by their consequences. If positive consequences result, the probability is high that the behavior will occur again. If negative consequences occur, the probability is low that the behavior will be repeated. Positive reinforcement (reward) rather than negative reinforcement (removal of an aversive condition) or punishment (aversive experience) provides the most effective motivation for behavioral change. When self-modification is the focus of an intervention, clients select the behavior they will change and the rewards they desire to receive for change. Behaviors that are to be reinforced must be clearly identified and a plan or contract for change negotiated either between the client and the health care provider or between the client and significant others.

If a client wishes to increase the incidence of a specific health-promoting behavior or decrease the incidence of a health-damaging behavior, one strategy is to obtain an initial frequency count of the target behavior (baseline data) so that extent of progress toward the desired change can be accurately assessed. An example of a daily record of smoking behavior is presented in Figure 2–4.

Benefits are classified as tangible, social, or self-generated and serve to reinforce desired behavior. Tangible benefits include objects or activities, such as making a purchase of a desired object or participating in a favorite activity. Social benefits include spending time with friends or family. Self-generated benefits

Behavior to Be Observed:	Smoking		
Observation Categories:	Morning Afternoon Evening		
Method of Coding Behavior:		E = Smoking after or during eating and drinking	
		S = Smoking while nervous in a social situation	
		D = Smoking while driving the car	
		O = Smoking at other times	

Smoking Record

Date: Tuesday, August 26		
Morning	Afternoon	Evening
E E D O S S E	O S S D S E E E	E O

Date: Wednesday, August 27		
Morning	Afternoon	Evening
E E E D D S E E	S S S S D D E E E E	S E O

FIGURE 2–4 Self-Observation Sheet *Source:* From Watson/Tharp. *Self-Directed Behavior*, 1E. © 1974 Wadsworth, a part of Cengage Learning, Inc. Reproduced by permission. www.cengage.com/permissions.

include self-praise and self-compliments. The time frame for application of reinforcement is critical. Immediate and continuous reinforcement is highly desirable, particularly in the early phases of change, as it promotes rapid learning of the desired behaviors. Intermittent reinforcement applied later stabilizes the behavior and makes it resistant to extinction.

Many behaviors are too complex to be acquired all at once. Gradually shaping desired behaviors is an effective approach to make permanent changes in lifestyle. An example of shaping is the following:

- Brisk walk for 15 minutes 2 days the first week
- Brisk walk for 20 minutes 3 days the second and third weeks
- Brisk walk for 30 minutes 3 days the fourth and fifth weeks
- Brisk walk for 45 minutes 4 days the sixth and seventh weeks
- Brisk walk for 60 minutes 5 days the eighth and ninth weeks

Each step toward the final behavior should be mastered before the next step is attempted.

After the client starts engaging in a desired behavior, the intrinsic rewards, such as losing weight, feeling more relaxed, or feeling more energetic, have reinforcing properties. When the behavior begins to offer its own reward, the nurse counsels the client that extrinsic rewards to enhance the benefits of the behavior may no longer be necessary.

Modifying the Environment

Modifying the environment to support behavior change is an important tenet of social cognitive theory (Levin, 1999). Stimulus control includes structuring multiple environments to elicit the desired behavior. Internal prompts coupled with external prompts encourage action; for example, "feeling good after brisk walking" coupled with "the invitation from spouse to take a walk." Synergistically, this provides powerful stimuli for behavior change. Table 2–2 presents an overview of possible stimulus configurations that prompt health-promoting and prevention behaviors.

Individuals define relevant environmental changes to make based on past knowledge and experiences. Reconfiguring environmental stimuli augments conditions for desirable behaviors or decreases conditions for undesirable behaviors.

TABLE 2–2   Possible Cues for Health-Promoting Preventive Actions

Internal Cues

Bodily states; e.g., feeling good, feeling energetic, recognizing aging, fatigue, cyclical discomfort

Affective states; e.g., enthusiasm, motivation for self-preservation, high level of self-esteem, happiness, concern

External Cues

Interactions with significant others; e.g., family, friends, colleagues, nurse, and physician

Impact of communication media; e.g., motivational messages from television, radio, newspapers, advertisements, and special mailings

Visual stimuli from the environment; e.g., passing a diabetic screening clinic, billboards, attendance at a health fair, passing a gym or exercise center, or viewing others participating in target activity

---

Specific approaches to stimulus reconfiguration include cue elimination, cue restriction, and cue expansion. In *cue elimination* environmental cues for undesired behaviors are decreased to zero. Examples include eating meals only with nonsmokers if cessation of smoking is the goal. In successful cue elimination, extinction of the behavior results.

Frequently, cues cannot be totally eliminated but can be reduced or restricted. In *cue restriction*, for example, the cues to eating may be reduced to one room in the house, the kitchen or dining room. By localizing the cues that activate behavior, arrangements for limited encounter with these cues are possible. In *cue expansion*, the number of prompts to desired behaviors is increased. For example, whereas personal preparation of food at home in one's own kitchen may prompt small servings of meats, fruits, and vegetables, the environment of a restaurant may prompt selection of rich entrées and desserts. In *cue expansion*, a menu at a restaurant provides cues for looking only at salad and vegetable options as opposed to scanning the dessert section. By expanding the range of cues that elicit specific responses, desirable behaviors may occur more frequently and with greater regularity. Controlling the environment conducive to the behavior through the elimination, restriction, or expansion of cues assists clients in creating internal and external conditions to support positive health practices.

Managing Barriers to Change

Barriers to change are central constructs in the health belief model and the health promotion model. The nurse facilitates the preparation, action, and maintenance stages of behavior change by minimizing or eliminating barriers to action. It is futile to encourage clients to take actions that are highly likely to be blocked or cause frustration.

Internal barriers to self-modification include the following:

- Unclear short-term and long-term goals
- Lack of skills needed to make change
- Perceptions of lack of control
- Lack of motivation

Barriers such as these often reflect insufficient attention to the preparation stage of behavior change.

The interaction of level of readiness and barriers to action is depicted in Table 2–3. Consequences and appropriate nursing interventions are also presented. When clients have a high level of readiness to engage in health-promoting or preventive behaviors and barriers are low, a low-intensity cue is sufficient to activate behavior. A high-intensity cue under these conditions may actually be a negative force. When readiness is high and barriers to action are also formidable, barriers must be reduced or eliminated. When both readiness and barriers are low, readiness to act should be increased in order to initiate action. When readiness is low and barriers high, both factors should be addressed, or behavior change is unlikely to occur.

Significant others often serve as barriers to health actions. When family members or other persons disagree or are neutral or apathetic toward health behaviors, the constraints created for the client depends on the following factors:

- Relevance of disagreeing persons
- Attractiveness of disagreeing persons

TABLE 2–3   Interrelationships among Level of Readiness to Take Health Actions, Barriers, Consequences for Clients, and Nursing Interventions

Level of Readiness	Barriers to Action	Consequences for Client	Nursing Interventions
High	Low	Action	Support and encouragement; provide low-intensity cue
High	High	Conflict	Assist client in lowering barriers to action
Low	Low	Conflict	Provide high-intensity cue
Low	High	No action	Assist client in lowering barriers to action and then provide high-intensity cue

- Extent of disagreement of relevant persons
- Number of persons relevant to the client who disagree with behavior
- Extent to which client is self-directed rather than other dependent

Membership in self-help or self-change groups may be critical at this point, because the group often provides needed support not provided by family or friends to identify barriers likely to be encountered in making changes, and various strategies to overcome these constraints.

TAILORING BEHAVIOR CHANGE INTERVENTIONS

Tailoring print and interactive computer communications in health promotion and prevention offers exciting opportunities for nurses to engage in development, testing, and implementation of individualized behavior-change strategies. The computer provides the nurse–client team with more power to collect and process information, collaboratively set goals, and tailor strategies to assist individuals and families in achieving health goals. "One-size-fits-all" health education materials are rapidly becoming outdated as information technology expands the range of possibilities for using complex, interactive behavior change strategies that are relevant to clients, practical for providers, and cost-effective for health care systems. The one-size-fits-all approach cannot address the range of details that vary from person to person and influence individuals' health-related decisions and health behaviors.

Tailoring is a process for creating individualized communication to meet the unique needs of an individual (Rimer & Kreuter, 2006). Tailored health materials are personalized, based on characteristics unique to that person, related to the outcome of interest, and derived from an individual assessment. Tailored materials are considered more effective than generic or targeted communication in terms of engaging individuals, building self-efficacy, and improving health behaviors, and they are more likely to be read, remembered, and viewed as personally relevant (Kreuter, Caburnay, Chen, & Donlin, 2004). Generic communication is not personalized in any way, and targeted communication messages are developed for a certain segment of the population. The potential to reach large numbers of persons through computer-based tailoring has great promise.

Tailored interventions must be theoretically based (Noar, Benac, & Harris, 2007). If the transtheoretical model with its stages of change is the basis for the intervention, interventions must be tailored to the stages that are most likely to be the most effective for changing behaviors. In addition, the core concepts of the theory should be tailored to the individual. Tailored intervention with the HBM would involve tailoring information based on clients' perceived threats as well as their perceived benefits and barriers to changing behavior. A tailored intervention using the TPB would target the individual's attitudes, subjective norms, and perceived behavioral control. Social cognitive theory–tailored interventions would focus on changing efficacy expectations to meet the individual's desired outcomes (outcome expectations), as well as relevant components of the environment. The selected theory provides the conceptual structure for designing the communication message to match client characteristics to individually tailored interventions. Tailored messages may be delivered through many channels: print, interactive computer programs, telephone, audio, video, or the Internet.

Current evidence supports the advantage of tailored interventions. In a meta-analytic review of tailored print health behavior change interventions, the effectiveness of such interventions was supported for behavior change (Noar et al., 2007). The strongest print tailored messages targeted preventive or screening behaviors; generated pamphlets, magazines, or newspapers; used more than one intervention contact; had shorter periods between intervention and follow-up; recruited participants from households rather than clinics or health centers; tailored on four to five theoretical concepts as well as behavior and demographics; and used one of the behavior change theories as a basis for the intervention. These findings provide useful information for tailoring interventions using print materials.

Web-based tailored programs offer many advantages, including the ability to be delivered to wider audiences and overcome geographical and temporal barriers. Two reviews support the application of computers to deliver tailored interventions. A review of computer-tailored health interventions delivered over the Web found that the interventions have a large diversity of formats and features (Lustria, Cortese, Noar, & Glueckauf, 2009). Interventions varied in level of sophistication, ranging from computer-assisted health risk assessments with immediate feedback to customized complex health programs of longer term with multiple opportunities for program access. Most programs were self-guided with minimal contact with the experts and consistently focused on four areas: health behavior, stage of change, risk factors, and information needs and were delivered by print, CD-ROM based applications, computer kiosks, or the Internet. The authors concluded that clearer guidance is needed for tailoring, and health outcomes must be evaluated. In a meta-analysis of 75 randomized controlled trials of computer-delivered interventions of health promotion and risk reduction, participants who received the computer-delivered interventions improved in antecedents of health behavior and health behaviors (nutrition, tobacco use, substance use, safer sexual behavior) (Portney, Scott-Sheldon, Johnson, & Carey, 2008). The authors concluded that computer–based interventions can lead to improvements in health-related knowledge, attitudes, intentions, and health behaviors immediately post-intervention.

Mobile telephones have also been effective for behavior change interventions. Mobile telephones allow for instantaneous delivery of short messages at any time, place, or setting; can be tailored to individuals; allows for quantifiable interaction between the participant and the interventionist; and is more cost-effective than other telephone or print-based interventions (Fjeldsoe, Marshall, & Miller, 2009). The potential use of the mobile telephone is significant, as the higher-frequency user groups are adolescents, young people, socioeconomically disadvantaged populations, less educated, and people who rent and change addresses frequently. Of 33 mobile telephone studies identified, 14 met inclusion criteria for review (Fjeldsoe et al., 2009). Significant positive behavior changes were noted in eight studies, and positive changes occurred in 13 of the 14 studies. Important features of the interventions included how the intervention was initiated, how the short messages were initiated, origin of the content, and interactivity. The mobile telephone has positive short-term behavioral outcomes. However, the quality of the studies must improve to allow the full potential to be explored.

Tailored interventions have been implemented to provide information about cancer risks (Albada, Ausems, Bensing, & van Dulmen, 2009); promote mammography screening (Sohl & Moyer, 2007); reduce fat intake (Kroeze, Oenema, Campbell, & Brug, 2008); and promote physical activity in adolescents (Haerens et al., 2009). In general, a consistent improvement has been reported in health outcomes with these interventions.

MAINTAINING BEHAVIOR CHANGE

Maintenance of health behavior raises special challenges for the client. Changes in behavior that are transient accomplish little to enhance one's health status. The behavior must be sustained in the environment in which it is learned, and the behavior must also be generalized to other situations. Factors important for continuation of positive health behaviors are similar to those necessary for initiating behavior change and include the following:

- Extent of personal skill to carry out the behavior
- Number of personal beliefs and attitudes that support the target behavior including beliefs about self-efficacy
- Extent of positive emotional response (positive affect) and cognitive commitment (intention) to perform the behavior
- Ease of incorporating behavior into lifestyle
- Absence of environmental constraints (barriers) to performing the behavior
- Extent to which the new behavior is intrinsically rewarding
- Extent to which there is social support for the behavior
- Consistency of behavior with self-image
- Personal attractiveness of incompatible action (Fishbein, Bandura, & Triandis, 1991)

The maintenance phase of health behavior extends from beginning stabilization of the new behavior throughout the client's life span. Habit formation facilitates maintenance of behaviors. Habits are behaviors that become automatic with little conscious effort (see discussion of habits in extended TPB). Habit formation results in stable patterns of behavior. For example, a client who has incorporated exercise into the daily routine, such as exercising each noon in the company fitness center, three to five days a week, is likely to continue to exercise as routinely as brushing teeth or showering.

ETHICS OF BEHAVIOR CHANGE

The Ottawa Charter for Health promotion is the ethical cornerstone for world health promotion (Mittelmark, 2007). The Ottawa Charter (WHO, 2006) defines *health promotion* as the process of enabling people to increase control over and improve their health.

Caring, holism, and ecology are essential issues in developing health promotion strategies, and a guiding principle is that individuals should become equal partners in each phase of planning, implementing, and evaluating health promotion activities (WHO, 2006). Allowing clients to assume leadership in modifying their lifestyles is an ethical, nonmanipulative approach to improving the health of all.

OPPORTUNITIES FOR RESEARCH WITH HEALTH BEHAVIOR THEORIES AND MODELS

All of the behavior change models described in this chapter need further testing to understand the mechanisms that promote behavior change. The following are suggestions for avenues of research:

1. Develop theory-based interventions to test the causal process underlying the relationship between the model antecedents and behavior outcomes.
2. Identify and test new concepts to extend the social cognition models.
3. Develop and test the effectiveness of tailored interventions customized to target perceived internal and external barriers to change.
4. Extend individual theories and models to incorporate long-term behavior change.
5. Explore the potential of incorporating biologic concepts into behavior change models.

Research requires collaboration of scientists from multiple disciplines to design and test the effectiveness of behavior-change interventions that are culturally and developmentally sensitive. Information about funding for health promotion and prevention intervention research is available on the National Institute of Health Web site.

CONSIDERATIONS FOR PRACTICE IN MOTIVATING HEALTH BEHAVIOR

Knowledge of individual theories and models of health behavior enables the nurse to select the most appropriate model for behavior change. Choice of theory must take into account the needs of the individual. For example, barriers such as discomfort, travel, or cost may be significant for a woman who needs to obtain mammography. In contrast, self-efficacy may be important to address for individuals who desire to develop healthy food preparation and eating patterns. The emerging availability of interactive information technology augments the efforts of the nurse to assist clients in assessing their health beliefs and health behaviors.

Intervention strategies vary for different stages of change. For example, raising consciousness has been shown to be an effective strategy in making clients aware of the benefits of behavior change. This strategy is more effective in the early stages of behavior change such as pre-contemplation, contemplation, or preparation. Restructuring the environment is more effective in the adoption and maintenance stages of change when cues for behavior must be abundant to trigger the behavior on a regular basis. Having healthy foods, such as fruits and vegetables, available in the house serves as a trigger for healthy family eating. Smoke-free environments are triggers for tobacco avoidance. Walking paths in the community are visible cues for individuals and families to develop regular walking habits.

Existing theories, models, and related strategies enable the nurse to engage in evidence-based counseling and implement tailored interventions for health promotion and prevention. Tailoring interventions to fit each individual, family, or community will enhance the quality of health promotion and preventive care for culturally diverse groups. For more information on evidence-based counseling strategies, visit the Agency for Health Care Research and Quality (AHRQ) Web site.

Summary

This chapter presents an overview of models and theories relevant to individual health behaviors. Continuing development of theories that incorporate a wider range of powerful explanatory and predictive variables for effective health promotion and prevention interventions is imperative. Examples of theory-based behavior-change strategies are also described. These strategies can be implemented to assist individuals, families, and communities to promote desired changes and provide clients with skills for continuing self-change and self-actualization. Health promotion interventions empower clients to engage in a wide array of behavior changes to improve their health and well-being.

Learning Activities

1. Choose one of the theories described in the chapter and use it to develop an intervention to address a selected behavior change for yourself.
2. Describe barriers that you will face in maintaining your behavior change and strategies to overcome them.
3. Using the social cognitive concepts described in the chapter, develop an intervention to change an unhealthy behavior, such as a high fat diet, for a client.

Selected Web Sites

Agency for Healthcare Research and Quality: Guide to Clinical Preventive Services
http://www.ahrq.gov/clinic/prevenix.htm

American Medical Association: Guidelines for Adolescent Preventive Services
http://www.ama-assn.org/adolhlth/recommend/monogrf1.htm

Bureau of Maternal/Child Health: Bright Futures
http://www.brightfutures.org

Healthy People 2020
http://www.healthypeople.gov/HP2020/

National Institute of Nursing Research
http://www.nih.gov/ninr

References

Ajzen, I. (1991). The theory of planned behavior. *Organizational Behavior and Human Decision Processes, 50*, 179–211.

Albada, A., Ausems, M., Bensing, J. M., & van Dulmen, S. (2009). Tailored information about cancer risk and screening: A systematic review. *Patient Education and Counseling, 77*(2), 155–171.

Armitage, C. J., & Conner, M. (2000). Social cognition models and health behavior: A structured review. *Psychology and Health, 15*, 173–189.

Aveyard, P., Massey, L., Parsons, A., Maneski, S., & Griffin, C. (2009). The effect of Transtheoretical Model based interventions on smoking cessation. *Social Science & Medicine, 68*, 397–403.

Bandura, A. (1985). Model of causality in social learning theory. In M. J. Mahoney & A. Freeman (Eds.), *Cognition and psychotherapy* (pp. 81–99). New York: Plenum Publishing Corporation.

——— (1986). *Social foundations of thought and action: A social cognitive theory.* Englewood Cliffs, NJ: Prentice Hall.

——— (1997). *Self-efficacy: The exercise of control.* New York: WH Freeman.

——— (2004). Health promotion by social cognitive means. *Health Education & Behavior, 31*(2), 143–164.

Blanchard, C. M., Kupperman, J., Sparling, P. R., Nehl, E., Rhodes, R., Courneya, K. S., et al. (2009). Do ethnicity and gender matter when using the theory of planned behavior to understand fruit and vegetable consumption? *Appetite, 53,* 15–20.

Champion, V. L., & Skinner, C. S. (2008). The health belief model. In K. Glanz, B. Rimer, & K. Viswanath (Eds.), *Behavior and Health Education* (4th ed., pp. 45–66). San Francisco: Jossey-Bass.

Conner, M., & Norman, P. (1998). Health behavior. *Comprehensive Clinical Psychology*, 2–29.

de Bruijin, G., Kremers, S., Singh, A., van den Putte, B., & van Mechelen, W. (2009). Adult active transportation, adding habit strength to the theory of planned behavior. *American Journal of Preventive Medicine, 36,* 189–194.

de Bruijin, G., Kroeze, W., Oenema, A., & Brug, J. (2008). Saturated fat consumption and the theory of planned behavior: Exploring additive and interactive effects of habit strength. *Appetite, 51,* 318–323.

de Bruijin, G., & van den Putte, B. (2009). Adolescent soft drink consumption, television viewing and habit strength, investigating clustering effects in the theory of planned behavior. *Appetite, 53*(1), 66–75.

Di Noia, J., & Prochaska, J. O. (2009, June 3). Mediating variables in a transtheoretical model dietary intervention program. *Health Education & Behavior, EPub, PMD 1949057.*

Eschiti, V. S. (2008). A model of CAM use by women with female-specific cancers. *Journal of Psychosocial Nursing, 46,* 50–53.

Everson, S. S., Daley, A. J., & Ussher, M. (2007, April). The theory of planned behavior applied to physical activity in young people who smoke. *Journal of Adolescence, 30*(2), 347–351.

Feather, N. T. (Ed.) (1982). *Expectations and actions: Expectancy-value models in psychology.* Hillsdale, NJ: Lawrence Erlbaum Associates, Inc.

Fishbein, M. & Ajzen, I. (1975). *Belief, attitude, intention and behavior: An introduction to theory and research.* Boston: Addison-Wesley Publishing Co., Inc.

Fishbein, M., Bandura, A., & Triandis H. (1991, October). Factors influencing behavior and behavioral change: Final report of theorist's workshop in AIDS-related behavior. In M. Fishbein (Chair), *Adherence to treatment.* Symposium conducted at the meeting of the National Institute of Mental Health, NIH, Washington, DC.

Fjeldsoe, B. S., Marshall, A. L., & Miller, Y. D. (2009, February). Behavior change interventions delivered by mobile telephone short-message service. *American Journal of Preventive Medicine, 36*(2), 165–173.

Haerens, L., Maes, L., Vereecken, C., de Henauw, S., Moreno, L., & de Bourdeaudhuij, H. (2009). Effectiveness of a computer tailored physical activity intervention in adolescents compared to a generic advice. *Patient Education and Counseling, 77*(1), 38–41.

Honkanen, P., Olsen, S. O., & Verplanken, B. (2005, October). Intention to consume seafood—the importance of habit. *Appetite, 45*(2), 161–168.

Hounton, S. H., Carabin, H., & Henderson, N. J. (2005). Towards an understanding of barriers to condom use in rural Benin using the health belief model: A cross sectional survey. *BMC Public Health, 5,* 8.

Janis, I. L., & Mann, L. (1977). *Decision making: A psychological analysis of conflict, choice and commitment.* New York: The Free Press.

Kreuter, M. W., Caburnay, C. A., Chen, J. J., & Donlin, M. J. (2004, January). Effectiveness of individually tailored calendars in promoting childhood immunization in urban public health centers. *American Journal of Public Health, 94*(1), 122–127.

Kroeze, W., Oenema, A., Campbell, M., & Brug, J. (2008, July–August). The efficacy of web-based and print-delivered computer-tailored interventions to reduce fat intake: Results of a randomized, controlled trial.

Journal of Nutrition Education Behavior, 40(4), 226–236.

Levin, P. F. (1999). Test of the Fishbein and Ajzen models as predictors of health care workers' glove use. *Research in Nursing & Health, 22*, 295–307.

Lewin, K., Dembo, T., Festinger, L., & Sears, P. S. (1944). Level of aspiration. In J. Hunt (Ed.), *Personality and the behavioral disorders: A handbook based on experimental and clinical research* (Vol. 1, pp. 333–378). Ronald, NY: Ronald Press.

Lustria, M. L., Cortese, J., Noar, S. M., & Glueckauf, R. L. (2009). Computer-assisted health interventions delivered over the Web: Review and analysis of key component. *Patient Education and Counseling, 74*, 156–173.

Martin, M. Y., Person, S. D., Kratt, P., Prayor-Patterson, H., Kim, Y., Salas, M., et al. (2008, July). Relationship of health behavior theories with self-efficacy among insufficiently active hypertensive African-American women. *Patient Education and Counseling, 72*(1), 137–145.

McClure, J. B., Ludman, E. J., Grothaus, L., Pabiniak, C., & Richards, J. (2009). Impact of a brief motivational smoking cessation intervention: The get PHIT randomized controlled trial. *American Journal of Preventive Medicine, 37*(2), 116–123.

Mittelmark, M. B. (2007). Setting an ethical agenda for health promotion. *Health Promotion International, 23*, 78–85.

Montano, D. E., Kasprzyk, D., & Taplin, S. H. (2002). The theory of reasoned action and the theory of planned behavior. In K. Glanz, F. M. Lewis, & B. K. Rimer (Eds.), *Health behavior and health education theory, research and practice* (3rd ed., pp. 85–112). San Francisco: Jossey-Bass Publishers.

Morowatisbarifabad, M., & Karimzadeh, K. (2007). Determinants of oral health behaviors among preuniversity (12th grade) students in Yazd (Iran): An application of the health promotion model. *Family and Community Health, 30*, 342–350.

Noar, S. M., Benac, C. N., & Harris, M. S. (2007). Does tailoring matter? Meta-analytic review of tailored print health behavior change interventions. *Psychological Bulletin, 133*, 873–893.

Noar, S. M., Chabot, M., & Zimmerman, R. S. (2008, March). Applying health behavior theory to multiple behavior change: Considerations and approaches. *Preventive Medicine, 46*(3), 275–280.

Norman, P., & Brain, K. (2005). An application of an extended health belief model to the prediction of breast self examination among women with a family history of breast cancer. *British Journal of Health Psychology, 10*, 1–16.

Oettingen, G., Pak, H., & Schnetter, K. (2001). Self-regulation of goal setting: Turning free fantasies about the future into binding goals. *Journal of Personality and Social Psychology, 80*, 736–753.

Padula, C. A., & Sullivan, M. (2006). Long-term married couples' health promotion behaviors. *Journal of Gerontological Nursing, 32*(11), 37–46.

Parrott, M. W., Tennant, L. K., Olejnik, S., & Poudevigne, M. S. (2008). Theory of planned behavior: Implications for an email-based physical activity intervention. *Psychology of Sports & Medicine, 9*, 511–526.

Pender, N. J. (1996). *Health promotion in nursing practice* (3rd ed.). Stamford, CT: Appleton & Lange.

Pender, N. J., Murdaugh, C. L., & Parsons, M. A. (2002). *Health promotion in nursing practice* (4th ed.). Upper Saddle River, NJ: Prentice Hall.

Pender, N. J., Walker, S. N., Sechrist, K. R., & Frank-Stromborg, M. (1990). Predicting health-promoting lifestyles in the workplace. *Nursing Research, 38*, 326–332.

Plotnikoff, R. C., Pickering, M. A., Flaman, L. M., & Spence, J. C. (June 8, 2009). The role of self-efficacy on the relationship between workplace environment and physical activity: A longitudinal mediation analysis. *Health Education & Behavior,* doi:10.177/109019810933.

Plotnikoff, R. C., Trinh, L., Courneya, K. S., Karunamunit, N., & Sigal, R. J. (2009). Predictors of aerobic physical activity and resistance training among Canadian adults with type 2 diabetes: An application for the protection motivation theory. *Psychology of Sport and Medicine, 10*, 320–328.

Portney, D. B., Scott-Sheldon, L., Johnson, B. T., & Carey, M. P. (2008). Computer-driven interventions for health promotion and behavioral risk reduction: A meta-analysis of 75 randomized controlled trials, 1988–2007. *Preventive Medicine, 42*, 3–16.

Prochaska, J. O., & DiClemente, C. C. (1983). Stages and processes of self-change of smoking: Toward an integrative model of change. *Journal of Consulting and Clinical Psychology, 51*, 390–395.

Prochaska, J. O., Johnson, S., & Lee, P. (2009). The transtheoretical model of change. In S. Shumaker, J. Ockene, & K. Riekert (Eds.), *The handbook of behavior change* (3rd ed., pp. 59–84). New York: Springer Publishing Co.

Rimer, B. K., & Kreuter, M. W. (2006) Advancing tailored health communication: A persuasion and message effects perspective. *Journal of Communication, S6*, S184–S201.

Rise, J., Thompson, M., & Verplanken, B. (2003). Measuring implementation intentions in the context of the theory of planned behavior. *Scandinavian Journal of Psychology, 44*, 87–95.

Rogers, R. W. (1983). Cognitive and physiological process in fear appraisals and attitude change: A revised theory of protection motivation. In J. Cacioppo & R. Petty (Eds.), *Social psychophysiology: A sourcebook* (pp. 153–176). New York: The Guilford Press.

Ronis, D. L., Hong, O., & Lusk, S. L. (2006). Comparison of the original and revised structures of the health promotion model in predicting construction workers' use of hearing protection. *Research in Nursing & Health, 29*, 3–17.

Rosenstock, I. M. (1960). What research in maturation suggests for public health. *American Journal of Public Health, 50*, 295–301.

Rosenstock, I. M., Stretcher, V. J., & Becker, M. H. (1988). Social learning theory and the health belief model. *Health Education Quarterly, 15*(2), 175–183.

Shin, K. R., Kang, Y., Park, H. J., Cho, M., & Heitkemper, M. (2008). Testing and developing the health promotion model in low-income, Korean elderly women. *Nursing Science Quarterly, 2*, 173–178.

Siela, D., & Wieseke, A. (2000). Stress, self-efficacy, and health. In V. Rice (ed.), *Handbook of stress, coping and health* (pp. 495–515). Thousand Oaks, CA: Sage Publications.

Smith, A. B., & Bashore, L. (2006). The effect of clinic-based health promotion educating on perceived health status and health promotion behaviors of adolescents and young adult cancer survivors. *Journal of Pediatric Oncology, 23*, 326–334.

Sohl, S. J., & Moyer, A. (2007). Tailored intervention to promote mammography screening: A meta-analytic review. *Preventive Medicine, 45*, 252–261.

Sullivan, K. A., White, K. M., Young, R., Chang, A., Roos, C., & Scott, C. (2008). Predictors of intention to reduce stroke risk among people at risk of stroke: An application of an extended health belief model. *Rehabilitation Psychology, 53*, 505–512.

Sutton, S. (2004). Health behavior: Psychosocial theories. *International Encyclopedia and Social and Behavioral Science, 6499*–6506.

Turner-McGrievy, G. M., & Campbell, M. K. (2009). Nutrition information to the desktop: A pilot online nutrition course on saturated fat for public librarians increases knowledge, expectancies, and self-efficacy. *Journal of Nutrition Education and Behavior, 1*, 188–193.

Tuuri, G., Zanovec, M., Silverman, L., Geaghan, J., Solman, M., Holston, D., et al. (2009, April). "Smart Bodies" school wellness program increased children's knowledge of health nutrition practices and self-efficacy to consume fruit and vegetables. *Appetite, 52*(2), 445–451.

Van Zundert, R. M. P., Nijhof, L. M., & Engels, R. C. M. E. (2009, March). Testing social cognitive theory as a theoretical framework to predict smoking relapse among daily smoking adolescents. *Addictive Behaviors, 34*(3), 281–286.

Vassallo, M., Saba, A., Arvola, A., Dean, M., Messina, F., Winkelman, M., et al. (2009). Willingness to use functional breads: Applying the health belief model across four European countries. *Appetite, 52*, 452–460.

Verplanken, B., & Melkevik, O. (2008). Predicting habit: The case of physical exercise. *Psychology of Sport and Exercise, 9*, 15–26.

von Wagner, C., Semmler, C., Good, A., & Wardle, J. (2009, June). Health literacy and self-efficacy for participating in colorectal cancer screening: The role of information processing.

Patient Education and Counseling, 75(3), 352–357.

Wai, C. T., Wong, M. L., Ng, S., Cheok, A., Tan, M. H., Chua, W., et al. (2005). Utility of the health belief model in predicting compliance of screening in patients with chronic hepatitis B. *Alimentary Pharmacology & Therapy, 21*, 10.

Weinstein, N. D., Rothman, A. J., & Sutton, S. R. (1998, May). Stage theories of health behavior. *Health Psychology, 17*(3), 290–299.

Weinstein, N. D., Sandman, P. M., & Blalock, S. J. (2008). The precaution adoption process model. In K. Glanz, B. Rimer, & K. Viswanath (Eds.), *Health behavior and health education* (4th ed., pp. 123–148). San Francisco: Jossey-Bass.

Wilson, M. (2005). Health-promoting behaviors of sheltered homeless women. *Family and Community Health, 28*, 51–63.

World Health Organization (WHO). (2006). *Ottawa charter for health promotion, 1986*. Geneva, Switzerland: WHO. Retrieved from http://www.euro.who.int/aboutWHO/Policy/20010827_2

CHAPTER 3

Community Models to Promote Health

OBJECTIVES

1. Describe commonalties and differences in the various definitions of communities.
2. Discuss the key concepts and features of social ecological models of health promotion.
3. Describe the characteristics of social capital and the role of social support in this approach.
4. Define the steps in the PRECEDE–PROCEED model in planning health promotion programs.
5. Compare and contrast the diffusion of innovation and social marketing models as effective models for health communication.

Outline

- The Concept of Community
- Community Interventions and Health Promotion
- Community Ecological Models and Theories
  A. Social Ecological Model
  B. Social Capital Theory
- Community Planning Models for Health Promotion
  A. The PRECEDE–PROCEED Model
- Community Dissemination Models to Promote Health
  A. Diffusion of Innovations Model
  B. Social Marketing Model
- Opportunities for Research with Community-Based Models
- Considerations for Practice Using Community Models of Health
- Summary
- Learning Activities
- Selected Web Sites
- References

ealth professionals' attention to community-based approaches to promote
health and prevent disease has dramatically increased in recent years. The
increased emphasis is due to many factors, including a greater understanding of
the complex etiologies of health problems, an appreciation of the relationship of individuals with their environment, and recognition of the limits of focusing only on individual behaviors to promote health. A greater understanding of the role of the environment in achieving health has resulted in multiple approaches to promoting wellness. Individual approaches to health promotion identify a finite number of lifestyle areas that can be quantified and targeted for intervention. Community-based models move beyond individual lifestyles to distal factors that influence health, such as social conditions. In a community-based view, the social, political, institutional, legislative, and physical environments in which behavior occurs can be targeted for change to promote health. Community approaches emphasize populations and communities as clients, as opposed to individual health, and acknowledge that the greater environment influences individual health behaviors.

Although health care professionals now recognize that attention to the social, physical, and political environment is necessary for health promotion, community-based models are not intended to neglect the individual. Individuals make up communities, so although the community may be targeted, individuals play a critical role in providing leadership. Community-based strategies for health promotion place control with individuals who reside in the community. The focus of this chapter is to introduce the concepts in community models and provide an overview of the major community models and theories in the literature.

THE CONCEPT OF COMMUNITY

Community has been defined in multiple ways. It is commonly defined as a collective body of individuals identified by geography, common interests, concerns, characteristics, or values (World Health Organization [WHO], 1974). A community can be considered an association, a self-generated gathering of common people or citizens who have the creativity and capacity to solve problems (McKnight, 2002). The definition has evolved from a structural focus on geographic boundaries to a functional focus of people interacting in social units and sharing common interests. Whatever the definition of *community*, residents must share values and are linked together for common goals or other purposes. Members must also have a sense of community, or a sense of identity, shared values, social norms, communication modes, and helping patterns and identify themselves as being of the same community.

The community in which individuals live, work, and play is critical to health promotion and prevention. The community context refers to the interdependence that exists between selected aspects of a given environment or setting. The context includes personal, physical, cultural, and social aspects of environments and the relationship between them that may influence an individual's mental and physical health, opportunities, achievement, and developmental outcomes (Clitheroe & Stokols, 1998). The relationship between individuals and the context or social system in which they interact is reciprocal, as individuals may work to change their neighborhood context, just as the context influences the individual. For example, lack of street lighting may limit persons from walking later in the evening. However, individuals may work to have appropriate lighting installed in their community to facilitate safe walking.

The context encompasses social institutions and resources within a community, surroundings, and social relationships (Matthews, 2008). Social institutions include cultural and religious organizations, economic systems, and political structures. Surroundings include neighborhoods, workplaces, towns, and cities; and social relationships include position in the social hierarchy, social group, and social networks. All of these aspects enable health care professionals to understand the relationship between the context and health.

A risk environment is an example of a context in which factors interact to increase the chances of unhealthy behaviors and harm. Risk environments have two key dimensions: the type of environmental influence (i.e., physical, social, economic, or policy) and level of environmental influence (i.e., micro or macro) (Rhodes, 2004). Examples of the physical environment that may increase risks or decrease health promotion efforts include lack of running water, poor transportation, and heavy street traffic with noise and air pollution. Micro level influences that may increase risk and decrease health-promoting efforts include social networks, social norms, values and rules, peer and social influence, and the social setting in which one functions. Macro level influences take into account one's economics, gender, ethnicity, and culture, as well as the legal and policy environment, including state and federal laws. Micro and macro level influences intersect with the environment to either increase risks or enable individuals to promote health. Knowledge of the environmental context is necessary to create an enabling environmental context in which potential risks are reduced to maximize healthy behavior change.

The client becomes the community when the focus is on the collective of the common good of the population instead of the individual (Shuster & Goeppinger, 2004). In the community models discussed in this chapter, the nurse works with individuals and groups. However, the outcomes of health promotion programs are expected to affect the entire community. For example, the nurse may work with parents to get safe walking tracks for adults and recreational parks for children. These changes improve the health of the community. In community health promotion, change must occur at multiple levels, beginning with the individuals and moving to the community as a whole (Shuster & Goeppinger, 2004). Policy changes may be necessary at the societal level for community-wide change to occur. When the community is the client, the nurse and the community work together to achieve mutual goals, as community members are actively involved in all steps of the process.

COMMUNITY INTERVENTIONS AND HEALTH PROMOTION

Community interventions differ from interventions within a community (Green & Kreuter, 2005). Community interventions target either the majority of the population in a community or the community as a whole, as the goal is to change the entire setting. Community interventions have multiple advantages. First, they have the potential to make population changes. Interventions based on community models focus on both high-risk persons and the larger community to promote health, and the interventions are relevant for the population in the community (Eriksson, 2002). Other benefits include a high level of exposure to the intervention and increased generalizability of the intervention to other communities. Second, the interventions are likely to be valuable in the development of public health policies. Community changes are integrated into existing structures within the community, thereby changing the system that influences health behaviors.

Community models are based on four underlying assumptions (Minkler, Wallerstein, & Wilson, 2008). First, communities shape individual behaviors through community values and norms. Second, communities can be mobilized to change individual behaviors by legitimizing the desirable behaviors and changing environments to facilitate the new behaviors. The third assumption is that participation of community leaders is crucial for community ownership; and last, members of the community must have a sense of responsibility and control over the planned change. In other words, they must own the planned change for it to be successful. People are more likely to commit to and sustain change if they participate in identifying the problem, and developing and implementing the program to address the problem (Green & Kreuter, 2005). Community interventions engage participants to promote successful behavior change. Members are involved early in the planning process to identify needs, develop priorities, and plan programs to promote change. Community-based models take into consideration individuals in interaction with their families, cultures, and social structures, as well as the actual physical environment. The "twin pillars" of community-based health promotion programs are community empowerment and community participation (Robertson & Minkler, 1995).

Community empowerment is a social action process by which people and communities are enabled to participate and act to transform their lives and their environments (Minkler, 2000). The concept of empowerment refers to a process by which people and communities gain mastery over their lives. Empowerment principles are essential components of participatory research in health promotion. Empowered communities are visible when people within the community participate in equal partnership with health professionals in defining their health problems and developing solutions. In addition, community members receive the benefits of the interventions and are partners in evaluation of the effectiveness of the intervention. Community empowerment is not new in public health; public health practitioners have long recognized the need for community members to take control of the health of their community.

Community participation is the process of taking part in activities, programs, or discussions to promote planned change or improve the community. Community participation is a basic principle in health education and has been the major focus of chronic disease prevention. Community participation is expected to empower individuals and communities through group decision making and knowledge of resources, as well as creating new networks and opportunities. Participation of community members results in greater buy-in, higher numbers involved and greater sustainability. Empowerment and community participation go hand in hand, as empowered members participate in the health agenda for the community.

COMMUNITY ECOLOGICAL MODELS AND THEORIES

An overview of systems theory is helpful to understand ecological models. Systems theory was originally described in the biological sciences as a complex of elements mutually interacting (von Bertalanffy, 1975). These elements are considered multiple aspects of the physical environment and the social environment as well as personal attributes of the individual. Some of the major terms used in systems theory include *boundary, adaptation, entropy, negentropy, equifinality*, and *feedback*. In social ecological models, communities are open systems in which there are interactions within a community among its members, as well as between community members and their environment. A community is made of many interrelated and independent parts that are organized to function for the good of the community (Lowry & Martin, 2004; Shuster & Goeppinger, 2004). These parts include school systems, health care systems, churches, welfare systems, law enforcement, economics, and recreational areas. The functions of these parts are interrelated: A change in one part affects other parts of the community. Functions require energy to carry out their activities. Communities have geographical boundaries that determine the external borders as well as internal boundaries within the community, such as isolated neighborhoods of poverty or wealth. Communities experience change within their environments, which is managed through the process of adaptation. Adaptation occurs when members of the community make changes, or changes occur within the community environment. *Negentropy* refers to energy used by the system for maintenance or growth. *Negentropy* is the positive aspect of a community that promotes well-being, such as adequate social support systems, jobs, good health. *Entropy* is the tendency of the system to break down. It is an indicator of disorder in the system. Entropy refers to negative aspects that do not contribute to the well-being of a community, such as deteriorating conditions seen in communities of poverty. As open systems, communities have inputs, throughputs, and outputs. *Inputs* take energy into the system. Inputs come from sources outside the system as well as members within the community. *Throughput* refers to the process of using inputs, such as community activities and *outputs* are the results of these activities. Feedback occurs through communication of the subparts of the community as they interact to facilitate effective functioning of the whole.

The term *ecology* has its roots in biology and refers to the interrelations between organisms and their environments. The concept has evolved to provide an understanding of the interactions of people with their physical and sociocultural environments (Stokols, 2000). Ecological models emphasize the social, institutional, and cultural contexts of people–environment relations.

Social Ecological Model

Stokols (2004) expands the concept of an ecology model to a social ecological approach to health promotion. He describes certain core assumptions about human health and the development of strategies to promote personal and collective well-being. First, the healthfulness of a situation and the well-being of its individuals are assumed to be influenced by both the physical and social environments as well as personal attributes of the individual. Second, environments are multidimensional and complex and can be described in physical and social terms; as objective or subjective (perceived), proximal or distal, and other attributes, such as noise, group size, and so on; or as constructs, such as social climate. Third, individuals within an environment can be described at multiple levels, such as individuals; families; groups or organizations, such as schools; and populations. Finally, system theory concepts—including interdependence, homeostasis, and feedback—help understanding of the interrelationships between people and their environments. Environments are viewed as complex systems, and efforts to promote well-being must take into account the interdependence among all components and levels of the environment.

In an ecological perspective, health promotion interventions target multiple levels: intrapersonal, interpersonal, organizational, community, and public policy. At the community level, community participation is necessary to build community capacity, as the change process is cultural as well as social (Dressendorfer et al., 2005). Community participation facilitates the development, implementation, and maintenance of health promotion programs. The socio-ecological perspective suggests that the effectiveness of health promotion interventions can be increased through multilevel interventions, which combine multiple behavioral and environmental strategies. In a social ecological approach to health promotion, the interplay between environmental resources and the health habits and lifestyles of individuals within that environment are analyzed to identify features of the environment that promote or hinder well-being. Identifying these interdependent links helps define both environmental components and individual characteristics that must be targeted to promote healthy lifestyles. For example, Lopez, Bryant, & McDermott (2008) use the socio-ecological framework to describe the perceptions that either facilitate or impede physical activity in Latina adults between 24 and 54 years. Both individual (work outside the home, education, attitudes about physical activity, social comparisons) and environmental factors (neighborhood safety, access to facilities) were associated with physical activity.

Ecological models go beyond a focus solely on environmental factors to include transactions of the individual and groups with the environment. This is a major strength, as strategies for behavior change are integrated with environmental change strategies. However, it is also a challenge to identify the critical determinants that can be realistically targeted for change.

Sallis, Owens, and Fisher (2008) formulate seven principles to guide social ecological approaches for interventions and research. The authors developed these principles after a review of ecological concepts and are listed in Table 3–1. Ecological models have been applied to research with physical activity, tobacco use, and substance abuse (Elder et al., 2007; Kim, Subramanian, Gortmaker, & Kawachi, 2006; Kliewer & Murrelle, 2007). An ecological intervention, in which community residents participated in urban renewal, was successful in improving sense of community and improving mental health and social capital (Semenza, March, & Bontempo, 2006).

TABLE 3–1   Principals of Ecological Approaches for Health Behavior Change

1. Multiple levels of factors have an influence on health behaviors.
2. Multiple types of environment have an influence on health behaviors.
3. Behavior-specific ecological models can guide interventions to target specific health behaviors.
4. Multilevel interventions that combine individual, community, and environmental components are more effective.
5. A multidisciplinary approach is more effective to implement multilevel interventions.
6. Ongoing process evaluations are needed to monitor implementation of multilevel interventions.
7. Ecological interventions can be hindered by political agendas.

Source: von Bertalanffy, L., 1975, Used with permission.

Evidence to date indicates that a multilevel ecological approach that incorporates intrapersonal, sociocultural, and environmental policy components—although complex—is promising for health promotion. Further development and testing of ecological models is a high priority for nurse researchers, as interventions using these models is limited.

Social Capital Theory

The theory of social capital focuses on resources available to individuals and groups in their community network and how access to and use of such resources benefit the actions of individuals within the community (Yip, et al., 2007). *Resources* are defined as valued goods in a society. The theory focuses on actions taken to either maintain or gain valued resources.

Although a definition of social capital lacks consensus, in all definitions, trust and reciprocity are central components (Kreuter & Lezin, 2002). Putnam's classic research on the efficiency of local governments in Italy popularized the social capital concept (Putnam, 2000). He suggests the core elements of social capital, trust and cooperation, are learned behaviors, indicating that social capital can be created. Putnam defines the characteristics of social capital, which include (1) measures of community organizational life or human interactions, such as clubs, churches, and other group organizations; (2) measures of engagement in civic affairs such as participation of people in presidential elections; (3) measures of community voluntarism; (4) measures of reciprocity or mutual help among members of a community; and (5) measures of social trust. Putnam also distinguishes between bonding (within groups) social capital and bridging (across groups) social capital. Bonding social capital refers to the reinforcement of links between similar people. It builds strong ties but can also build higher walls to exclude those who are different. Bonding social capital is assumed to be a critical factor in creating and nurturing group solidarity seen in close neighborhoods and ethnic groups. Bridging social capital refers to building connections between heterogeneous groups. Bridging social capital facilitates linkages among different agencies and organizations in a community around a common purpose. Behavioral scientists have begun to study the link between the social capital dimensions of bonding and bridging. In studies of the relationship between bonding and bridging neighborliness, both were associated with better self-rated health (Beaudoin, 2009; Nogueira, 2009). Although these studies measure bonding and bridging with different questions, they indicate positive results for both dimensions of social capital.

A key ingredient of social capital is social support, as this is the initial informal link among individuals. It is important to note the difference between social support, a component of social capital, and social capital, as some authors believe they are the same (Kritsotakis & Gamarnikow, 2004). Social capital is a property of communities, and social support is a property of individuals. More work is needed to differentiate the two concepts and their influence on the health of the community. Debate continues over the extent to which social capital represents a new concept, because social support and social competence, as well as community competence, have been in the literature for many years (Wakefield & Poland, 2005).

The social support component of social capital draws attention to the significant role of the family as a builder and source of social capital through its nurturance, caregiving, socialization, values, attitudes, expectations, and habitual patterns of behavior (Bulboz, 2001). Building trust, a component of social capital, begins with the attachment process in infancy and continues throughout early life. Family relationships and behavior also help establish the principle of reciprocity, the idea of receiving and giving in return, which is another major component of social capital.

Research to test the relationship between social capital and community health promotion has expanded dramatically in the past 10 years. Descriptive studies provide evidence for a link between social capital and physical activity, adolescent risk taking, and physical health (Boyce, Davies, Gallupe, & Shelley, 2008; Fujiwara & Kawachi, 2008; Mummery, Lauder, Schofield, & Caperchione, 2008). In addition, findings from a randomized clinical trial in rural South Africa to strengthen social capital indicate that it is possible to do so (Pronyk, et al., 2008). Higher levels of structural (group membership) and cognitive (perceived levels of reciprocity and community support, perceived solidarity, and participation in collective action) social capital were found in the group that received financial credit for income-generating activities and a 12-month HIV educational training program to strengthen knowledge, communication skills, critical thinking, and leadership. An ongoing issue is the lack of consistency and limited measures of social capital. Clear definitions and accurate and valid measures are needed to test the theory. However, beginning evidence indicates that interventions can be developed to strengthen social capital.

COMMUNITY PLANNING MODELS FOR HEALTH PROMOTION

The PRECEDE–PROCEED Model

The PRECEDE–PROCEED model was designed as a model to guide the planning and development of health education programs (Green & Kreuter, 2005). The model, which is shown in Figure 3–1, provides a structure to identify and implement the most appropriate intervention strategies. It can be considered a road map that provides all possible routes; in contrast, theories suggest which avenues to follow. Two fundamental propositions of the model are as follows: (1) Health and health risks have multiple determinants, and (2) efforts to change the behavioral, physical, and social environment must be multidimensional and participatory.

The PRECEDE framework builds on 40 years of work. The acronym stands for Predisposing, Reinforcing, and Enabling Constructs in Educational/Ecological Diagnosis and Evaluation. The PRECEDE model is based on the premise that an educational diagnosis should precede an intervention plan. PROCEED was added to the framework to account for the role of environmental factors in health. PROCEED recognizes forces outside the individual that can influence lifestyle behaviors. The acronym stands for Policy, Regulatory, and Organizational Constructs in Educational and Environmental Development.

The original planning process consisted of nine steps in sequential order. Planning begins with a social assessment to learn people's perceptions of their own needs and life quality. This step involves a community assessment, including problem-solving capacity, strengths, and readiness for change. In step 2, an epidemiologic assessment is performed to identify health problems that are most important. Secondary sources of data (e.g., state and national surveys) can be used to identify major health problems in the community. A behavioral and environmental assessment

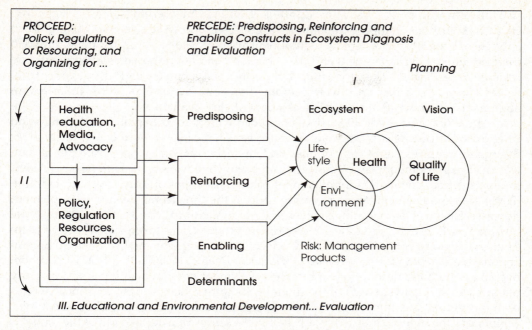

PROCEED:
Policy, Regulating
or Resourcing, and
Organizing for ...

PRECEDE: Predisposing, Reinforcing and
Enabling Constructs in Ecosystem Diagnosis
and Evaluation

Planning

Health education, Media, Advocacy

Predisposing

Ecosystem

Vision

Life-style

Health

Quality of Life

Reinforcing

Envi-ronment

Policy, Regulation Resources, Organization

Enabling

Risk: Management Products

Determinants

III. Educational and Environmental Development... Evaluation

FIGURE 3–1   The PRECEDE–PROCEED Model for Health Promotion Planning and Evaluation
Source: From Green, L. W., & Kreuter, M. W. (2005). The PRECEDE-PROCEED model of health program
planning and evaluation. In *Health Program Planning: An Educational and Ecological Approach*
(4th ed.) New York: McGraw-Hill. Reprinted by permission.

is performed in step 3 to identify factors that may contribute to the health problem. Behavioral factors include lifestyle behaviors of the individual at risk for the problem, and physical and social factors are environmental ingredients that may influence lifestyle behaviors. The community then ranks the identified factors that are amenable to change to prioritize their importance and changeability. During step 3, individual-level as well as community-level theories that may be useful are identified to guide interventions for the priority health problems. Step 4 consists of an educational and ecological assessment to identify the predisposing, reinforcing, and enabling factors that must be in place to initiate and sustain the proposed change. Predisposing and reinforcing factors target individual-level factors, whereas enabling factors focus on community-level factors such as programs, services, and resources needed. These factors are also prioritized for interventions, as in step 3. As in the prior stage, individual- and community-level interventions are also relevant to guide appropriate interventions. In step 5, administration and policy assessment intervention strategies and planning for implementation occurs. Policies and resources are identified that may facilitate or hinder program implementation. Resources needed, barriers to implementation, and organization policies that may affect implementation are assessed. In step 6, implementation of the planned intervention takes place, and both process and outcome evaluations are performed in steps 7–9. Objectives, which are written at each step, are the basis for evaluating accomplishments.

In 2004, the model was significantly streamlined by merging the nine steps into six phases without changing the data to be collected (Green & Krueter, 2005). Phase 1 consists of a social assessment and situational analysis. Steps 2 and 3 of the old model, the epidemiological assessment and the behavioral and environmental assessments, are combined for Phase 2. Therefore, Step 4, the educational and ecological assessment, becomes Phase 3; and Steps 5–9 were combined to form Phases 5, 6, and 7: Intervention alignment, administrative and policy assessment, and evaluation.

The PROCEDE–PRECEDE model has been widely used to plan health promotion programs. Despite its success, several weaknesses have been identified. Application of the model requires significant human and financial resources, as the model is data driven. The planning process is time intensive, which may dampen enthusiasm of community members who want to implement change strategies quickly. Cole and Horacek (2009) develop a consolidated version to shorten the time frame needed to implement the assessment. Demographic, behavioral, organizational, and administrative are obtained with a single survey instead of distinct steps. Focus groups, made up of planning and steering committee members, are conducted to obtain environmental, organizational and policy assessment data. The consolidated PRECEDE–PROCEED model overcomes the time needed to conduct the assessment while remaining a participatory planning model. The strength of the model is its comprehensiveness, as it incorporates both individual and community perspectives and can be used in a variety of settings. A bibliography of more than 900 published papers reporting application of the model is available (see http://www.lgreen.net/precede.htm).

COMMUNITY DISSEMINATION MODELS TO PROMOTE HEALTH

Diffusion of Innovations Model

The diffusion of innovations model was developed to help disseminate health behavior interventions that have been successfully tested into the mainstream for practical use (Rogers, 2003). The framework enables one to understand the process of innovation and the various stages involved in adopting a new idea, thereby narrowing the gap between what is known and what is put to use.

Diffusion has been defined as the process through which an innovation is communicated through certain channels, over time, among members of a social system (Rogers, 2003). It is a special kind of communication to spread messages about new ideas that might represent a certain degree of uncertainty to the individual or organization. Diffusion is a type of social change, as social changes may occur when new ideas are adopted. The terms *dissemination* and *diffusion* are used interchangeably in the diffusion of innovations model.

The four main elements of diffusion of new ideas are (1) innovation, (2) communication channels, (3) time, and (4) social system. These elements, shown in Figure 3–2, are found in every diffusion program. An *innovation* is an idea or practice that is thought to be new. The innovation is broad and can be almost any new idea, ranging from a new program to the Internet. It does not matter if the idea is not new, as it is the perceived newness that decides how individuals will react to it.

Characteristics that help explain the relative speed of adoption of an innovation include relative advantage, compatibility, complexity, trialability, and observability.

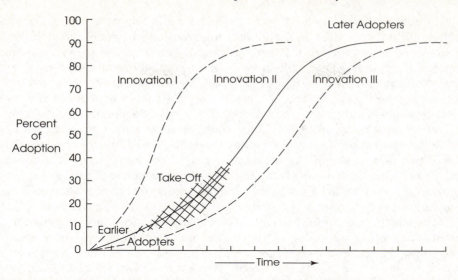

FIGURE 3–2   The Diffusion Process   *Source:* Adapted with the permission of The Free Press, a Division of Simon & Schuster, Inc. *Diffusion of Innovations,* 5th edition by Everett M. Rogers. Copyright © 1955, 2003, by Everett M. Rogers. Copyright © 1962, 1971, 1983 by the Free Press. All rights reserved.

Relative advantage is the degree to which the innovation is perceived to be better than the current, older idea. It does not matter if the innovation has no true advantage. What matters is whether an individual thinks the innovation will be better. Relative advantage may be perceived in economic terms or as social prestige, convenience, or satisfaction. *Compatibility* is the degree to which an innovation is perceived to fit with existing values and past experiences. Innovations that are consistent with the existing values and norms of the social system are more likely to be adopted. For example, an incompatible innovation might be the use of contraceptives in a traditionally Catholic community, as it is unlikely that the majority would adopt it. *Complexity* is the degree to which the innovation is thought to be difficult to understand or use. In general, new ideas that are simple to understand are more easily adopted than complex ones. *Trialability* is the extent to which the innovation may be considered tentative for a limited time period. Ideas that can be tried in installments are usually adopted more quickly than those that cannot be divided. Last, *observability* is the degree to which the results of the innovation are visible to others. The easier it is to see results, the more likely the idea will be adopted. Relative advantage and compatibility have been found to be the most important in the rate of adoption of an innovation. Additional characteristics include the influence of the innovation on social relationships, the ability to reverse the innovation, the ability to easily communicate the innovation, time and commitment needed to adopt the innovation, and the ability to modify the innovation over time (Olderburg & Glanz, 2008).

Communication must take place for an innovation to spread. Mass media channels are used to reach large audiences to provide initial information of the innovation. Since diffusion is a process of people talking to people, interpersonal or face-to-face communication channels are effective in forming and changing attitudes toward a new idea.

Innovativeness refers to the degree to which individual, organizations, or systems adopt new ideas or practices. Five adopter categories have been described: innovators, early adopters, early majority, late majority, and laggards. These patterns of adoption have been shown to be predictable in a variety of populations and settings. *Innovators* are active information seekers and can cope with high levels of uncertainty about a new idea. They are open to taking risks and the first to adopt a new idea. Innovators are role models for others in the social system. *Early adopters* have the greatest degree of opinion leadership in most social systems and are considered the person to check with before adopting the innovation. The *early majority* may deliberate before adopting, so they seldom lead in adoption of the idea. The *late majority* view innovations with skepticism and may only adopt because of increasing pressure from peers, or they feel it is safe to adopt. The *laggards* tend to be suspicious of innovations and change. They must be sure that the innovation will not fail before they will adopt and often slow down the innovation diffusion process. Identification of adopter categories facilitates implementing new health behavior programs or behaviors, as it is important to know that everyone will not accept the change in the same time frame. Laggards, for example, will need more time and evidence that the change is effective and safe. Early adopters, the opinion leaders in a social system who can influence others, need to be identified, as they will facilitate change.

Preventive innovations are defined as new ideas that require action at one point in time to avoid unwanted consequences at a future point in time (Rogers, 2002). The rewards of adopting a preventive innovation are delayed and intangible, and unwanted consequences may never occur, resulting in a low relative advantage of the innovation. Because relative advantage is one of the most important predictors of the rate of adoption of an innovation, it is understandable why preventive innovations may be slow or fail to be adopted. To increase the rate of adoption of a preventive innovation, perceived relative advantages of the preventive innovation should be identified and made visible as much as possible. For example, the relative advantage of dietary changes for those at risk for hypertension is low, as hypertension does not have immediate or obvious symptoms. Perceived relative advantages, such as weight loss, or less need for medications, should be identified and communicated. Strategies to speed up the adoption of preventive innovations include increasing the relative advantage, using role models to devote their personal influence to promote the innovation, changing the system norms through peer support, placing educational ideas in entertainment messages, and activating peer communication networks.

The innovation diffusion model has been applied with varying success. Lack of successful outcomes has been attributed to focusing on the nature of the innovation without attending to resource constraints (Peterson, Rogers, Cunningham-Sabo, & Davis, 2007). Diffusion of an innovation is a complex, multilevel change process, as change must occur at multiple levels across different settings, using multiple change strategies to promote widespread behavior change. Understanding the diffusion process enables health care practitioners to implement behavior changes at multiple levels. The theory is based on many years of research in diffusion of innovations to change behaviors, programs, and policies to promote health. The theory incorporates strategies to promote widespread, long-term change. The theory also takes into account social structures and communication systems, as well as characteristics of the innovation to promote successful behavior change.

In recent years, the innovation diffusion model has been expanded to explain the research utilization process (Davis, Peterson, Helfrich, & Cunningham-Sabo, 2007). Davis, Peterson, Helfrich, and Cunningham-Sabo's five-stage model includes dissemination, intent to adopt, implementation, adaptation, institutionalization, diffusion, and replication. The model can be used as a road map for dissemination of evidence for health promotion practice.

It has been suggested that the innovation diffusion model could be further modified to capture current Internet communication trends (Lillie, 2008). The diffusion innovations model presents communication channels as either mass media or interpersonal. However, communication channels that capture current communication trends, such as YouTube, could lead to new forms of health interventions. The benefits of technology to promote health have been seen with telephone- and computer-based messages. However, the increasing importance of new Internet communication channels point to the need for applying hybrid communication channels (e.g., YouTube, FaceBook) into models of health promotion communication.

Social Marketing Model

In a social marketing model, commercial marketing technologies are applied to plan, implement, and evaluate programs to change the behavior of target audiences to improve health (Morris & Clarkson, 2009). Marketing practices that have traditionally been used in business advertising are applied to social purposes to adopt an idea, product, or behavior. Core principles are adhered to in social marketing (Mah, Deshpandé, & Rothschild, 2006; Morris & Clarkson, 2009). These include (1) a consumer orientation, (2) knowledge of competition, (3) mutual exchange of tangible or intangible goods, (4) segmentation of populations and careful selection of target audiences, and (5) marketing and intervention mix. A marketing approach goes beyond education to change behavior, as social marketers attempt to increase the attractiveness of the desired behavior so that consumers will desire the new behavior. Efforts are made to provide immediate effects, as immediate reinforcement has a greater potential to shape behavior.

The social marketing model is a set of principles rather than a theory. The framework considers the "Four P's": product, price, place, and promotion (Kotler & Roberto, 1989). The *product* is the desired health behavior change, such as eating five fruits and vegetables daily. *Price* refers to the social, emotional, and monetary costs associated with adoption of the program or behavior. Higher priced products are more difficult to implement than less expensive ones. *Place* is the distribution point or location of the intervention program. The more convenient the place, such as exercise facilities, the more likely the adoption. *Promotion* refers to the behavior being promoted and strategies used to persuade adoption of the desired behavior. Both mass media and interpersonal communication channels are used to promote the change. An additional concept is the product's competition, or the existing behavior that must be changed.

The interrelated components and basic principles described here serve as guides to design implementation strategies for target populations. The product must provide a solution to problems that consumers believe is important to them. Consumers are confronted with making a choice between the new behavior and the current risk behavior, so the new behavior (product) must outweigh the benefits of the current behavior. Price, from the consumer's perspective, is the cost, such as the cost of a joining a health club to exercise. Costs may also be time, effort, and emotional discomfort in changing behaviors such as smoking cessation. Place is also an important component for consumers, and social marketers must assess when and where the target audience will be most receptive to messages, or where and when they are ready to purchase products. Promotion to motivate change includes communication objectives for the target audience; strategies for designing attention-getting, effective messages; and credible, trustworthy spokespersons. Strategies may include mass communication, public information, consumer education, direct mail, public relations, and printed materials. Additional promotion strategies that may be implemented include service delivery enhancements, policy changes, and use of coupons to attract consumers. Two additional approaches are the idea of "edu-entertainment," or the use of traditional entertainment media for educational purposes, and media advocacy, and the strategic use of mass media to increase public support to address the change.

The consumer orientation in social marketing distinguishes it from other approaches in health promotion. In a consumer orientation, one must understand the consumer's perception of product benefits, price, the competition's benefits and costs, and others factors that may influence consumer behavior. Research findings are used to identify recommendations for health promotion programs. Recommendations based on research defining what works best assist in planning marketing strategies.

Social marketing uses audience segmentation to select target audiences, a process of dividing the population into distinct segments based on characteristics that might influence their response to the marketing program. Segments identify smaller groups that may require different marketing strategies. Group profiles help health care providers decide who to target and the best way to reach the targeted segment.

In social marketing, programs are monitored continuously to evaluate their effectiveness in promoting change. Continuous monitoring also enables one to identify activities that should be revised as well as activities that are most effective. The target audience is constantly checked for their responsiveness to the intervention.

Social marketing models of dissemination have been successfully used to change behavior. A six-month POWER social marketing campaign to increase condom use found that the amount of exposure to the media channels determines condom use (Bull et al., 2008). Social marketing was also used with success to improve the intention and consumption of iron-fortified soy sauce in China (Sun, Guo, Wang, & Sun, 2007). Purchase and use increased in rural and urban interventions groups 30% more than in control groups.

Social marketing has also been used to deliver health messages to children and youth. The VERB™ campaign delivered messages through mass media, school and community promotions, and national and community partnerships to encourage children to be physically active (Wong, Greenwell, Gates, & Berkowitz, 2008). The campaign had an important impact on physical activity in the population. Increased awareness and understanding were noted to be the factors that led to behavior change in youth aged 9–13 years. Six communities were selected for "high" doses of advertising and promotion activities. At two-year follow-up, youth in these communities reported higher awareness and understanding, higher self-efficacy, and greater free time physical activity (Bauman et al., 2008; Berkowitz, Huhman & Nolin, 2008; Huhman, Bauman, & Bowles, 2008).

In, 2008, antismoking messages, known as TRUTH, were targeted to youth (Farrelly, Nonnemaker, Davis, & Hussin, 2009). The influence of television commercials on smoking initiation was found to be associated with a decreased risk of smoking initiation. Factors that were negatively associated with initiation were race (African American), ethnicity (Hispanic), and living with both parents.

The social marketing model is a valuable model to assist in disseminating results of health promotion programs. As with other models, it requires time and resources. However, a consumer orientation is worth the effort, as it has the potential to promote healthy communities by promoting physical activity in communities, healthy choices when eating out, as well as other larger-scale environmental changes.

OPPORTUNITIES FOR RESEARCH WITH COMMUNITY-BASED MODELS

The limited success of individual-level theories and models to achieve long-term changes in health behavior has led to an exploration of the role of community theories and models in health promotion. Community-level theories and models are not new. However, these models have only recently been used to guide health promotion interventions to facilitate community change; therefore, many questions still must be answered. Research is needed to test and refine these theories. Application of the models will open avenues to develop effective interventions to guide behavior change for communities. Because the individual, group, and community are of interest in community health promotion, models that include all of these levels are needed. Multilevel models are complex and need further development and testing. Additional research in the following areas is recommended:

1. Identify the most parsimonious and effective socio-ecological concepts to target for health promotion.
2. Develop and test reliable and valid measures of social capital.
3. Identify sensitive and measurable community outcomes of health promotion.
4. Develop and test programs that target community change.
5. Test the effectiveness of the diffusion models to produce community-level changes in health behaviors.

CONSIDERATIONS FOR PRACTICE USING COMMUNITY MODELS OF HEALTH

Although community models of health promotion have been limited in their application, the concepts are important for practice. Communities also must be assessed prior to implementing health promotion programs. For example, assessment of an individual's physical and social environment as well as social capital will provide helpful information about facilitators and barriers to healthy lifestyle practices in the community. Knowledge of the physical environment will shed light on the resources (or lack thereof) in a neighborhood, such as safe walking areas and access to grocery stores or transportation, that influence one's ability to implement the proposed change. The diffusion of innovations model, as well as social marketing approaches, can be used to facilitate change within a community. Learning to identify characteristics of adopters will enable the nurse to choose specific strategies that must be stressed for successful change, depending on, for example, whether one is an innovator or laggard. Social marketing strategies that target specific populations and behaviors offer exciting opportunities for large-scale health promotion. As the nurse gains a broader under-standing of the role of the community and greater social system in promoting health, interventions can be developed to target changes that are realistic, feasible, and likely to be successful for individuals and communities.

Summary

The increased interest in community-based models to promote healthy behaviors has occurred because of a greater need to understand the complex etiologies of health problems, an appreciation of the interrelationship between individuals and their social and physical environment, and recognition of the limits of individual models to promote health. Community-based models focus on contextual factors that influence health, such as social conditions, and the political, institutional, legislative, and physical environments in which behavior occurs. Tests of community-level interventions show positive results. Additional research is needed to identify the most effective models to guide health promotion interventions. Diffusion of innovations and social marketing models have the potential to promote widespread change.

Learning Activities

1. Describe three ways in which people in communities can be empowered to participate in their health.
2. What elements in a community would you assess using a social ecological model for health behavior?
3. Apply the nine steps in the PRECEDE—PROCEED model to design a program to improve a specific health behavior such as physical activity for adolescents. Which individual and community theories would you choose to implement the program?
4. Using the "Four P's" of the social marketing framework, choose and design a behavior change intervention for a specific segment of the population, such as women between the ages of 25 and 40 years or men over the age of 50 years. How would you evaluate the effectiveness of the change?

Selected Web Sites

CDC Social-Ecological Model for Prevention
http://www.cdc.gov/ncipc/dvp/social-ecological-model_ DVP.htm

Resources fo Studying Social Capital
http://www.socialcapitalgateway.org

Social Marketing Institute
http://social-marketing.org

PRECEDE–PROCEED Model
http://www.lgreen.net/precede.htm

References

Bauman, A., Bowles, H. R., Huhman M., Heitzler, C. D., Owen, N., Smith, B. J., et al. (2008). Testing a hierarchy-of-effects model: Pathways from awareness to outcomes in the VERB™ campaign. *American Journal of Preventive Medicine, 34*(6S), S249–S256.

Beaudoin, C. E. (2009). Bonding and bridging neighborliness: An individual-level study in the context of health. *Social Science & Medicine, 68*(12), 1–8.

Berkowitz, J. M., Huhman, M., & Nolin M. J. (2008). Did augmenting the VERB™

campaign advertising in select communities have an effect on awareness, attitudes, and physical activity? *American Journal of Preventive Medicine, 34*(6S), S257–S266.

Boyce, W. R., Davies, D., Gallupe, O., & Shelley, D. (2008). Adolescent risk taking, neighborhood social capital and health. *Journal of Adolescent Health, 43,* 246–252.

Bulboz, M. M. (2001). Family as source, user and builder of social capital. *Journal of Socio-Economics, 30,* 129–131.

Bull, S. S., Posner, S. F., Ortiz, C., Beaty, B., Benton, K., Lin, L., et al. (2008). POWER for reproductive health: Results from a social marketing campaign promoting female and male condoms. *Journal of Adolescent Health, 43,* 71–78.

Clitheroe, H. C., & Stokols, D. (1998). Conceptualizing the context of environment and behavior. *Journal of Environmental Psychology, 18,* 3–12.

Cole, R. E., & Horacek, T. (2009). Applying PROCEDE–PRECEED to develop an intuitive eating nondieting approach to weight management pilot program. *Journal of Nutrition Education and Behavior, 41,* 120–126.

Davis, S. M., Peterson, J. C., Helfrich, C. D., & Cunningham-Sabo, L. (2007). Introduction and conceptual model for utilization of prevention research. *American Journal of Preventive Medicine, 35*(1S), S1–S5.

Dressendorfer, R. J., Raine, K., Dyck, R. C., Colins-Nakai, R. L., McLaughlin, W. K., & Ness, K. (2005). A conceptual model of community capacity development for health promotion in the Alberta Heart Health Project. *Health Promotion Practice, 6,* 31–36.

Elder, J. P., Lytle, L., Sallis, J. F., Young, D. R., Steckler, A., Simons-Mortin, D., et al. (2007). A description of the social-ecological framework used in the trial of activity for adolescent girls (TAAG). *Health Education Research, 22,* 155–165.

Eriksson, C. (2002). Learning and knowledge production for public health: A review of approached to evidenced-based health. *Scandinavian Journal of Public Health, 28,* 298–308.

Farrelly, M. C., Nonnemaker, J., Davis, K. C., & Hussin, A. (2009). The influence of the national truth campaign on smoking initiation. *American Journal of Preventive Medicine, 35,* 379–384.

Fujiwara, T., & Kawachi I. (2008). Social capital and health a study of adult twins in the U.S. *American Journal of Preventive Health, 35,* 139–144.

Gielen, A. C., & McDonald, E. M. (2002). Using PRECEDE–PROCEED planning model to apply health behavior theories. In K. Glanz, B. K. Rimer , & F. M. Lewis (Eds.), *Health behavior and health education theory, research and practice* (3rd ed., pp. 490–536). San Francisco: Jossey Bass.

Green, L. W., & Kreuter, M. W. (2005). *Health promotion program planning: An educational and ecological approach* (4th ed.). Boston: McGraw Hill.

Huhman M., Bauman, A., & Bowles, H. R. (2008). Initial outcomes of the VERB™ campaign. *American Journal of Preventive Medicine, 34*(6S), S241–S248.

Kim, D., Subramanian, S. V., Gortmaker, S. L., & Kawachi, I. (2006). U.S. state and county level social capital in relation to obesity and physical inactivity: A multilevel, multivariable analysis. *Social Science & Medicine, 63*(4), 1045–1059.

Kliewer, W., & Murelle, L. (2007). Risk and protective factors for adolescents' substance use: Finding from a study in selected Central American countries. *Journal of Adolescent Health, 40*(5), 448–455.

Kotler, P., & Roberto, E. (1989). *Social marketing strategies for changing public health.* New York: The Free Press.

Kreuter, M. W., & Lezin, N. (2002). Social capital theory: Implications for community based health promotion. In R. J. DiClemente, R. A. Crosby, & M. C. Kegler (Eds.), *Emerging theories in health promotion practice and research* (pp. 228–254). San Francisco: Jossey Bass.

Kritsotakis. G., & Gamarnikow, E. (2004). What is social capital and how does it relate to health? *International Journal of Nursing Studies, 41,* 43–50.

Lillie, S. E. (2008). Diffusion of innovation in the age of YouTube. *American Journal of Preventive Medicine, 34,* 267.

Lopez, I. A., Bryant C. A., & McDermott, R. J. (2008). Influences on physical activity participation among Latinas: an ecological perspective. *American Journal of Health Behavior, 32*(6), 627–639.

Lowry, L. W., & Martin, K. S. (2004). Organizing frameworks applied to community health nursing. In M. Stanhope & J. Lancaster (Eds.), *Community and Public Health Nursing* (pp. 194–219). St. Louis, MO: Mosby.

Mah, M. W., Deshpandé, S., & Rothschild, M. I. (2006). Social marketing: A behavior change technology for infection control. *American Journal of Infection Control, 34,* 452–457.

Matthews, S. A. (2008). The salience of neighborhood. *American Journal of Preventive Medicine, 34,* 257–259.

McKnight, J. L. (2002). Two tools for well-being: Health systems. In M. Minkler (Ed.), *Community organizing and community building for health* (pp. 20–29). New Brunswick, NJ: Rutgers University Press.

Minkler, M. (2000). Health promotion at the dawn of the 21st century: Challenges and dilemma. In M. S. Jamner & D. Stokols (Eds.), *Promoting human wellness* (pp. 349–377). Berkeley: University of California Press.

Minkler, M., Wallerstein, N. B., & Wilson, N. (2008). Improving health through community organization and community building. In K. Glanz, B. K. Rimer, & K. Viswanath (Eds.), *Health behavior and health education theory, research and practice* (4th ed., pp. 279–311). San Francisco: Jossey Bass.

Morris, Z. S., & Clarkson P. J. (2009). Does social marketing provide a framework for changing healthcare practice? *Health Policy, 91*(2), 135–141.

Mummery, W. K., Lauder, W., Schofield, G., & Caperchione, C. (2008). Associations between physical inactivity and a measure of social capital in a sample of Queensland adults. *Journal of Science and Medicine in Sport, 11,* 308–315.

Nogueira, H. (2009). Healthy communities: The challenge of social capital in the Lisbon metropolitan area. *Health & Place, 15*(1), 133–139.

Olderburg, B., & Glanz, K. (2008). Diffusion of innovations. In K. Glanz, B. K. Rimer, & K. Viswanath (Eds.), *Health behavior and health education theory, research and practice* (4th ed., pp. 312–334). San Francisco: Jossey Bass.

Peterson, J. C, Rogers, E. M., Cunningham-Sabo, L., & Davis, S. M. (2007). A framework for research utilization applied to seven case studies. *American Journal of Preventive Medicine, 33*(1S), S21–S34.

Pronyk, P. M., Harpham T., Busza, J., Phetia, G., Morison, L. A., Hargreaves, J. R., et al. (2008). Can social capital be intentionally generated? A randomized trail from rural South Africa. *Social Science & Medicine, 67*(10), 1559–1570.

Putnam, R. (2000). *Bowling alone: The collapse and revival of American community.* New York: Simon & Schuster.

Rhodes, J. (2004). The 'risk environment': A framework for understanding and reducing drug-related harm. *International Journal of Drug Policy, 12,* 85–94.

Robertson, A., & Minkler, M. (1995). The new health promotion movement: A critical examination. *Health Education Quarterly, 21*(3), 295–312.

Rogers, E. M. (2002). *Theory of innovation.* In N. J. Smelser & P. B. Batles (Eds.), *International encyclopedia of the social & behavioral science* (pp. 7540–7543). St. Louis, MO: Elsevier.

Rogers, E. M. (2003). *Diffusions of innovations* (5th ed., pp. 5–34). New York: The Free Press.

Sallis, J. F., Owens, N., & Fisher, E. B. (2008). Ecological models. In K. Glanz, B. K. Rimer, & K. Viswanath (Eds.), *Health behavior and health education theory, research and practice* (4th ed., pp. 464–484). San Francisco: Jossey Bass.

Semenza, J., March, T., & Bontempo B. (2006). Community-initiated urban development: an ecological intervention. *Journal of Urban Health, 84*(1), 8–20.

Shuster, G. F. & Goeppinger, J. (2004). Community as client: Assessment and analysis. In M. Stanhope & J. Lancaster (Eds.), *Community and public health nursing* (pp. 342–375). St. Louis, MO: Mosby.

Stokols, D. (2000). The social ecological paradigm of wellness promotion. In M. S. Jamner & D. Stokols (Eds.), *Promoting human wellness* (pp. 21–37). Berkeley: University of California Press.

———— (2004). Ecology and health. In N. J. Smelser & P. B. Bolten (Eds.) *International encyclopedia of the social and behavioral sciences* (pp. 4030–4035). St. Louis, MO, Elsevier, Ltd.

Sun, X., Guo, Y., Wang, S., & Sun, J. (2007). Social marketing improved the consumption of iron-fortified soy sauce among women in China. *Journal of Nutrition Education Behavior, 39*, 302–310.

von Bertalanffy, L. (1975). General systems theory. In B. D. Ruben & J. Y. Kim (Eds.), *General systems theory and human communication.* Rochelle Park, NJ: Hayden Book Co.

Wakefield, S. E., & Poland, B. (2005). Family, friend or foe? Critical reflections on the relevance and role of social capital in health promotion and community development. *Social Science & Medicine, 60*, 2819–2832.

Yip, W., Subramanian, S. V., Mitchell, A. D., Lee, D. T. Wang, J. & Kawachi, I. (2007). Does social capital enhance health and well-being? Evidence from rural China. *Social Science & Medicine, 64*(3), 35–49.

Wong, F. L., Greenwell, B. A., Gates, S., & Berkowitz, J. M. (2008). It's what you do! Reflections on the VERB™ campaign. *American Journal of Preventive Medicine, 34*(6S), S175–S182.

World Health Organization (WHO). (1974). *Community health nursing: report of a WHO expert committee* (Report No. 559). Geneva, Switzerland: WHO.

PART 2

Planning for Health Promotion and Prevention

CHAPTER 4

Assessing Health and Health Behaviors

OBJECTIVES

1. Describe the expected outcomes of a nursing health assessment.
2. Discuss the criteria for conducting a screening in the community.
3. Identify the components of a nursing health assessment conducted for an individual client.
4. Describe life span, language, and culturally appropriate nursing health assessment tools for children, adults, and older adults.
5. Discuss the similarities and differences among the various approaches to assessing the family.
6. Discuss the similarities and differences among the various approaches to assessing the community.

Outline

- Nursing Frameworks for Health Assessment
- Guidelines for Preventive Services and Screenings
- Assessment of the Individual Client
  - A. Physical Fitness
  - B. Nutrition
  - C. Life Stress
  - D. Spiritual Health
  - E. Social Support Systems
  - F. Lifestyle
- Assessment of the Family
- Assessment of the Community
- Opportunities for Research in Health Assessment
- Considerations for Practice in Assessment of Health and Health Behavior
- Summary

- Learning Activities
- Selected Web Sites
- References

A thorough assessment of health and health behaviors is the foundation for tailoring a health promotion-prevention plan to a given client. Assessment provides the database for making clinical judgments about the client's health strengths, health problems, nursing diagnoses, and desired health or behavioral outcomes, as well as the interventions likely to be effective. This information also forms the nature of the client–nurse partnership. The portfolio of assessment measures depends on characteristics of the client, including developmental stage and cultural orientation. The nurse should assess age, language, and cultural appropriateness of the various measures. *National Standards for Culturally and Linguistically Appropriate Services in Health Care* (U.S. Department of Health and Human Services, 2001) provides a practical guide for nurses to offer culturally and linguistically sensitive care. Understanding of one's own cultural characteristics and how they may interface with the client's culture—as well as recognizing that diversity exists in all cultures based on educational level, socioeconomic status, religion, rural/urban residence, and individual and family characteristics—will ensure a more successful encounter.

The use of the electronic health record (EHR) is another strategy to involve the individual client in developing a dynamic, tailored database. The EHR allows storage and almost instantaneous access to data while improving quality and efficiency in health care and improving communication among providers, insurers, and consumers (Figure 4–1). For EHRs to be fully integrated into the health sector, important issues that must be addressed include cost, security, privacy, consumer and provider

EHR Backbone of Care Management Effectiveness

Utilizing EHR to Improve Care Delivery and Coordination

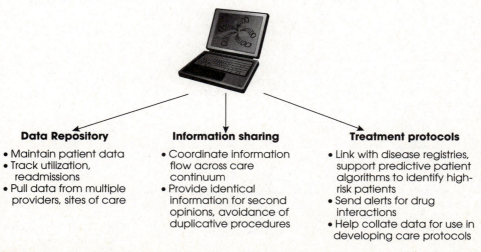

Data Repository	**Information sharing**	**Treatment protocols**
• Maintain patient data • Track utilization, readmissions • Pull data from multiple providers, sites of care	• Coordinate information flow across care continuum • Provide identical information for second opinions, avoidance of duplicative procedures	• Link with disease registries, support predictive patient algorithms to identify high-risk patients • Send alerts for drug interactions • Help collate data for use in developing care protocols

FIGURE 4–1 EHR: Backbone of Care Management Effectiveness *Source: Future of Care Management,* Health Care Advisory Board, 2008, p. 58. Reprinted by permission of the Health Care Advisory Board.

education, and user-friendly systems. To overcome some of the current issues, researchers are investigating tamper-resistant and portable health folders (Anciaux et al., 2008), Web-based portal links for consumers to view and modify health data and interact with providers (Schnipper et al., 2008), and evidence-based designs to evaluate consumer health informatics (McDaniel, Schutte, & Keller, 2008).

Promising developments in EHR are facilitating more widespread usage. Research findings; cooperation among health care providers and technology companies to create interoperability standards for seamless communication, regardless of vendor; cost subsidization of implementing EHRs to encourage physician usage; and incentives offered by Centers for Medicare and Medicaid Services (CMS), will increase widespread adoption of the EHR.

The personal health record (PHR) is the next generation of applications to help consumers take charge of their health, improve care, lower costs and help clients manage and obtain the care they need (Robert Wood Johnson Foundation, 2008) (Figure 4–2). Medicare initiated a pilot PHR program in 2009 for patients to add supplemental information to their health record, authorize access to third parties such as family members, and track and view claims. The PHR belongs to the user and is distinct from physician records. For information about this pilot program and additional issues that must be addressed for it to succeed, go to the Web site listed at the end of this chapter.

In the near future, nursing clinics, community health centers, and primary care centers will use EHRs, PHRs, and new cell phone technology (Figure 4–3) to offer comprehensive resources, including easily customized and self-managed online portfolios. Tailored health information, delivered through these new informatics interventions, enhances self-efficacy, decision making, and healthy behaviors, and fosters self-care (McDaniel et al., 2008).

PHRs Allowing Patients to Actively Manage Their Data

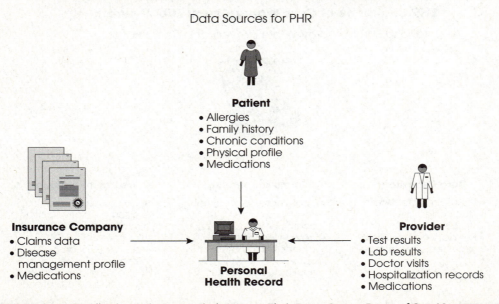

Data Sources for PHR

Patient
- Allergies
- Family history
- Chronic conditions
- Physical profile
- Medications

Insurance Company
- Claims data
- Disease management profile
- Medications

Personal Health Record

Provider
- Test results
- Lab results
- Doctor visits
- Hospitalization records
- Medications

FIGURE 4–2 PHRs: Allowing Patients to Actively Manage Their Data *Source: Future of Care Management,* Health Care Advisory Board, 2008, p. 64. Reprinted by permission of the Health Care Advisory Board.

New Cell Phone Technologies Fostering Self-Care
Remotely Assisted Exercise Prescription Care

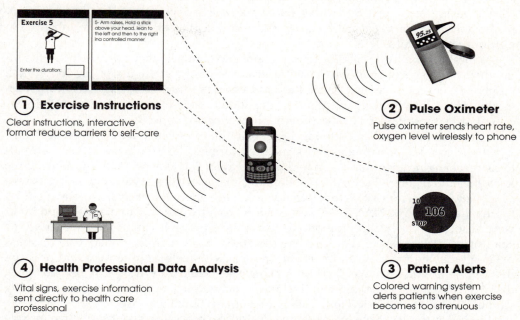

(1) Exercise Instructions

Clear instructions, interactive format reduce barriers to self-care

(2) Pulse Oximeter

Pulse oximeter sends heart rate, oxygen level wirelessly to phone

(4) Health Professional Data Analysis

Vital signs, exercise information sent directly to health care professional

(3) Patient Alerts

Colored warning system alerts patients when exercise becomes too strenuous

FIGURE 4–3   New Cell Phone Technologies Fostering Self-Care   *Source:* Adapted from Marshall, A. et al., "Use of a Smartphone for Improved Self-Management of Pulmonary Rehabilitation." *International Journal of Telemedicine and Applications* in *Future of Health Care Management*. Health Care Advisory Board, 2008, p. 69. Reprinted by permission of the Health Care Advisory Board.

The potential for consumers to be involved in the ownership and maintenance of their health record with "cradle-to-grave" information is especially relevant for computer users and technology-savvy consumers who interface with providers and health systems that have electronic systems. Non–computer users and vulnerable populations are at risk, which may exacerbate health disparities (Shields et al., 2007) unless a safeguard system is put in place to protect these groups. Age is the most significant discriminator of computer/Internet usage, with a much lower percentage of older people using the Internet for health information compared with young adults. However, the overall percentage of Internet users has grown substantially (Madden, 2006).

NURSING FRAMEWORKS FOR HEALTH ASSESSMENT

Health assessment performed by the nurse is a collaborative partnership with the client that promotes mutual input into decision making and planning to improve the client's health and well-being. The desired outcomes are to describe (1) health assets, (2) health problems, (3) health-related lifestyle strengths, (4) key health-related beliefs, (5) health behaviors that put the client at risk, and (6) desired changes to improve quality of life. The initial assessment provides a valuable baseline against which subsequent assessments can be compared.

Several frameworks for nursing assessment and diagnosis are available. At this point, it is important to differentiate between nursing assessment and nursing diagnosis as they are used in this book. *Nursing assessment* is systematic collection of data about a client's health status, beliefs, and behaviors relevant to developing a health promotion-prevention plan. *Nursing diagnosis* is the identification of assets that may be enhanced to maximize health status.

Nursing diagnostic classification systems (taxonomies) focus primarily on the individual and aspects of illness. Positive health states or strengths of the individual, family, or community are not adequately addressed in these taxonomies. As health promotion and prevention knowledge has expanded, taxonomies have developed new definitions supportive of a health promotion/wellness perspective.

The North American Nursing Diagnosis International (NANDA-I) (2009) provides nursing diagnosis taxonomy structured around the nine human response patterns: exchanging, communicating, relating, valuing, choosing, moving, perceiving, knowing, and feeling. The NANDA-I defining characteristics of each diagnosis, as well as related factors and risk factors, provide guidance about the critical assessment areas for the diagnosis. The NANDA-I classification provides one way to diagnose and intervene in some of the health promotion and wellness processes and problems across the span of nursing practice (Popkess-Vawter, 2008). For example, a diagnosis of stress overload may be made when the client presents with feelings of tension and pressure that interfere with effective decision making and results in physical or psychological distress. Potential interventions, including active listening and decision-making support, should be recorded in the assessment plan (Lunney, 2006).

Other examples of wellness nursing diagnoses/processes (client strengths) include nutrition, adequate to meet or maintain body requirements; exercise level, appropriate to maintain wellness state; and spiritual strength. Case studies and sample care plans illustrate how diagnostic statements provide direction for health promotion-prevention care planning (Carpenito-Moyet, 2005).

Gordon (2006) groups the NANDA-I diagnoses into 11 functional health patterns to assist in classifying nursing diagnoses, including: health perception–health management, nutritional–metabolic, elimination, activity–exercise, sleep–rest, cognitive–perceptual, self-perception–self-concept, role–relationship, sexuality–reproductive, coping–stress tolerance, and value–belief.

Gordon's work provides guidelines to conduct a nursing history and examination to assess clients' functional health patterns. As assessment proceeds, diagnostic hypotheses are generated to direct targeted or more detailed data collection. Refer to Gordon's *Manual of nursing diagnoses* (2006) for recommended formats to assess functional health patterns in infants and young children, adults, families, and communities.

The Omaha Visiting Nurse Association System is a useful guide for community health nursing practice, a method of documentation, and a framework for information management (Martin, 2005). The Omaha System incorporates the needs of individuals and families in categories of environment, psychosocial, physiological, and health behavior needs. These categories are referenced by key words such as *individual*, *family*, or *health promotion* in the individual and family categories. Nurse researchers have shown its usefulness in quantifying nursing practice in community health, rural nursing practice, primary care, and wellness centers (Keyzer, 2008; Leonardo, Resick, Bingman, & Strotmeyer, 2004). The Omaha System is useful for target populations, such as at-risk groups for obesity. One difficulty in developing nursing classification systems for communities is that nursing diagnoses/problem classifications focus on nursing practice, whereas community problems are more interdisciplinary.

The Nursing Interventions Classification (NIC), a system that generates standardized nursing actions and interventions for providing care, is relevant for community health because nursing services are categorized and linked to direct reimbursement (Westra, Delaney, Konicek, & Keenan, 2008). However, NIC does not have categories for the health behavior of communities. The Nursing Outcomes Classification (NOC) system was developed to measure the responses of an individual, family, and community behavior/perception to a nursing intervention (Moorhead, Johnson, & Maas, 2004). The NOC system can be used in all settings and with individuals, families, and communities.

The next phase of knowledge generation in nursing is the integration of terminologies into EHR information systems to support care of clients across settings. Research using data from information systems embedded with nursing standards and terminology will help build nursing knowledge and document the contribution of nursing to health care (Westra et al., 2008).

GUIDELINES FOR PREVENTIVE SERVICES AND SCREENINGS

An increasing emphasis on the prevention of disease has resulted in the development of varying sets of guidelines for the delivery of preventive services to individuals, families, and communities across the life span. These guidelines focus on clinical care directed toward prevention of specific diseases such as HIV disease and behavioral morbidity such as substance abuse.

The Guide to Clinical Preventive Services, 2007 (Agency for Healthcare Research and Quality [AHRQ], 2007) is an authoritative source for making decisions about preventive services. Screenings are conducted to detect a particular, unrecognized health problem in individuals who are members of a group at risk for a certain disease or health problem.

Information from screenings is an important component of the community assessment. Community screenings can uncover health problems in an efficient and economically feasible manner. However, screenings should be conducted only if the following factors are present: (1) The specific population has a high prevalence of the disease or health problem, (2) the problem can be successfully treated, (3) treatment is available if the condition is identified, and (4) screening instruments are valid and reliable (AMA Council on Scientific Affairs, 2002).

The cost of conducting screenings must be considered in the decision to offer large-scale screenings. For example, conducting a screening to detect osteoporosis requires special equipment, and the cost may be high due to the number of machines needed to screen in a timely, efficient manner.

Elective Preventive Services Selector (ePSS) is an application designed to help health care providers identify screening services that are appropriate for particular clients. The information is based on recommendations of the U.S. Preventive Services Task Force and can be searched by specific client characteristics, such as age, sex, and behavioral risk factors (AHRQ, 2007).

Nurses in settings in which primary care is delivered should be familiar with the *Guide to Clinical Preventive Services* (AHRQ, 2007) and *Bright Futures: Guidelines for Health*

Supervision of Infants, Children, and Adolescents (American Academy of Pediatrics, 2008) to ensure that clients benefit from state-of-the-art preventive services. These publications provide recommendations and rationale for a wide array of preventive measures.

ASSESSMENT OF THE INDIVIDUAL CLIENT

Assessment of the individual client in the context of health promotion expands beyond physical assessment to include a comprehensive examination of other health parameters and health behaviors. The components of health assessment are (1) functional health patterns, (2) physical fitness, (3) nutrition, (4) life stress, (5) spiritual health, (6) social support systems, (7) health beliefs, and (8) lifestyle. Components are addressed based on the purpose of the assessment, setting, functional health, culture, and age. Functional assessment of patterns comprises a health history, including hereditary and family characteristics, and physical assessment. Assessment components that focus on individuals and have particular relevance for health promotion-prevention are described.

Physical Fitness

Physical activity is an important part of personal health status and is discussed in detail in Chapter 6. Evaluation of physical fitness is a critical part of the nursing assessment because a sedentary lifestyle, for many individuals, begins early in childhood and continues into adulthood. The assessment is applicable to clients of all ages, with restrictions on some components for individuals who are physically compromised. It is important to differentiate between skill-related physical fitness and health-related physical fitness. Skill-related fitness is defined by qualities that contribute to successful athletic performance: agility, speed, power, and reaction time. Health-related fitness qualities found to contribute to one's general health include cardio-respiratory endurance, muscular endurance, body composition, and flexibility (American College of Sports Medicine [ACSM], 2005).

CARDIO-RESPIRATORY ENDURANCE.   Fitness reflects the ability of the circulatory and respiratory (CR) systems to efficiently adjust to and recover from exercise. A number of approaches are used to assess CR endurance. For example, the President's Challenge Physical Fitness test, the 1-mile walk/run, may be used for children and adolescents between 6 and 17 years of age. The individual is asked to walk or run 1 mile at a steady pace over the entire distance. One mile can be measured on either an outdoor or indoor track. Youths are encouraged to practice the day before and warm up just before the walk or run. Health fitness standards for a 10-year-old boy range from 9 to 11:30 minutes; for a 16-year-old boy, 7 to 8:30 minutes. The range for girls of the same ages is 30 seconds to one minute more in each category (Freedson, Cureton, & Heath, 2000).

Another assessment approach is the step test, which is a field version of the laboratory stress test for adults. If the step test is conducted in a clinical setting, the electrocardiogram may be monitored. A physician should be available for emergency backup if the client is over 40 years of age, is obese, or has a history of cardiovascular problems. The step test is not as physiologically stressful as the laboratory stress test, but caution must be taken in individuals with high-risk profiles for cardiovascular disease. For the step test, a step 16- to 17-inchess high is recommended. The step rate should be 24 steps per minute for men and 22 steps per minute for women. Each step consists of the following sequence: left foot up; right foot up; left foot down; right foot down. Apical or carotid pulse rates are measured after stepping for three minutes at the prescribed cadence. With the client comfortably seated in a chair following step testing, pulse rates are counted for 15 seconds in immediate recovery (5–20 seconds) and multiplied by 4 to obtain recovery heart rate. Recovery rate of 140 for women and 124 for men is in the low-risk range of recovery; a recovery rate of 184 for women and 178 for men is in the high-risk range of recovery (ACSM, 2005).

MUSCULAR ENDURANCE. Bent-knee sit-ups are used as a test of muscular endurance for children, youths, and adults (Figure 4–4). The number of sit-ups per minute is counted. The fitness standard for 10–17 year olds is 9–12 sit-ups in one minute (ACSM, 2005). Adults 50 years of age and older and those with cardiovascular disorders must be observed carefully for fatigue during endurance testing. Sit-ups should be terminated if signs of distress occur. Men aged 36–45 years are rated excellent if they can perform 42 or more sit-ups; and women if they can perform 39 or more sit-ups per minute. Men and women in this age range are below average if they can only perform 21 and 12, respectively. Men aged 46 years and older are rated excellent if they can perform 38 or more sit-ups, and women if they can perform 24 or more sit-ups. Men and women are below average if they can perform only 18 and 11, respectively (ACSM, 2005). Sit-ups must be performed accurately to prevent injury.

Timed sit-ups may not adequately measure abdominal strength or endurance because the hip flexor muscles are involved in addition to the abdominal muscles. The push-up muscular endurance test and the bench press test are also used to evaluate muscle endurance. Procedures for conducting these endurance tests are found in the *ACSM resource manual for guidelines for exercise testing and prescription* (2009)

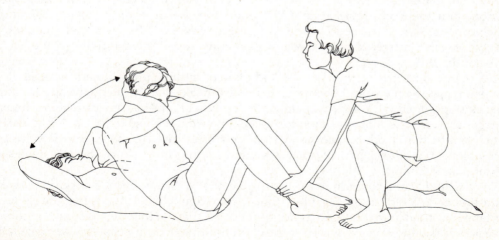

FIGURE 4–4   Bent-Knee Sit-Ups

and *ACSM guidelines for exercise testing and prescription* (2005) and Freedson et al.'s (2000) work on fitness testing in children and youth. The nurse must decide which muscular endurance test to use based on the client's health history and current field-testing reports.

BODY COMPOSITION.   Estimates of body fat can be done using several methods. Hydrostatic underwater weighing is considered the gold standard, or most accurate, estimate of indirect body fat. However, it is seldom used in the clinical setting because of the complex and expensive equipment required and the time and potential anxiety involved in the underwater experience.

Bioelectrical impedance analysis (BIA) is named most frequently in published studies for estimating body fat (Buchholz, Bartok, & Schoeller, 2004). BIA is measured when a small, safe electrical current passes through the body, carried by water and electrolytes of the fluid spaces. Impedance is greatest in fat tissue, which contains only 10–20% water, whereas muscle tissue, which contains 70–75% water, allows the signal to pass more easily. Using a person's height and weight, body type, gender, age, and fitness level, and BIA measurement, it is possible to calculate the percentage of body fat, muscle mass, and hydration level (ACSM, 2005).

BIA is recommended for use in healthy, young, normally hydrated adults and for monitoring this population for changes in body fat composition over time. The procedure recommended for use in research studies consists of the client lying in the supine position with sensor electrodes placed at the standard locations on the right wrist and right ankle. The single frequency parallel BIA has been demonstrated to be a better predictor of total body fat than the bioelectrical impedance spectroscopy serial model (Buchholz et al., 2004). BIA can also be measured in easy and convenient methods using body fat scales (similar to bathroom scales) and handheld body fat analyzers, both available at reasonable costs.

BIA has been compared with hydrostatic weighting in a sample of 418 male and female volunteers in a normal hydrated state and found to be simple, reliable, and accurate (Girandola & Contarsy, 2004), and a better predictor of body fat composition than the Body Mass Index (BMI) and the use of anthropometric methods including skin-fold measures and waist circumference (Nooyens et al., 2007). However, circumference measurement equations added substantially to the accuracy of the BIA.

Anthropometric methods are still advocated by some practitioners because they are simple, convenient, and inexpensive. It is estimated that the predictive accuracy of the skin-fold method is approximately ±5% body fat. Skin-fold measurement should not be used in assessing and monitoring obese clients (Girandola & Contarsy, 2004). The combination of weight, anthropometric methods, and BIA has been shown to be an excellent predictability of total body fat composition (Buchholz et al., 2004; Girandola & Contarsy, 2004).

Skin-fold and circumference measurements to assess body composition may continue to be used in some settings. Since approximately half of the body fat is subcutaneous, total body fat can be estimated by this method. A pair of skin-fold calipers is used to take measures at the chest, mid-axillary, triceps, sub scapular, abdomen, supra iliac, and thigh sites (Figure 4–5). Duplicative measures are taken at

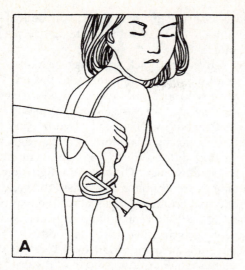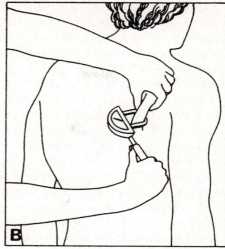

FIGURE 4–5   Skin-Fold Sites: A. Triceps. B. Sub Scapula

each of the sites to ensure accuracy. All measurements should be taken on the right side to conform to standard measurement technique. The sum of the sub scapula and the triceps skin-folds or the calf and triceps skin-folds are used to obtain a measure of body fat in children and youth.

Results above or below the values found in Table 4–1 mean that further assessment is needed to identify either too much or too little nutrient intake for body requirements. In absence of a more accurate and affordable field test to measure body fat, skin-fold measurements must be performed with the knowledge of its limitations. Error may be reduced by adhering to standards, using high-quality skin-fold calipers, and recognizing that body types are different.

FLEXIBILITY.   Flexibility, the ability to move muscles and joints through their maximum range of motion, is also an important component of physical fitness. Flexibility may decrease with age or as a result of chronic illness. The lack of ability to

TABLE 4–1	Triceps Skin-Fold Thickness Indicating Obesity (mm)	
Age (yr)	Males	Females
5	≥12	≥15
10	≥13	≥17
15	≥15	≥20
20	≥16	≥28
25	≥20	≥29
30 and above	≥23	≥30

flex or extend muscles or joints often reflects poor health habits, such as sedentary lifestyle, poor posture, or faulty body mechanics. Loss of flexibility greatly decreases one's ability to move about with ease and comfort.

Trunk flexion measures the ability to stretch the low back and thigh or hamstring muscles. The sit-and-reach test is the most commonly used test to measure flexion. The client sits on a floor mat or flat examining table with legs fully extended and feet flat against a box (Figure 4–6). Arms and hands are extended forward as far as possible and held for a count of three. With a ruler, the distance that the client can reach beyond the proximal edge of the box is measured in inches. If the client cannot reach the edge, the distance of the fingertips from the edge is measured and recorded as a negative number. Normal values for trunk flexion vary among men and women. The desired range for men is $+1$ to $+5$ inches; for women, $+2$ to $+6$. Some researchers have challenged the validity of this test because one's arm-to-leg length ratio may influence one's reach (Freedson et al., 2000). Individual differences must be taken into consideration. Despite limitations of the sit-and-reach test, it may provide a reasonably accurate measure of flexibility.

A physical fitness evaluation assists in planning an appropriate exercise or physical activity program. Careful attention to assessment will optimize the fit of the exercise prescription to the physical capabilities of the client.

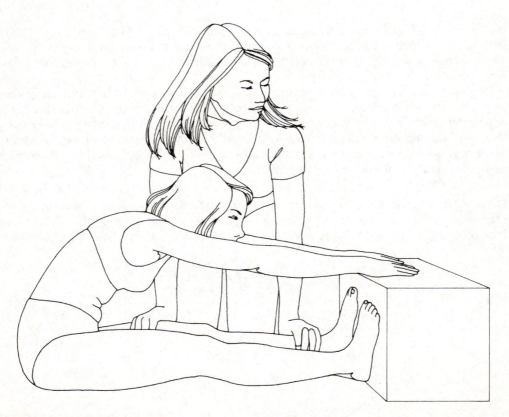

FIGURE 4–6 Trunk Flexion

Nutrition

Effective planning for health promotion requires evaluation of the nutritional status of clients. Anthropometrical measurements and/or BIA analysis, laboratory values, and dietary habits are used to establish a baseline.

Anthropometrics assessment measures include height and weight, circumference of various areas of the body, and skin-fold thickness. Height is measured wearing 1-inch heels. Weight is taken with lightweight clothing. BMI is the best method to assess healthy weight (ACSM, 2005). BMI does not assess body fat composition or fat distribution, but it is a useful screening tool for overweight or obesity. In a study of 2,610 children ages 2–17 years who were followed to ages 18–37 years, childhood BMI was found to be associated with adult adiposity; however, it was dependent on the relative fatness of children (Freedman et al., 2005). This result was supported by a longitudinal study of 168 men and 182 women, in which adolescent skin-fold thickness was a better predictor of overweight in adulthood than BMI (Nooyens et al., 2007).

The BMI table for adults is shown in Table 4–2, and the classification of overweight and obesity by BMI, waist circumference, and associated disease risks standards for adults are in Table 4–3. Healthy and unhealthy weight guidelines are found in Table 4–4. Deviations from any of the norms on the measurements are recorded.

The waist-to-hip ratio is used to assess the amount of fat distributed in the abdomen versus fat distributed below the waist. The ratio is the waist circumference over the hip circumference. The higher the value of the waist-to-hip ratio, the greater the risk of health problems for the client (ACSM, 2005).

Biochemical analyses of blood and urine are used to identify nutritional deficiencies. In addition to laboratory tests for cholesterol, triglycerides, glucose, and high-density lipoproteins, tests for protein (creatinine index, serum protein, serum albumin, total lymphocyte count, blood urea nitrogen, and uric acid), serum or plasma vitamin levels (water-soluble, fat-soluble), and minerals (calcium, sodium, potassium, iron, phosphorus, and magnesium) are used to assess nutritional status. Three values that are particularly important in assessing nutritional status are serum albumin less than 3.5 g/dL, total lymphocyte count less than 1800 mm, and an involuntary loss of body weight greater than 15%. These three indicators have repeatedly been shown to correlate with nutritional status (McVay-Smith, 2001).

One common measure to assess nutritional status is a dietary diary. Clients who have computer access can go to the Web site My Pyramid Tracker at www.mypyramid .gov (U.S. Department of Agriculture Human Nutrition Information Service, 2006), click on *Assess Your Food Intake*, and complete the online dietary assessment. After the client enters a day of dietary information, the intake will be evaluated with current nutritional guides. The client can track dietary intake for up to one year.

With a paper option, clients are instructed to keep a record of everything eaten for three days during the week prior to their office or home visit. Food intake is best kept on a form that list types of foods and amounts consumed during regular meals and snacks. Daily food choices are compared with published daily food guides or one of the computerized dietary analysis packages available. When usual dietary patterns have been identified, the nurse can provide needed nutritional assistance (see Chapter 7). The nurse and nutritionists work together to prepare educational materials and/or recommend Web sites to ensure that the client has the latest and most accurate research

TABLE 4–2 Body Mass Index Table

BMI	19	20	21	22	23	24	25	26	27	28	29	30	31	32	33	34	35
Height								Weight (in pounds)									
4'10" (58")	90	96	100	105	110	115	119	124	129	134	138	143	148	153	158	162	167
4'11" (59")	94	99	104	109	114	119	124	128	133	138	143	148	153	158	163	168	173
5' (60")	97	102	107	112	118	123	128	133	138	143	148	153	158	163	168	174	179
5'1" (61")	100	106	111	116	122	127	132	137	143	148	153	158	164	169	174	180	185
5'2" (62")	104	109	115	120	126	131	136	142	147	153	158	164	169	175	180	186	191
5'3" (63")	107	113	118	124	130	135	141	146	152	158	163	169	174	180	186	191	197
5'4" (64")	110	116	122	128	134	140	145	151	157	163	169	174	180	186	192	197	204
5'5" (65")	114	120	126	132	138	144	150	156	162	168	174	180	186	192	198	204	210
5'6" (66")	118	124	130	136	142	148	155	161	167	173	179	186	192	198	204	210	216
5'7" (67")	121	127	134	140	146	153	159	166	172	178	185	191	198	204	211	217	223
5'8" (68")	125	131	138	144	151	158	164	171	177	184	190	197	203	210	216	223	230
5'9" (69")	128	135	142	149	155	162	169	176	182	189	196	203	209	216	223	230	236
5'10" (70")	132	139	146	153	160	167	174	181	188	195	202	209	216	222	229	236	243
5'11" (71")	136	143	150	157	165	172	179	186	193	200	208	215	222	229	236	243	250
6'(72")	140	147	154	162	169	177	184	191	199	206	213	221	228	235	242	250	258
6'1" (73")	144	151	159	166	174	182	189	197	204	212	219	227	235	242	250	257	265
6'2" (74")	148	155	163	171	179	186	194	202	210	218	225	233	241	249	256	264	272
6'3" (75")	152	160	168	176	184	192	200	208	216	224	232	240	248	256	264	272	279

Source: Data from the *Evidence Report of Clinical Guidelines on the Identification, Evaluation, and Treatment of Overweight and Obesity in Adults*, 1998. NIH/National Heart Lung, and Blood Institute [NHLBI].

TABLE 4–3 **Classification of Overweight and Obesity by BMI, Waist Circumference, and Associated Disease Risk***

	BMI (kg/m²)	Disease Risk* Relative to Normal Weight and Waist Circumference	
		Men ≤ 40 in. Women ≤ 35 in.	Men > 40 in. Women > 35 in.
Normal[†]	18.5 – 24.9	—	—
Overweight	25.0 – 29.9	Increased	High
Obesity	30.0 – 34.9	High	Very High

*Disease risk for type 2 diabetes, hypertension, and CVD.

[†]Increased waist circumference can also be a marker for increased risk even in persons of normal weight.

Source: Adapted from *Preventing and Managing the Global Epidemic of Obesity.* Report of the World Health Organization Consultation of Obesity. WHO, Geneva, June 1997. http://www.nhlbi.nih.gov/guidelines/obesity/e_txtbk/txgd/411.htm

findings about nutritional supplements, including vitamins and minerals (e.g., calcium, iron), as well as proteins or complex carbohydrates.

To review dietary assessment measures for use in primary care, see "Practical nutrition assessment in primary care settings: A review" (Calfas, Zabinski, & Rupp, 2000), *Instruments for Clinical Health-Care Research* (Frank-Stromborg & Olsen, 2004), and research instruments developed by Stanford Patient Education Research Center and available at http://patienteducation.stanford.edu/research/

Poor eating patterns, obesity, and malnutrition occur in all cultures and socioeconomic levels. In addition, dietary risk factors for chronic disease are widespread. Assessment of nutritional status and dietary habits is a critical part of a comprehensive health assessment for individuals, families, and specific target groups, such as high-school students, pregnant women, and the elderly. An analysis of assessment data determines which interventions are necessary to improve the nutritional status of the client.

Life Stress

Stress is a potential threat to mental health and physical well-being and is associated with illnesses such as cardiovascular disease, cancer, and gastrointestinal disorders. Life stress should be evaluated as a part of comprehensive health assessment. Stress is typically evaluated with questionnaires that ask about difficulties or negative life experiences. The next sections describe several of these instruments. In addition, *Instruments for Clinical Health-Care Research* (Frank-Stromborg & Olsen, 2004) provides a review of instruments on stress, coping, and anxiety and relevance of each measure for nursing.

STRESS SCALES.   Assessing a person's vulnerability to stress and strength to cope provides an essential measure of mental and physical well-being. The Derogates Stress Profile (Derogatis & Fleming, 1997) is used to assess personal and professional stress in adolescents and adults. The 77-item instrument is designed to screen response to stress related to time pressure, driven behavior, attitude, relocation, work environment, family relationships, hostility, anxiety, depression, and health. The Perceived Stress Scale (Cohen, Kessler, & Gordon, 1997) measures moods and feelings about life stressors and is considered a measure of global stress. The 10-item scale is easy to administer and score.

TABLE 4–4 Healthy and Unhealthy Weight Guidelines

Are you at a healthy weight?

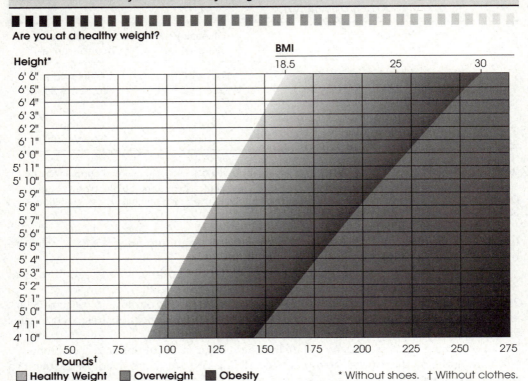

Healthy Weight   Overweight   Obesity   * Without shoes. † Without clothes.

The BMI (weight-for-height) ranges shown above for adults. They are not exact ranges of healthy and unhealthy weights. However, they show that health risk increases at higher levels of overweight and obesity. Even within the healthy BMI range, weight gains can carry health risks

Directions: Find your weight on the bottom of the graph. Go straight up from that point until you come to the line that matches your height. Then look to find your weight group.

BMI of 25 defines the upper boundary of healthy weight

BMI of higher than 25 to 30 defines overweight

BMI of higher than 30 defines obesity

Source: http://www.cnpp.usda.gov/Publications/DietaryGuidelines/2000/2000DGCommitteeReport.pdf, p. 11

HASSLES AND UPLIFTS. Hassles are defined as the irritating, frustrating, distressing demands such as traffic jams, losing items, and arguments that may characterize everyday life. Uplifts, the counterpart of hassles, are defined as the positive experiences or joys of life, such as getting a good night's rest, receiving a letter from a friend, or spending time with a pet. Assessment of daily hassles and uplifts may be a better approach to the prediction of health or illness outcomes than the usual assessment of life events. Negative experiences such as hassles cause neuroendocrine changes that predispose to illness, while positive experiences such as uplifts may buffer stress disorders.

The Adolescent Hassle Scale (AHS) was used to examine personal, psychosocial, sociocultural, and environmental predictors of tobacco use for 1,671 Arab-American adolescents (Rice et al., 2006). The AHS is a 28-item tool specifically developed to measure stressors of family, school, friends, and leisure. Initiation of cigarette smoking in the study population was highly influenced by use of tobacco by family and friends.

In a study of the relationship among daily hassles, uplifts, and depressive symptoms in college students, results showed that minor uplifts were associated with decreases in depressive symptoms. Daily hassles were predictive of depressive symptoms. Minor negative events were perceived more severely than minor positive events, or students gave negative events much more weight than they did minor positive events (Armstrong, Davis, & Dixon, 2005).

ANXIETY INVENTORY.   Anxiety may also be assessed as part of the life-stress review. The State-Trait Anxiety Inventory consists of 20 items that assess the extent of anxiety one feels at that moment (state anxiety) and 20 items that assess how one generally feels (trait anxiety) (Spielberger, Gorsuch, Lushene, & Vagg, 1983). A State-Trait Anxiety Inventory is available for children ("How I Feel Questionnaire," Spielberger et al., 1983). Both instruments and administration manuals are available from Mind Garden, Palo Alto, California. The State-Trait Anxiety Inventories provide an efficient, reliable method to assess feelings of anxiety experienced by children and adults.

STRESS WARNING SIGNALS INVENTORY.   Clients should understand how they respond to stress and be aware of symptoms of an elevated stress level. When clients are aware of their own stress signals, they can use stress-management techniques (see Chapter 8) more effectively. Symptoms of stress may be physical, behavioral, emotional, or cognitive, as shown in Figure 4–7.

COPING MEASURES.   Coping is defined as an individual's ongoing efforts to manage specific internal and external demands that are appraised as exceeding personal resources. Coping is a process and changes over time in relation to changing stressful events in one's life. The interaction of an individual with the environment determines how a stressful event is appraised and managed. Coping efforts, in response to a stressful encounter, are described as either problem focused or emotion focused.

Coping is commonly measured with the Ways of Coping Questionnaire developed by Folkman and Lazarus (1988). The scale measures both the emotion- and problem-focused coping strategies an individual uses when responding to a stressful situation.

The Schoolager's Coping Strategies Inventory is used to measure the type, frequency, and effectiveness of children's stress-coping strategies. The scale was used to study fears and coping of 79 healthy children in Nepal and their parents' perceptions of their children's fears and coping strategies (Mahat & Scoloveno, 2003). Significant differences were found between levels of fear by children and parents. Children reported less effective coping strategies than their parents' perceptions of the effectiveness of the children's coping strategies. Information is needed from both children and their parents to accurately assess coping in children.

Mastery is defined as a human response to difficult or stressful circumstances in which a person gains competence and control over the stressful experience. In a study of the relationship of negative events and age-related decline in mastery, results showed that loss of personal and social resources may be the reason older adults handle stress more poorly than younger adults (Cairney & Krause, 2008).

Stress Warning Signals

PHYSICAL SYMPTOMS

- ☐ Headaches
- ☐ Indigestion
- ☐ Stomachaches
- ☐ Sweaty palms
- ☐ Sleep difficulties
- ☐ Dizziness

- ☐ Back pain
- ☐ Tight neck, shoulders
- ☐ Racing heart
- ☐ Restlessness
- ☐ Tiredness
- ☐ Ringing in ears

BEHAVIORAL SYMPTOMS

- ☐ Excess smoking
- ☐ Bossiness
- ☐ Compulsive gum chewing
- ☐ Attitude critical of others

- ☐ Grinding of teeth at night
- ☐ Overuse of alcohol
- ☐ Compulsive eating
- ☐ Inability to get things done

EMOTIONAL SYMPTOMS

- ☐ Crying
- ☐ Nervousness, anxiety
- ☐ Boredom—no meaning to things
- ☐ Edginess—ready to explode
- ☐ Feeling powerless to change things

- ☐ Overwhelming sense of pressure
- ☐ Anger
- ☐ Loneliness
- ☐ Unhappiness for no reason
- ☐ Easily upset

COGNITIVE SYMPTOMS

- ☐ Trouble thinking clearly
- ☐ Forgetfulness
- ☐ Lack of creativity
- ☐ Memory loss

- ☐ Inability to make decisions
- ☐ Thoughts of running away
- ☐ Constant worry
- ☐ Loss of sense of humor

Do any seem familiar to you?

Check the ones you experience when under stress. These are your stress warning signs.

Are there any additional stress warning signals that you experience that are not listed? If so, add them here.

_____

_____

_____

_____

_____

FIGURE 4–7   Stress Warning Signals   *Source:* From *The Wellness Book* by H. Benson & Eileen M. Stuart. Copyright © 1992 Herbert Benson & Eileen M. Stuart. All rights reserved. Reprinted by arrangement with Citadel Press/Kensington Publishing Corp.

Spiritual Health

Spiritual health is defined as the ability to develop one's inner being to its fullest potential. Spiritual health includes the ability to discover and articulate one's basic purpose in life; to learn how to experience love, joy, peace, and fulfillment; and to help oneself and others achieve their fullest potential. The appraisal of spiritual health is critical in a holistic approach to health assessment because spiritual beliefs affect a client's interpretations of life events and health. Spirituality, religion, and health are factors that need more research, and standards to assess delivery and evaluation of spiritual care are needed as well. The supportive approach may be the best one for nurses to use, because "to routinize spiritual care" carries risks (Taylor, 2007). Measures of spirituality are discussed next. Additional measures are found in *Instruments in clinical health-care research* (Frank-Stromborg & Olsen, 2004).

The Spiritual Involvement and Beliefs Scale (SIBS) was designed to be used across religious traditions to access actions as well as beliefs. The 26-item scale is easy to administer and score and avoids the use of cultural and religious bias (Hatch, Burg, Naberhaus, & Hellmich, 1998). Using the revised scale (SIBS-R), Litwinczuk and Groh (2007) measured the relationship between a patient's spirituality, purpose in life, and well-being in 46 HIV-positive men and women. Spirituality was significantly correlated with purpose in life but not with well-being. Further study of the relationship between spirituality and well-being is needed.

The Spiritual Perspective Scale (SPS) is a 10-item instrument that measures one's perceptions of the extent to which one's spiritual beliefs and one's daily interactions are consistent. Reed (1992), the developer of the SPS, proposes that spirituality throughout one's life and especially during the later stages may help one manage life stresses more effectively. In a study using the SPS, results indicate that nurses were able to define spiritual activities, perspectives, and attitudes in nursing care (Cavendish et al., 2003).

Areas of spirituality to be assessed include relationship with a higher being, relationship with self, and relationships with others (Chung, Wong, & Chan, 2007). Questions related to spiritual assessment are usually asked toward the end of the interview when the client and nurse are more at ease with each other. Clients should be informed that assessing their spiritual well being is integral to evaluating overall health.

Social Support Systems

Two approaches for reviewing the social support networks of clients are useful in providing the client and nurse increased insight into existing support resources. When assessing the adequacy of support systems, it is important to be cognizant of factors that may cause the assessments to vary. Such things as the client's culture, age, social context (e.g., school, home, work), and role context (e.g., parent, student, professional) influence perceived and received support. People's use of the Internet to expand their social contacts is increasing in popularity and should also be included in assessing the client's social support system. Definitive measures for assessing social support are abundant in the literature. They can also as be found on the Web at http://patienteducation.stanford.edu/research/.

SUPPORT SYSTEMS REVIEW.   One straightforward, useful approach to assess support systems is to ask the client to list individuals who provide informational, emotional, appraisal, or instrumental support. The client is then asked to indicate the relationship of the persons listed, such as family members, friends, fellow workers, or social acquaintances. Next, persons who have been sources of support for five years or more are identified. This list enables the client to become aware of the stability of personal support systems. Last, the frequency and types of contact are identified. The type of

List individuals who provide support to you. Next indicate the following relationships: Family member (FM); Fellow worker (FM); or Social Acquaintance (A). Frequency of Contact: Daily (D); Weekly (W); Monthly (M); or Rarely (R). Types of Contact: Face-to-Face (F); Telephone (T); or Email (EM). If individual has been supportive for 5 years or more, place the number 5.

Individual	Relationship	Frequency	Type	Time
John	FM (husband)	D	F	5
Peter	FM (son)	D	F	5
Helen	FM (daughter)	D	F	5
Ted	FM (father)	W	T	5
Andrew	FW	D	F	-
Frances	FW	W	F	-
Rose	FW	W	T	5
Elsa	A	M	E	-
Jack	A	M	E	5

Ask the client to identify the type of support provided by individuals in the list. They may provide more than one type of support.

Sources of Emotional Support

FAMILY	WORK	SOCIAL GROUP
John	Frances	Elsa
Peter	Rose	Jack
Helen	Andrew	
Ted		

Sources of Instrument Support

FAMILY	WORK	SOCIAL GROUP
John	Andrew	Jack
Ted		

Sources of Information Support

FAMILY	WORK	SOCIAL GROUP
John	Andrew	Jack
Ted	Rose	

Sources of Appraisal Support

FAMILY	WORK	SOCIAL GROUP
John	Rose	Elsa

FIGURE 4–8 Support System Review: Social Network and Type of Support

contact may be face-to-face or telephone and email communication. Examining the social network enables the client and nurse to mutually assess the adequacy of support. If it is inadequate, strategies are generated to enhance existing social networks. Figure 4–8 shows a sample support system for a hypothetical client.

After reviewing the client's social support systems, the following questions can be explored:

- In what areas do you need more support: informational, emotional, instrumental, appraisal?
- Who within your present support system might provide the needed support?

- Who else do you think needs to become a part of your support system?
- What can you do to add the people you believe you need to your support system?

Answers to these questions suggest actions the client can take to expand sources of personal support.

EMOTIONAL SUPPORT DIAGRAM.   Sources of emotional support can also be diagrammed to assess the strength of support available. Figure 4–9 presents a sample emotional support diagram that is coded to indicate strong, moderate, and weak sources of support, as well as current conflicts with supportive individuals. The length of each line is used to indicate geographic proximity to the client. This approach is particularly appropriate for clients who need a visual presentation of their emotional support system to take action to sustain or enhance emotionally satisfying relationships.

Review of sources of social support is an integral part of the assessment. A review enables the client to recognize current sources of support and identify barriers in social relationships that may block desirable health actions. The nurse must always be alert to client situations in which social support is minimal or nonexistent. Extensive review of support systems may cause anxiety and depression. In this case, a more informal, nonthreatening approach should be used.

Social support instruments represent the broad spectrum of measures used in clinical settings as well as research. The Social Support Questionnaire is a six-item

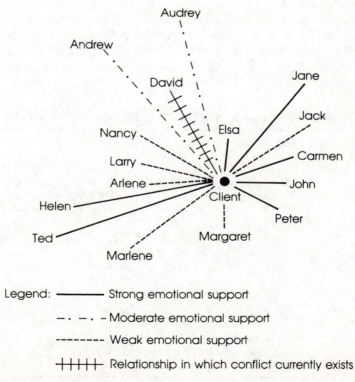

Legend: ——— Strong emotional support

—·—·— Moderate emotional support

-------- Weak emotional support

+|+|+|+ Relationship in which conflict currently exists

FIGURE 4–9   Emotional Support Diagram for Client

measure of perceived social support and satisfaction with social support. Each item presents a specific scenario for which respondents are asked to list the people who would be available for support in that situation. Respondents are also asked to rate their satisfaction with the support available (Sarason, Shearin, Pierce, & Sarason, 1987).

The Medical Outcomes Study Social Support Survey is a self-administrated, 19-item scale that assesses emotional, informational, and tangible support; positive social interaction; and affection (Sherbourne & Stewart, 1991).

Lifestyle

In the context of health, *lifestyle* is defined as discretionary activities that are a regular part of one's daily pattern of living and significantly influence health status. Health-promoting behavior is an expression of the human actualizing tendency that is directed toward optimal well-being, personal fulfillment, and productive living. The 52-item Health-Promoting Lifestyle Profile II (HPLP-II), a revision of the original instrument, consists of six subscales to measure major components of a health-promoting lifestyle: health responsibility, physical activity, nutrition, interpersonal relations, spiritual growth, and stress management. Scores are obtained for each subscale, or a total scale score is calculated to measure overall health-promoting lifestyle (Sechrist, Walker, & Pender, 1987). The HPLP-II provides important information about a client's lifestyle. Sample items for each of the subscales are in Table 4–5. A HPLP-II profile provides information to develop an individualized health promotion plan that identifies lifestyle strengths and resources as well as areas for further growth. A Spanish language version of the HPLP-II is available. The Adolescent Lifestyle Profile (ALP) measures seven domains of health-promoting lifestyle (Hendricks, Murdaugh, & Pender, 2006). The ALP was modeled after the HPLP-II.

TABLE 4–5   Health-Promoting Lifestyle Profile II: Subscales and Sample Items

Subscale	Sample Item
Health responsibility	Read or watch TV programs about improving my health.
	Question health professionals in order to understand their instructions.
Physical activity	Exercise vigorously for 20 or more minutes at least three times a week (brisk walking, bicycling, aerobic dancing, using a stair climber).
	Get exercise during usual day activities (such as walking during lunch, using stairs instead of elevators, parking car farther away from destination and walking).
Nutrition	Choose a diet low in fat, saturated fat, and cholesterol.
	Eat 2 to 4 servings of fruit each day.
Interpersonal relations	Spend time with close friends.
	Settle conflicts with others through discussion and compromise.
Spiritual growth	Feel connected with some force greater than myself.
	Am aware of what is important to me in life.
Stress management	Take some time for relaxation each day.
	Pace myself to prevent fatigue.

TABLE 4–6   True–False Statements for Assessing States of Behavior Change

1. I currently do not (specify exact behavior, e.g., exercise 30 minutes three times a week, eat 2 to 4 servings of fruit daily) and do not intend to start in the next 6 months. (Precontemplation)
2. I currently do not (specify behavior), but I am thinking about starting to do so in the next 6 months. (Contemplation)
3. I have tried several times to (specify behavior) but am seriously thinking of trying again in the next month. (Planning)
4. I have (specify behavior) regularly for less than 6 months. (Action)
5. I have (specify behavior) regularly for more than 6 months. (Maintenance)

Sources of additional lifestyle instruments can be found in the literature and at http://patienteducation.stanford.edu/research/.

STAGE OF CHANGE ASSESSMENT.   Clients may be at one of several stages in relation to any given behavior change. The transtheoretical model (see Chapter 2) proposes that stage of readiness will determine the intervention plan that is most effective. Stages of change for positive health behaviors may be assessed with the true–false questions presented in Table 4–6. Recognizing the different stages of the client in relation to various health behaviors allows for more precise tailored interventions.

ASSESSMENT OF THE FAMILY

The family is the primary social structure for health promotion, as health-promoting as well as health-damaging behaviors and lifestyles are learned within the context of the family. The family also acts as a powerful mediating factor in determining how its members cope with health concerns and challenges. The family is a logical unit of assessment and intervention for health promotion, because it has the primary responsibility for (1) developing self-care and dependent-care competencies of its members, (2) fostering resilience of family members to include shared values and shared goals, (3) providing social and physical resources to the family group, and (4) promoting healthy individuals while maintaining family cohesion (Peace & Lutz, 2009; Tyler & Horner, 2008). Although women generally carry the major responsibility for health decision making and health education for the family, the task of fostering health and healthy behaviors should be "mainstreamed" as an integral part of family functioning.

The milieu for health promotion is likely to differ significantly across families, depending on their composition, structure, socioeconomic status, living environment, cultural context, and family history. A family history is a window to one's health and an invaluable insight into the risk of inheriting specific diseases, shared environmental factors, and individual health concerns. The nurse can encourage clients to visit My Family Health Portrait at www.familyhistory.hhs.gov to complete the history online, download the form, or print a copy for the family to complete. As noted by Peace and Lutz (2009), the limitation of this traditional family history representation is evident when applied to diverse families. Genepro (www.genopro.com) is a commercial application for drawing genograms and may be more useful for assessing a nontraditional family unit.

Healthy family traits can be expressed in many different ways, and family strengths can have many different modes of expression. One-parent families, blended families, unmarried parents with children, and gay and lesbian families must all be taken into consideration. When conducting a family assessment, the nurse must be attuned to this wide variation among families as well as variations produced by transitions in family life. This section briefly describes some approaches to assessment that can be used in all types of families.

Using a systems approach to family, five assessment categories are described, including (1) individual members, (2) subsystems (developmental, biological, psychological, and social characteristics), (3) interactional patterns (relationships, communication patterns, roles, and attachment patterns), (4) family processing, and (5) change or adaptive abilities (Kaakinen, Hanson, & Birenbaum, 2004). Three categories of processes that underlie a systems model of family assessment are (1) those that regulate exchanges with the environment, (2) processes designed to prevent an overload of the system, and (3) internal processes that regulate the family's ability to adapt and change (Clark, 2003).

In a structural–functional approach to family assessment, the family is viewed as a system with communication patterns, power structure, role structure, family values, affective function, socialization patterns, health care function, family stress, coping, and adaptation mechanisms (Friedman, 2003; Friedman, Bowden, & Jones, 2003). Assessment based on systems theory provides insight about the internal processes of the family as well as the relationship of the family to the environment and larger social system. Family decision-making patterns in relation to health are identified in assessing power structure and health care function.

The Calgary Family Assessment Model has been adapted for nurses to use to assess families (Wright & Leahey, 2000). This model consists of family structural assessment, family developmental assessment, and family functional assessment. In structural assessment, the family is analyzed in terms of both its internal and external structure. Aspects of the internal structure include family composition, rank order, subsystem, and boundary, and components of the external structure are culture, religion, socioeconomic level, mobility, environment, and extended family.

To assess family development, the model reviews the current stage of the family in relation to family developmental history. Family development focuses primarily on the traditional family developmental cycle, but it also includes assessment of alterations in the family developmental life cycle brought about by separation, divorce, single parenthood, and remarriage.

Family functional assessment is dichotomized as instrumental functioning and expressive functioning. *Instrumental functioning* refers to the routine activities of everyday living, whereas *expressive functioning* connotes emotional communication, verbal communication, nonverbal communication, circular communication, problem solving, roles, control, beliefs, alliances, and coalitions. (See Wright & Leahey 2000 for more discussion of family functional assessment.)

Sawin, Harrington, and Wood (1995) prepared an excellent compilation of approximately 20 measures of family functioning that is useful in practice. Instruments include the Feetham Family Functioning Survey, Family Adaptability and Cohesion

Scale, and the Family Hardiness Index. The compilation includes a description of each instrument with sample items, psychometric properties, cross-cultural uses, gender sensitivity, applicability to variant family structures, list of selected studies using the instrument, critique, and source for accessing the instrument.

A significant gap in family assessment is lack of instruments that measure family dimensions of a health-related lifestyle. Nurse scientists should develop valid and reliable measures to assess families' aggregate health behaviors. As nurses continue to find limitations with these measures, they have an opportunity to develop computer-based applications. Suggested assessment areas are in Table 4–7.

TABLE 4–7 Components of Family Assessment

Nutrition

1. Meals prepared in the home are generally consistent with the food guide pyramid.
2. Healthy snacks are consumed in the home.
3. Knowledge about healthy eating habits is shared among family members.
4. Mutual assistance occurs among family members for maintenance of recommended weights and avoidance of overweight and underweight.
5. Family members praise each other for healthy eating.
6. Family members encourage each other to drink 6 to 8 glasses of water per day.
7. Family members base purchase decisions on nutritional labels on food.

Physical Activity

1. Many family outings consist of vigorous or moderate physical activity.
2. Exercise equipment is available within the home.
3. Use of home exercise equipment is part of "family time."
4. Family members expect each other to be physically active.
5. A family membership is held in recreational facilities or programs.
6. Time together is seldom spent watching television or playing video games.
7. Family prefers to spend as much time out of doors as possible.

Stress Control and Management

1. Family manages time well to minimize stressful demands on members.
2. Family often relaxes, shares stories, and laughs together.
3. Emotional expression is encouraged within the family.
4. Family members share stressful experiences with each other.
5. Family members offer each other assistance with difficult tasks.
6. Family members seldom criticize each other.
7. Periods of relaxation and sleep are considered important by the family.

Health Responsibility

1. A schedule for preventive care visits is maintained by the family.
2. Family often discusses news and articles about health topics.
3. Family members are encouraged to seek health care early if a problem develops.
4. Personal responsibility for health is encouraged by the family.
5. Family feels a sense of responsibility for the health of the family and each member.
6. Health professionals are consulted about health promotion as well as care in illness.
7. Appropriate protective behaviors are openly discussed and encouraged (abstinence, use of condoms, hearing protection, eye protection, sunscreen, helmets).

TABLE 4–7 (Continued)

Family Resilience and Resources

1. Worship or spiritual experiences are a regular part of family activities.
2. Family members share a sense of "togetherness" despite difficult life events.
3. Family has a common sense of purpose in life.
4. Family members encourage each other to "keep going" when life is difficult.
5. Growth in positive directions is mutually encouraged within the family.
6. Health is nurtured as a positive family resource.
7. Personal strengths and capabilities are nurtured.

Family Support

1. Family has a number of friends or relatives that they see frequently.
2. Family is involved in community activities and groups.
3. Family members frequently praise each other.
4. In times of distress, the family can call on a number of other families or individuals for help.
5. Disagreements are settled through discussion rather than verbal abuse or physical violence.
6. Family members model healthy habits for each other.
7. Professional support services are sought when needed.

Family assessment complements individual assessment; thus, the two must be considered interrelated processes. To provide further guidance, Chapter 5 presents a format for developing a family health promotion-prevention plan.

ASSESSMENT OF THE COMMUNITY

A third essential component of health assessment is community analysis or appraisal. Community analysis is the process of assessing and defining needs, opportunities, and resources involved in initiating community health action programs. A community analysis is done *with* the community, not *on* or *for* the community. Local citizens and organizations are involved in the assessment process so that they can have "ownership" of the program and build widespread commitment to community action.

Five approaches have been identified for collecting data about communities: (1) informant interviewing (directed conversation with community members), (2) participant observation (sharing in community life activities), (3) mobile survey (observation while driving about), (4) secondary analyses (use of preexisting data), and (5) community surveys (organized data collection efforts) (Shuster & Goeppinger, 2008). Because community members constitute a critical primary data source, informant interviewing should always be used as one approach to data collection. An assessment methodology that combines at least three to four of the data collection methods is more likely to provide a holistic picture of the community than an assessment that relies on only one or two approaches.

One approach to community assessment is to collect information about the following community subsystems and their interrelationships: values and culture, politics, education, recreation, transportation, religion, communications and media, welfare, economics, utilities, business and labor, social life, safety and protection, and health. Population growth patterns, functional activity status, nutritional status, dominant lifestyle patterns, coping ability, community stressors, goal setting and achievement capabilities, and risk factors should be assessed in addition to traditional indices of morbidity, mortality, and accessibility of health care resources.

The nature of the assessment is based on the time available and how the information will be used. Comprehensive assessment includes all relevant information about the community that is synthesized from existing documents and primary data collection. This approach is costly and time-consuming and is not recommended unless such a comprehensive study is absolutely essential before high-priority program goals are addressed. A familiarization assessment is more efficient and provides a broad rather than in-depth overview of the community at large. The windshield survey is an example. In a windshield survey, the nurse drives through the community and identifies multiple dimensions, including housing quality, recreation facilities, and the people residing in the area (Anderson & McFarlane, 2006).

A problem-oriented assessment begins with a single problem and assesses the community in terms of the problem—for example, neighborhood violence. Aspects of the community relevant to the health issue are assessed to determine their contributory, ameliorative, or preventive effects. Subsystem assessment is focused on a particular sector of the community and permits an in-depth assessment of that sector. For example, the subsystem might be assessed to evaluate the impact of educational programs on the health and productivity of the community (Shuster & Goepinger, 2008).

Data collection methods are numerous and varied. Existing records can be examined to obtain as much information as possible before data collection is instituted. Key informants who are knowledgeable about the community are another important data source. When primary data collection is necessary, focus group interviewing is the method of choice because of the rich interactive data that can be obtained. Survey data can also be important, as information from a large segment of the population is provided.

Community assessment provides information about a community's health status from which community diagnoses are derived. The assessment is a primary building block for planning, implementing, and evaluating community health promotion-prevention programs. The components of a community assessment have been identified, organized, and further expanded in Table 4–8. Examples of assessment instruments are available in most community health textbooks (e.g., Anderson & McFarlane, 2006; Shuster & Goepinger, 2008).

Assessment of communities is a complicated and time-consuming task. Collaboration is required among many individuals in the community as well as health professionals. However, such assessments are critical to identify community strengths and resources as well as diagnose community problems and/or deficits. Successful implementation of community health promotion-prevention programs depends in large part on accurate assessment of community characteristics.

TABLE 4–8   Components of Community Assessment

Human Biology

1. Composition of population by age, gender, and race
2. Population patterns of longevity
3. Genetic inheritance patterns by gender and race
4. Disease incidence and prevalence compared to prior years, and to state and national statistics
5. Health status indicators (immunization levels, nutritional status, mobility)

Environment

1. Physical environment (urban/rural/suburban, housing, water supply, parks and recreation, climate, topography, size, population density, aesthetics, natural or manmade resources, goods and services, health risks)
2. Psychologic environment (productivity level, cohesion, mental health status, communication networks, intergroup harmony, future orientation, prevalence of stressors)
3. Social environment (income and education levels, employment, family composition, religious affiliations, cultural affiliations, language[s] spoken, social services, organization profile, leadership and decision-making structures)

Community Lifestyles

1. Consumption patterns (e.g., nutrition, alcohol)
2. Occupational groups
3. Leisure pursuits
4. Comunity health attitudes and beliefs
5. Patterns of health-related behaviors in aggregates
6. History of participation in community health action

Health System

1. Health care services available (health promotion, prevention, primary care, secondary care, tertiary care, mental health)
2. Accessibility of promotive and preventive care (low income, homeless, varying racial and ethnic groups)
3. Financing plans for health care

Source: Clark, Mary Jo, *Community Health Nursing: Caring for Populations,* 4th Edition, © 2003. Reproduced by permission of Pearson Education, Inc., Upper Saddle River, New Jersey.

OPPORTUNITIES FOR RESEARCH IN HEALTH ASSESSMENT

Research that develops and tests assessment instruments for health and health behaviors of aggregates from diverse racial, cultural, and socioeconomic backgrounds is a high priority. Reliable and valid instruments, based on theory and research, are needed to perform meaningful assessments. Community interventions should be developed and tested in subgroups. Accurate knowledge of the client, family, and community will facilitate the development and implementation of successful health promotion interventions.

CONSIDERATIONS FOR PRACTICE IN ASSESSMENT OF HEALTH AND HEALTH BEHAVIOR

Nurses must be able to use assessment measures to document areas for improvement to enhance the health status of individuals, families, and communities. Assessment data about health status and behaviors provide the basis for clinical judgments and help plan appropriate individual, family, and community interventions. Nurses must use their knowledge and influence to ensure that a portfolio of conceptually congruent assessment instruments is available and used in the work setting. The nurse must know how to administer assessment measures and articulate the value of conducting systematic assessments to the client. The busy work environment may discourage the use of detailed assessments because they require time to administer and follow up. One strategy to manage the time issue is to seek innovative ways to communicate with clients through videotapes loaned to clients and brochures that explain assessment procedures. Information technology has made computerized assessment possible. Thus, clients may be able to complete self-assessments at home as time allows, with transmission of the information by computer prior to health care visits.

Practicing nurses must keep up-to-date about new assessment measures and strategies that can be quickly implemented and yield accurate data. Nurses influence the quality of the health promotion plan of the individual, family, and community through a commitment to thorough assessment of health and health behaviors (Rice & Wicks, 2007).

Summary

Health assessment is conducted at the individual, family, or community levels. Assessment is time intensive, so measures must be carefully selected according to client characteristics and presenting health issues. The nurse and client must mutually decide which assessments are needed to establish a relevant plan for health promotion.

Learning Activities

1. Go to My Family Health Portrait at www.familyhistory.hhs.gov and record a traditional family health portrait. Examine the differences between My Family Health Portrait and the commercial application at Genepro.
2. Develop an assessment plan based on age-specific instruments for a child, young adult, and older adult.
3. Using Table 4–4, determine your percentage of body fat and outline a personal goal based on the results.
4. Investigate one approach to assessing a family and discuss its strengths and weaknesses for use in the clinical setting.
5. Identify the relationship between family and community assessments and how they affect the health outcomes of the family and community.
6. Discuss factors to consider in a community assessment including those influencing the extent of assessment to be conducted.

Selected Web Sites

Personal Health Record
http://www.cms.hhs.gov/apps/media/press/release.asp?Counter=3232
The PHR belongs to the user and is distinct from physician records.

Elective Preventive Services Selector (ePSS)
www.epss.ahrq.gov

Preventive Services Guidelines
http://www.ahrq.gov/clinic/pocketgd.htm and
http:/brightfutures.aap.org/clinical_practice.html

My Pyramid Tracker
www.mypyramid.gov

North American Nursing Diagnosis International (NANDA-I)
http://www.nanda.org/
The NANDA-I provides nursing diagnosis structured around the nine human response patterns: exchanging, communicating, relating, valuing, choosing, moving, perceiving, knowing, and feeling.

Research Instruments Developed by Stanford Patient Education Research Center
http://patienteducation.stanford.edu/research/

Mind Garden
www.mindgarden.com/products/mlq.htm
Research instruments and administration manuals are available from Mind Garden, Palo Alto, California.

Instruments for Clinical Health-Care Research
http://patienteducation.stanford.edu/research/
A definitive source of measurement tools for assessing social support as well as additional lifestyle instruments is found in *Instruments for Clinical Healthcare Research.*

My Family Health Portrait
www.familyhistory.hhs.gov

Genepro
www.genopro.com

References

Agency for Healthcare Research and Quality (AHRQ). (2007). *The guide to clinical preventive services, 2007: Recommendations of the U.S. Preventive Services Task Force.* Retrieved from http://www.ahrq.gov/clinic/pocketgd07/pocketgd07.pdf

Allender, J. A., & Spradley, B. W. (2004). *Community health nursing: Promoting and protecting the public's health* Philadelphia: Lippincott Williams & Wilkins.

AMA Council on Scientific Affairs. (2002). *Report 7 of the Council on Scientific Affairs (A-02) Full text.* Baltimore, MD: American Medical Association. Retrieved from http://www.ama-assn.org/ama/pub/category/13659.html

American Academy of Pediatrics. (2008). *Bright futures: Guidelines for health supervision of infants, children and adolescents* (3rd ed.). In J. F. Hagan, J. S. Shaw & P. Duncan (Eds.). Elk Grove Village, IL: American Academy of Pediatrics.

American College of Sports Medicine (ACSM). (2005). *ACSM's guidelines for exercise testing and prescription* (7th ed.). Baltimore, MD: Williams & Wilkins: A Waverly Company.

_____ (2009). *ACSM's resource manual for guidelines for exercise testing and prescription* (6th ed.). Baltimore, MD: Williams & Wilkins: A Waverly Company.

Anciaux, N., Berthelot, M., Braconnier, L., Bouganim, L., De la Blache, M., Gardarin, G., et al. (2008). A tamper-resistant and portable healthcare folder. *International Journal of Telemedicine and Application.* doi 10.1155/2008/763534.

Anderson, E. T., & McFarlane, J. M. (2006). *Community as partner: Theory and practice in nursing* (5th ed.). Philadelphia: Lippincott Williams & Wilkins.

Armstrong, N. L., Davis, A. M., & Dixon, W. A. (2005). An examination of the relationship among daily hassles, uplifts and depressive symptoms in a college population. *Psi Chi Journal of Undergraduate Research, 10*(4). Retrieved from http://www.psichi.org/Pubs/Articles/Article_530.aspx

Buchholz, A. C., Bartok, C., & Schoeller, D. A. (2004). The validity of bioelectrical impedance models in clinical populations. *Nutrition in Clinical Practice, 19*(5), 433–446.

Cairney, J., & Krause, N. (2008). Negative life events and age-related decline in mastery: Are older adults more vulnerable to the control-eroding effect of stress? *Journal of Gerontology: B Psychological Sciences and Social Sciences, 63*(3), S162–S170.

Calfas, K. J., Zabinski, M. F., & Rupp, J. (2000). Practical nutrition assessment in primary care settings: A review. *American Journal of Preventive Medicine, 18*(4), 289–299.

Carpenito-Moyet, L. J. (2005) *Nursing diagnosis: Application to clinical practice* (11th ed.). Philadelphia: Lippincott Williams & Wilkins.

Cavendish, R., Konecny, L., Mitzeliotis, C., Russo, D., Kraynyak Luise, B., et al. (2003). Spiritual care activities of nurses using Nursing Interventions Classification (NIC) labels. *International Journal of Nursing Terminologies and Classifications, 14*(4), 113–124.

Chung, L. Y., Wong, F. K., & Chan, M. F. (2007). Relationship of nurses' spirituality to their understanding and practice of spiritual care. *Journal of Advanced Nursing, 58*(2), 158–170.

Clark, M. J. (2003). *Community health nursing: Caring for populations.* Upper Saddle River, NJ: Prentice Hall.

Cohen, S., Kessler, R. C., & Gordon, L. U. (1997). *Measuring stress.* New York: Oxford Press.

Derogatis, L. R., & Fleming, M. P. (1997). *Evaluating stress. The Derogatis stress profile (DSP): A theory driven approach to stress measurement.* Lanham, MD: Scarecrow Press.

Folkman, S., & Lazarus, R. S. (1988). Coping as a mediator of emotion. *Journal of Personality and Social Psychology, 54*(3), 466–475.

Frank-Stromborg, M., & Olsen, S., (2004). *Instruments for clinical health-care research* (3rd ed.). Sudbury, MA: Jones & Bartlett Publishers.

Freedman, D. S., Khan, L. K., Serdula, M. K., Dietz, W. H., Srinivasan, S. R., & Berenson, G. S. (2005). The relation of childhood BMI to adult adiposity: The Bogalusa heart study. *Pediatrics, 115*(1), 22–27.

Freedson, P. S., Cureton, K. J., & Heath, G. W. (2000). Status of field-based fitness testing in children and youth. *Preventive Medicine, 31*, S77–S85.

Friedman, M. M. (2003). *Family nursing: Research theory and practice* (5th ed.). New York: Appleton Century-Crofts.

Friedman, M. M., Bowden, V. R., & Jones, E. (2003) *Family nursing: Research, theory and practice* (5th ed.). Upper Saddle River, NJ: Prentice Hall.

Girandola, R. N., & Contarsy, S. (2004). The validity of bioelectrical impedance to predict body composition. Retrieved from http://www.bioanalogics.com/validity.htm

Gordon, M. (2006). *Manual of nursing diagnosis: Including all diagnostic categories approved by the North American Nursing Diagnosis Association* (11th ed.). Sudbury, MA: Jones and Bartlett Publishers, Inc.

Hatch, R. L., Burg, M. A., Naberhaus, D. S., & Hellmich, L. K. (1998, June). The spiritual involvement and beliefs scale. Development and testing of a new instrument. *The Journal of Family Practice, 46*(6), 476–486.

Hendricks, C., Murdaugh, C., & Pender, N. (2006). The adolescent lifestyle profile: Development and psychometric characteristics. *Journal of National Black Nurses Association, 17*(2), 1–5.

Kaakinen, J. R., Hanson, S. M., & Birenbaum, L. K. (2004). Family development and family nursing assessment. In M. Stanhope & J. Lancaster (Eds.), *Community and public health nursing* (6th ed., pp. 562–593). St. Louis, MO: Mosby.

Keyzer, D. M. (2008). Patient classification systems and case mix funding: Implications for rural nursing practice. *Australian Journal of Rural Health, 2*(3), 5–9.

Leonardo, M. E., Resick, L. K., Bingman, C. A., & Strotmeyer, S. (2004). The alternatives for wellness centers: Drown in data or develop a reasonable electronic documentation system. *Home Health Care Management and Practice, 16*(3), 177–184.

Litwinczuk, K. M., & Groh, C. J. (2007). The relationship between spirituality, purpose in life, and well-being in HIV-positive persons. *Journal of the Association of Nurses in AIDS Care, 18*(3), 13–22.

Lunney, M. (2006). Stress overload: A new diagnosis. *International Journal of Nursing Terminologies and Classifications, 17*(4), 165–175.

Madden, M. (2006) *Internet penetration and impact, 2006.* Pew Internet & American Life Project. Retrieved February 10, 2009, from http://www.pewinternet.org/pdfs/PIP_Internet_Impact.pdf

Mahat, G., & Scoloveno, M. (2003). Comparison of fears and coping strategies reported by Nepalese school-age children and their parents. *Journal of Pediatric Nursing, 18*(5), 305–313.

Martin, K. S. (2005) *The Omaha system: A key to practice, documentation and information management* (2nd ed.). St Louis, MO: Elsevier.

McDaniel, A. M., Schutte, D. L., & Keller, L. O. (2008). Consumer health informatics: From genomics to population health. *Nursing Outlook, 56*(5), 216–223.

McVay-Smith, C. (2001). Nutrition assessment. *Nutrition, 17*(9), 785–786.

Moorhead, S., Johnson, M., & Maas, M. (2004). *Nursing outcomes classification* (NOC) (3rd ed.). St. Louis, MO: Mosby.

Nooyens, A. C. J., Koppes, L. L. J., Visscher, T. L. S., Twisk, J. W. R., Kemper, H. C. G., Schuit, A. J., et al. (2007). Adolescent skin fold thickness is a better predictor of high body fatness in adults than is body mass index: the Amsterdam Growth and Health Longitudinal Study. *American Journal of Clinical Nutrition, 85*(6), 1533–1539.

North American Nursing Diagnosis International (NANDA-I). (2009). *Nursing diagnoses: Definitions and classification, 2009* (11th ed.). Philadelphia: Wiley-Blackwell. Retrieved from http://www.nando.org/

Peace, J., & Lutz, K. (2009) Nursing conceptualizations of research and practice. *Nursing Outlook, 57*(5), 42–49.

Popkess-Vawter, S. (2008). Wellness nursing diagnoses: To be or not to be? *Terminologies and Classifications, 2*(1), 19–25.

Reed, P. G. (1992). An emerging paradigm for the investigation of spirituality in nursing. *Research in Nursing and Health, 15*, 349–357.

Rice, M. C., & Wicks, M. N. (2007). The importance of nursing advocacy for the health promotion of female welfare recipients. *Nursing Outlook, 55*(5), 220–223.

Rice, V., Weglicki, L., Templin, T., Hammad, A., Jamil, H., & Kulwicki, A. (2006). Predictors of Arab American adolescent tobacco use. *Merrill-Palmer Quarterly, 52*(2), 327–342.

Robert Wood Johnson Foundation. (2008). *The power of personal health records.* Retrieved from http://www.rwjf.org/pr/product.jsp?id=32412

Sarason, B. R., Shearin, E. R., Pierce, X. X., & Sarason, I. G., (1987). A brief measure of social support: Practical and theoretical implications. *Journal of Social and Personal Relations, 4*, 497–510.

Sawin, K. J., Harrington, M. P., & Wood, P. (1995). *Measures of family functioning for research and practice.* New York: Springer.

Schnipper, J. L., Gandhi, T. K., Wald, J. S., Grant, R. W., Poon, E. G., Volk, L. A., et al. (2008). Design and implementation of a Web-based patient portal linked to an electronic health record designed to improve medication safety: The Patient Gateway medications module. *Informatics in Primary Care, 16*(2), 147–155.

Sechrist, K. R., Walker, S. N., & Pender, N. J. (1987). Development and psychometric evaluation of the Exercise Benefits/Barrier Scale. *Research in Nursing Health, 10*, 357–365.

Sherbourne, C. D., & Stewart, A. L. (1991). The MOS Social Support Survey. *Social Science & Medicine, 32*(6), 704–714.

Shields, A. E., Shin, P., Leu, M. G., Levy, D. E., Betancourt, R. M., Hawkins, D., et al. (2007). Adoption of health information technology in community health centers: Results of a national survey. *Health Affairs, 26*(5), 1373–1383.

Shuster, G. F., & Goepinger, J. (2008). Community as client: Assessment and analysis. In M. Stanhope & J. Lancaster (Eds.), Public health nursing, 7th edition (pp. 389–422). St. Louis, MO: Mosby.

Spielberger, C. D., Gorsuch, R. L., Lushene, R., & Vagg, P. R. (1983). *Manual for state-trait anxiety inventory.* Palo Alto, CA: Consulting Psychologists Press Inc.

Taylor, E. J. (2007). Client perspectives about nurse requisites for spiritual caregiving. *Applied Nursing Research, 20*(1), 44–46.

Tyler, D., & Horner, S. D. (2008). Family-centered collaborative negotiation: A model for facilitating behavior change in primary care.

Journal of the American Academy of Nurse Practitioners, 20(4), 194–203.

U.S. Department of Agriculture Human Nutrition Information Service. (2006). *My Pyramid Tracker*. Retrieved from http://www .mypyramid.gov

U.S. Department of Health and Human Services. (2001). *National standards for culturally and linguistically appropriate services in health care, final report*. Washington, D.C.: DHHS.

U.S. Preventive Services Task Force. (2007). *Guide to clinical preventive services: Report of the U.S.* *Preventive Services Task Force.* Electronic Preventive Services Selector (ePSS). Retrieved from http://www.ahrq.gov/clinic/USpstfix .htm

Westra, B. L., Delaney, C. W., Konicek, D., & Keenan, G. (2008). Nursing standards to support the electronic health record. *Nursing Outlook, 56*(5), 258–266.

Wright, L. M., & Leahey, M. (2000). *Nurses and families: A guide to family assessment and intervention*. Philadelphia: FA Davis Co.

CHAPTER 5

Developing a Health Promotion-Prevention Plan

OBJECTIVES

1. Identify the nine steps in the health planning process.
2. Discuss barriers to overcome in developing an individual and family health plan.
3. Describe strategies to increase the client's "ownership" of a health behavior change plan.
4. Discuss strategies to ensure that the health plan is an interdisciplinary process.
5. Discuss barriers that hinder effective individual and family behavior change.
6. Describe how community-level plans and interventions influence individual and family health plans.

Outline

- Guidelines for Preventive Services and Screenings
- The Health-Planning Process
  - A. Review and Summarize Data from Assessment
  - B. Emphasize Strengths and Competencies of the Client
  - C. Identify Health Goals and Related Behavior-Change Options
  - D. Identify Behavioral or Health Outcomes
  - E. Develop a Behavior-Change Plan
  - F. Reinforce Benefits of Change
  - G. Address Environmental and Interpersonal Facilitators and Barriers to Change
  - H. Determine a Time Frame for Implementation
  - I. Formalize Commitment to Behavior-Change Plan
- The Revised Health Promotion-Prevention Plan
- Community-Level Health Promotion-Prevention Plan
- Opportunities for Research in Behavior Change

- Considerations for Practice in Health Planning
- Summary
- Learning Activities
- Selected Web Sites
- References

Clients must be active participants in planning and interpreting assessment data. Client collaboration with the nurse promotes positive perceptions of worth. It also affirms the ability of individuals, families, or communities to function on their own behalf to create conditions supportive of healthy lifestyles. The role of the nurse is to *assist* clients with health planning rather than to *control* the process. During assessment, the nurse and client develop a mutual understanding of the client's (1) health status, (2) current health-behavior patterns, (3) attitudes and beliefs that affect health and health-related behaviors, (4) expectations of important referent groups, (5) potentially available behavioral options, (6) social-ethnic-cultural background, (7) potential or actual barriers to health behavior change, and (8) existing support systems for health-promoting behaviors. Developing a systematic plan for behavior change provides an opportunity for the client to express purposeful ways to increase wellness and enhance life satisfaction.

Health planning is a dynamic process. Flexibility is critical to meet the changing needs of clients. The plan systematically lends direction but does not dictate goals that must be attained or behaviors that must be learned. The health promotion-prevention plan should be reasonable in terms of both demands on the client and the time frame allocated to accomplish desired health or health-related goals. Knowledge, skills, and strengths of the client should be taken into consideration in the planning process. Capitalizing on current positive health practices creates a sense of competence or efficacy essential to successful behavior change. Together, the nurse and the client should assess the behaviors the client wishes to modify. The nurse can then discuss strategies for change that are likely to be most effective. The plan should be revised as needed to make behavior change a positive growth experience. The ultimate goal of health planning and implementation is to make health promotion and prevention a way of life for individuals, families, and communities.

Innovative developments in information technology increasingly allow assessment and intervention protocols to be personalized to the unique characteristics and needs of individual clients. In addition, electronic health records will enable clients to share their health promotion plan with multiple care providers. Nurses must be cognizant of the increasingly significant role of computer technology for health assessments, as well as Web-based technology for health interventions, as they work with clients to develop and implement health promotion plans (Laustria, Cortese, Noar, & Glueckauf, 2009).

GUIDELINES FOR PREVENTIVE SERVICES AND SCREENINGS

The increased emphasis on disease prevention has resulted in helpful guidelines for the delivery of preventive services to individuals and families throughout the life span. These guidelines focus on clinical care to prevent specific conditions, such as HIV disease, or behavioral morbidity, such as substance abuse. The 2008 *Guide to Clinical Preventive Services* recommends screenings as an important component of prevention. The value and benefits of age-specific periodic screenings based on gender and individual risk factors are available in the guidelines. Counseling clients about their personal health habits is identified as one of the most important components of the health visit. Nurses in primary care settings should become familiar with the available guidelines to ensure that their clients benefit from "state-of-the-science" preventive services, including *The guide to Clinical Preventive services* (U.S. Preventive Services Task Force [USPSTF], 2008); *AMA Guidelines for Adolescent Preventive Services [GAPS]: Recommendations and rationale* (American Medical Association [AMA], 1997); *Women: Stay healthy at any age* (Agency for Healthcare Research and Quality [AHRQ], 2007a), and *Men: Stay healthy at any age* (AHRQ, 2007b). All of these guidelines are accessible on the Web. Preventive services that have the greatest health impact and best cost value are also available (Maciosek et al., 2006). These priorities undergo a systematic review on a regular basis (see http://www.prevent.org/ncpp).

THE HEALTH-PLANNING PROCESS

The process for developing a health promotion-prevention plan is outlined here, with each step in the process discussed separately. These nine steps actively involve both the client and the nurse in the health-planning process:

1. Review and summarize data from assessment.
2. Emphasize strengths and competencies of the client.
3. Identify health goals and related behavioral change options.
4. Identify behavioral or health outcomes that will indicate that the plan has been successful from the client's perspective.
5. Develop a behavior-change plan based on the client's preferences and on "state-of-the-science" knowledge about effective interventions.
6. Reinforce benefits of change and identify incentives for change from the client's perspective.
7. Address environmental and interpersonal facilitators and barriers to behavior change.
8. Determine a time frame for implementation.
9. Formalize a commitment to behavior-change goals and provide support needed to accomplish them.

Review and Summarize Data from Assessment

During assessment, the nurse obtains a wealth of data from the client. The information must be summarized in a format that is useful. The outcome of assessment activities should include information available in the following domains as a basis for planning and action:

1. Physical health status
2. Functional health patterns
3. Physical fitness
4. Nutritional status
5. Life stressors
6. Spirituality
7. Social support
8. Personal health behaviors

9. Family health practices
10. Environmental and community supports or constraints for health behaviors.

During one or more clinic appointments or home visits, the nurse and client review the assessment summary. Both should retain either a hard copy or an electronic copy for continuing reference during the health-planning process.

Emphasize Strengths and Competencies of the Client

Each individual or family has in place a system of health care practices compatible with the client's cultural orientation. Thus, the nurse and client should achieve consensus on areas in which the client is already taking informed and responsible health action as well as on areas for further development of self-care competencies. Clients bring unique strengths to the health-planning task. These assets should be identified, acknowledged, and reinforced. Individuals perform health behaviors according to their cultural beliefs, preferences, and current levels of knowledge and skill. Therefore, it is important to integrate existing cultural practices into the overall health plan. The client's sense of cultural or ethnic pride should be reinforced during the health-planning process.

Through teaching, guidance, and support, the nurse promotes existing competencies to enhance health practices. Self-care requirements and resources will vary according to the client's age, gender, developmental stage, and health status. The self-care needs of families will also vary by family composition, developmental tasks being confronted, and role demands. Although clients differ in their self-care and self-management competencies, it is important to emphasize each client's importance as the "primary self-care agent." However, promoting individual responsibility for health does not negate the importance of changing the larger social infrastructure to make health-promoting options more available to groups and communities. Personal change and social change are both essential for effective health promotion and prevention.

A sample health promotion-prevention plan for an individual is presented in Figure 5–1 and one for a family in Figure 5–2. In both plans, sections are provided in which client strengths can be identified.

Identify Health Goals and Related Behavior-Change Options

The next step in the planning process is to identify and prioritize personal or family health goals and review related behavior-change options. Systematically reviewing the range of changes that are possible to achieve health goals can assist clients in deciding the behavioral changes on which they will initially focus. Providing relevant options enables the client to prioritize behavior-change strategies. Clients should not be made to feel guilty about their current health practices. During health counseling sessions, the nurse should create enthusiasm and excitement about growth in positive directions and the benefits of new health-related experiences.

Many clients will initially place high priority on prevention behaviors for which the threat of illness is tangible and easily understood. Decreasing risk for specific chronic health problems fits the medical orientation to which most Americans have been socialized. A high level of client interest in reducing risk of disease indicates that prevention is likely the most meaningful area for emphasis in early health planning. Mastery of specific prevention measures will often motivate clients to consider making additional lifestyle changes directed toward health promotion to experience a

Designed for: ___James Moore_____

Home Address: ___714 George Street_____

Home Telephone Number: ___222–3333_____

Occupation (if employed): ___building services supervisor_____

Work Telephone Number: ___445-6666_____

Cultural Identification: ___African-American_____

Birth Date: ___3/14/59___ Date of Initial Plan: ___1/15/2005___

Client strengths:	Satisfactory peer relationships, spiritual strength, adequate sleep pattern
Major risk factors:	Elevated cholesterol, mild obesity, sedentary lifestyle, moderate life change, multiple daily hassles, few reported uplifts
Nursing diagnoses: (derived from assessment of functional health patterns)	Diversional activity deficit; altered nutrition: more than body requirements; caregiver role strain (elderly mother)
Medical diagnoses: (if any)	Mild hypertension
Age-specific screening recommendations: (derived from *Guide to Clinical Prev. Services*)	Blood pressure, cholesterol, fecal occult blood, malignant skin lesions, depression
Desired behavioral and health outcomes:	Become a regular exerciser (3x/week), lower my blood pressure, weigh 165 lb

FIGURE 5–1   Example of an Individual Health Promotion-Prevention Plan

higher level of health and well-being (Allegante, Peterson, Boutin-Foster, Ogedegbe, & Charlson, 2008).

Clients often give important emotional cues about the behaviors they wish to change. Examples of such cues include the following:

"I hate myself when I gorge on fattening foods!"
"I get mad at myself for being so uptight!"
"The only time our family is together is in front of the television."
"We need to stop eating at so many fast food places."
"We are very critical of each other."
"We don't participate in physical activities together."

Personal Health Goals (1 = highest priority)	Selected Behaviors to Accomplish Goals	Stage of Change	Strategies/ Interventions for Change
1. Achieve desired body weight	Begin a progressive walking program	Planning	Counter-conditioning Reinforcement management Patient contracting
	Decrease caloric intake while maintaining good nutrition	Action (eating 2 fruits and 2 vegetables daily; using low-fat dairy products for last 2 months)	Stimulus control Cognitive restructuring
2. Decrease risk for hypertension-related disorders	Change from high- to low-sodium snacks	Contemplation	Consciousness raising Learning facilitation
3. Learn to manage stress effectively	Attend relaxation classes and use home relaxation tapes	Contemplation	Consciousness raising Self-reevaluation Simple relaxation therapy
4. Increase leisure-time activities	Join a local bowling league	Contemplation	Support system enhancement

FIGURE 5–1   Continued

The more open an individual or family is in discussing health concerns with the nurse, the greater the probability of developing a meaningful health promotion-prevention plan. Areas that clients are most reluctant to discuss—such as marital relationships, human sexuality, spirituality, and family cohesiveness—are often the most crucial ones for behavior change. A "safe" climate should be created in which personal health issues can be discussed with assurance of confidentiality.

Identify Behavioral or Health Outcomes

Together, the nurse and client decide the desired health outcomes of the health promotion-prevention plan. Clear identification of outcomes both energizes and guides the client in

Designed for (family name): ___The Marshalls___

Home Address: _1718 Green Street_

Home Telephone Number: ___777-4444___

Occupations of Employed
Members of Household: _Mother—Dental assistant_

Work Telephone Number: ___883-7777___

Family Form: __One-parent family__

Cultural Identification: __Asian American__

Family Members: Position in Family   Birth Date   Occupation/
                                                          Student/Retired

                 Joan (Mother)   9/65   Dental assistant
                 Dana (Daughter)   4/87   Student
                 Tiffany (Daughter)   7/91   Student
                 Eric (Son)   1/94   Student

Date of Initial Plan: __1-15-2005__

Family strengths:	Open communication patterns, intrafamily cooperation, healthy snacks consumed at home
Major risk factors:	Mother recently divorced, oldest daughter has driver's license, high life change for family, minimal family physical activity
Nursing diagnoses:	Family coping: potential for growth
Medical diagnoses for family members:	None
Desired behavioral and health outcomes:	Active family outings, avoidance of early sexual activity and binge drinking among adolescent family members, injury prevention for children, adjustment to new family form

FIGURE 5–2 Example of a Family Health Promotion-Prevention Plan

changing or establishing new health behaviors. The client's perceptions about desired outcomes should guide the criteria used to evaluate the success of the plan and its implementation. "Have I reached my goal or made significant progress toward it?" is a critical question that the client must ask periodically to evaluate the relevance of the health promotion-prevention plan.

Research that documents the link between particular interventions and desired outcomes should be the basis for development of the plan. For example, factors or

Family Health Goals (1 = highest priority)	Selected Behaviors to Accomplish Goals	Stage of Change	Strategies/ Interventions for Change
1. Healthy adjustment to single-parent family status	Realign family responsibilities	Action (divorced 3 mo)	Social liberation Family process maintenance Caregiver support
	Increase spiritual resources (increase church attendance)	Contemplation	Spiritual support Helping relationships
	Discuss life purpose and goals among family members	Planning	Self-reevaluation Self-esteem enhancement Anticipatory guidance
2. Develop more active family lifestyles	Plan active family outings (biking, recreation center)	Planning	Exercise promotion Environmental reevaluation Modeling
3. Foster healthy sexuality among preadolescent and adolescents	Provide age-appropriate information	Action	Anticipatory guidance Parent education: adolescent stage
	Enhance self-esteem through praise, expression of affection, and assistance with skill development	Maintenance	Self-esteem enhancement Helping relationships

FIGURE 5–2 Continued

| 4. Encourage adolescents to avoid alcohol use | Hold family meetings to discuss binge drinking, drinking and driving, use of nonalcoholic alternatives | Contemplation | Parent education: adolescent stage Self-responsibility facilitation Substance use prevention |

FIGURE 5–2   Continued

strategies shown to increase the likelihood of maintaining a healthy diet should be integrated into the plan for persons wishing to address nutritional issues. Clients must be assisted in setting realistic outcomes. For example, a behavioral goal of eating only at meal times may be easier to attain than a goal of losing a certain number of pounds. Weight will most likely be reduced if the plan is followed, but realistic, tangible behaviors that are under the control of the client are easier to reinforce and manage. Success with long-term outcomes is achieved through a progressive set of short-term successes that move the client toward the desired outcome.

Develop a Behavior-Change Plan

A positive program of change is based on the client taking "ownership" of behavior changes. The client should be assisted in examining significant value–behavior inconsistencies that exist. Alternative actions that are both healthful and enjoyable should substitute for behaviors that are inconsistent with personal values. Many individuals and families prefer or value the American lifestyle, which is frequently considered detrimental to health. Clarifying the value and meaning of health is important to do prior to the development of an individual or family behavior-change plan (Allicock, Sandelowski, DeVellis, & Campbell, 2008).

Clients should select, from the available options, behaviors that are appealing and that they are willing to implement. The client's priorities for behavior change will reflect personal values, activity preferences, cognitive and psychomotor skills, affective responses to the various behavioral options, expectations for success, and ease with which the selected behaviors can be integrated into one's daily lifestyle.

Appropriate strategies and interventions to facilitate individual behavior can be found in the nursing and behavioral science literature (Aveyard, Massey, Parsons, Manaseki, & Griffen, 2009; Cameron, 2009; Hall & Rossi, 2008; Kennett, Worth, & Forbes, 2009; Williamson et al., 2008). As the expert health care provider, the nurse can assist the client in gaining the behavior-change skills needed to adopt and maintain positive health behaviors.

Reinforce Benefits of Change

Although clients are aware of the benefits of the desired change, the positive benefits should be frequently reinforced. A list of benefits should be kept in a highly visible place so they can be reviewed frequently, such as on the refrigerator, the bathroom mirror, the dashboard of the car, or the computer. Keeping health benefits in front of the client is a reminder that the behaviors in the health promotion-prevention plan are personally worthwhile and directed toward important life goals.

The benefits of change include both health-related and non-health-related outcomes. Sensitivity to non-health-related benefits of change such as increased popularity or more time with friends is important, as these may be central to the client's motivation to engage in health promotion-prevention planning and implementation.

Address Environmental and Interpersonal Facilitators and Barriers to Change

The features of the physical environment and interpersonal relationships supportive of positive change can be used to bolster efforts to modify lifestyle. For example, social networks help counter barriers to change. Encouragement from family and friends helps the client to persist when change efforts are difficult, or other demands or preferences compete for attention. All individuals and families experience barriers to changing behavior. Although some obstacles cannot be anticipated, others can be planned for and their potential negative impact considerably weakened. If the client is aware of possible barriers and has formulated plans for managing them, successful behavior change is more likely to occur.

Barriers to effective health behavior may arise from clients' internal conflicts, significant others, or the environment. Internal barriers to change include lack of motivation, fatigue, boredom, giving up, lack of appropriate skills, and disbelief that behavior can be successfully changed. Family members can impose considerable barriers if they encourage continuation of health-damaging behaviors' or if they actively discourage attempts at behavior change. Environmental barriers that can inhibit positive change include unsafe neighborhoods, such as heavy traffic or high crime rate; lack of facilities to support positive behaviors, such as access to parks or grocery stores; and inclement weather. The nurse should assist both the client and the community to work to address environmental barriers, as they are major challenges confronting behavior change.

Determine a Time Frame for Implementation

Developing healthy behaviors takes time as new behaviors must be learned, integrated into one's lifestyle, and stabilized. Attempting to change or initiate multiple new behaviors simultaneously may result in confusion, discouragement, and even abandonment of the health promotion-prevention plan. Whether the client is attempting to reduce risk for chronic diseases or to enhance health, gradual change is desirable. Just as health education for self-care must proceed at the pace of the learner, changes in behavior must be sequenced in reasonable steps appropriate for the client.

Developing a time plan for implementation allows appropriate knowledge and skills to be mastered before a new behavior is implemented. For example, it is difficult to warm up before brisk walking or jogging if the client is not aware of appropriate warm-up exercises. The time frame for developing a particular behavior may be several weeks or several months. Accomplishing short-term goals should be rewarded, as this provides encouragement to continue pursuit of long-term goals and desired outcomes. A meaningful plan requires that deadlines be set for accomplishing specific goals. Adherence to deadlines should be encouraged, with changes made only when the time frame must be shortened or lengthened to make it more conducive to permanent behavior change.

Formalize Commitment to Behavior-Change Plan

The client may be more motivated to follow through with selected actions if the personal commitment is formalized. A commitment to change can be formalized using one of the following options: (1) nurse–client contract agreements, as seen in Figures 5–3 and 5–4; (2) self-contracts, such as those shown in Figures 5–5 and 5–6; (3) public announcements to family members and friends of intentions to engage in new behaviors; (4) integration of new health behaviors into a daily or weekly calendar; and (5) purchase of necessary supplies (e.g., low-fat foods, exercise audiotapes) and equipment (e.g., exercise bike, walking shoes).

Behavioral contracts contain specific information about (1) the change to be made, (2) how the change will be accomplished, (3) the individual or family members who are to engage in the change, (4) the time frame for behavior change, and (5) the consequences of meeting or not meeting the terms of the agreement. A *nurse–client contract* provides direction through the identification of mutual objectives and the responsibilities of each party. Contracts enable clients to participate actively by choosing goals that can be realistically accomplished. Generally, the client is responsible for carrying out certain behaviors, whereas the nurse is responsible for providing information, training, counseling, and/or specific reinforcement rewards. The nurse bears the additional responsibility of providing helpful input and continuing feedback about the adequacy of performance of activities identified in the contract. It is critical for the nurse to be consistent and conscientious in managing the reinforcement-reward contingencies of the contract. Failure to fulfill this commitment will alter the trust and confidence placed in the nurse.

In a nurse–client contract with a family, the agreement may be made for family members to walk, jog, or bicycle together two to three times each week or to modify their nutritional practices, such as increasing vegetables at family meals. Family members serve as important sources of encouragement, reinforcement, and reward for one another because of their continuing contact and emotional bonding.

The effectiveness of the contract must be evaluated: Were the goals accomplished fully, partially, or not at all? If failure occurred, what were the reasons? How could the contract be rewritten to increase the probability of success? Should the contract be renegotiated? Should the contract be terminated? Careful analysis of the contracting process and evaluation of subsequent outcomes will enable the nurse and client to design contracts that successfully move clients toward desired health goals.

With a *self-contract*, the client is responsible for both the behavioral commitment and reinforcement of identified behaviors. Self-contracting is an effective approach to enhance one's control over behavior, thus creating a sense of independence, competence, and autonomy. The client does not become overly dependent on the nurse for reinforcement. Instead, individuals may choose extrinsic sources for rewards such as tangible objects (e.g., magazine, cosmetics) or experiences (e.g., warm bath, telephone call to a

---

Nurse–Client Contract and Agreement

Statement of Health Goal: _Decreased feelings of stress and tension_

I   _Jim Johnson_   promise to   _use progressive relaxation_
       (client)

techniques upon arriving home from work each day
                        (Client Responsibility)

for a period of   _one week_   , whereupon,

Kathy Turner   will provide _(1) guest_
       (nurse)

coupon for 2 Spruill Coffees   _(2) Complimentary message_
                        (Nurse Responsibility)

on   _Saturday, March 7th_   to me.
                        (date)

If I do not fulfill the terms of this contract in total, I understand that the designated reward will be withheld.

Signed: _____
                        (client)

           _____
                        (date)

           _____
                        (nurse)

           _____
                        (date)

FIGURE 5–3   Sample Nurse–Client Contract for an Individual Client

friend), or intrinsic rewards (e.g., self-praise, feelings of pride). Rewards selected should be highly desirable to have reinforcement value. A reward–reinforcement plan is illustrated in Figure 5–7.

Success in fulfilling contracts enhances the client's self-esteem and problem-solving abilities. The client gains increased confidence in meeting future health needs. In reality, it is the client who must learn to manage a self-reward system to support new positive health practices.

Nurse–Client Contract and Agreement

Statement of Health Goal: _____*Improve eating habits*_____

We _____*The Nichols*_____ promise to __*eat two servings of*__
                    (family)

_____*vegetables and two servings of fruit daily*_____
                    (family responsibility)

for a period of _____*1 week*_____ whereupon,

_____*Lana Buxton*_____ will provide _____*guest passes*_____
                    (nurse)

*to Riverbanks Zoo*_____
                    (nurse responsibility)

on _____*Friday, April 10th*_____ to us.
                    (date)

If we do not fulfill the terms of this contract in total, We understand that the
designated reward will be withheld.

            Signed: _____
                                    (family representative)

                            _____
                                            (date)

                            _____
                                            (nurse)

                            _____
                                            (date)

FIGURE 5–4   Sample Nurse–Client Contract for a Family

Publicly announcing intentions to engage in a new behavior to family members
and close friends is another way to increase one's commitment to a particular course of
action. The positive expectations of family members or friends often enhance motivation to change behavior.

Integrating new behaviors into one's calendar is another important strategy to incorporate them into daily routines. For example, exercise time may be scheduled during

---

Self-Contract

Personal Health Goal: _____ *Change dietary habits* _____

I _____ *Doris Downs* _____ promise myself that I will _*follow*_

_____ *the sample menus for a 1,200 calorie diet for breakfast, lunch, and*

_____ *dinner* _____ for a period of _____ *4 days* _____,

whereupon I will _____ *buy myself a new pair of earrings* _____

on _____ *Wednesday, June 8th* _____ .

Signed: _____

Date: _____

FIGURE 5–5   Sample Individual Self-Contract

Self-Contract

Family Health Goal: _____ *Get more exercise* _____

We _____ *The Stones* _____ promise each other that we will _____ *go* _____

_____ *swimming at the "Y" once a week* _____ for a period of _____ *3 weeks* _____

whereupon we will _____ *buy the newest version of Trivial Pursuit* _____

on _____ *Friday, February 10th* _____ .

Signed: _____

_____

_____

Date: _____

FIGURE 5–6   Sample Family Self-Contract

Behavior: Learn to Use Progressive Relaxation as One Approach to Handling Stress

Component of Behavior	Reward or Reinforcement
Attend first class session at 9 A.M. Saturday at the County Health Department	Watch the football game in the afternoon on TV
Use relaxation audiotape at home for 20 minutes of practice	
Sunday	Call John and visit for a while
Monday	Spend an hour at the driving range
Tuesday	Buy a new paperback novel
Wednesday	Praise myself for having practiced relaxation each day thus far
Thursday	Invite Harry and Jim over to play pool
Friday	Take my family to a movie
Attend second class session at 9 A.M. Saturday at the County Health Department	Take an orange juice break afterward with Bret, a class member
Practice relaxation techniques for 20 minutes providing my own cues rather than using the tape	
Sunday	Go for a short drive and enjoy the scenery
Monday	Spend 30 minutes reading my new novel
Tuesday	Buy myself a new bottle of aftershave lotion
Wednesday	Praise myself for persistence and successful practice
Thursday	Allow myself to linger in a warm shower longer than usual
Friday	Go biking with the family
Keep my weekly record of relaxation practice	The nurse will provide a copy of *Relaxation Response* by Herbert Benson

FIGURE 5–7   Reward–Reinforcement Plan

lunch hour. The appointment for exercise is then kept, just as an appointment with one's friend or coworker. Lack of time is a frequent excuse for being unable to follow through with newly adopted behaviors. When time is actually scheduled to accomplish health behaviors, the probability of their occurrence is significantly enhanced.

Purchasing necessary supplies and equipment is another strategy to help make a commitment to behavior change. When a monetary investment is made, clients are more likely to follow through with the desired behavior. For example, people who have exercise equipment and exercise videos in their home are more likely to be active than persons who do not.

THE REVISED HEALTH PROMOTION-PREVENTION PLAN

A schedule for periodic review of the health promotion-prevention plan should be established. Revisions can be made during counseling sessions, with both the client and the nurse contributing to the process. Impetus for changes in the plan may result from mastery of target behaviors, changes in client's values and priorities, or awareness of new options available to the client. Outdated plans fail to provide motivation or direction for change and thus become uninteresting and meaningless to the client. Periodic revisions and updates provide a systematic approach to assist the client in moving toward more positive health behaviors and a higher level of health.

COMMUNITY-LEVEL HEALTH PROMOTION-PREVENTION PLAN

Community-level plans and interventions may be the most effective way to engage members in improving their health. Important health concerns such as youth and family violence, substance abuse, unintended pregnancy in adolescents, and unintentional injuries may require broad-based planning and intervention. Evidence has validated the influence of the social and physical environments of the community on the health of its people. Wealth, access to health services, social inequity, race, and ethnicity are only a few of the factors that must be taken into account when assessing a community to plan for behavior change (Barnett, Anderson, Blosnich, Halverson, & Novak, 2005; Giles-Corti, 2006). The nurse must be knowledgeable of community initiatives and encourage client participation. The nurse may also serve as a consultant to communities to implement programs and be an advocate for community-based health plans and interventions.

OPPORTUNITIES FOR RESEARCH IN BEHAVIOR CHANGE

Nurses are in a pivotal position to address research questions about planning for health promotion and prevention and create new knowledge about the behavior-change planning process. Questions to be addressed include the following:

1. How can face-to-face and computerized feedback from health assessment be combined to optimize one's level of motivation for health promotion planning?
2. What interventions are most effective to reinforce clients' positive cultural health practices during health counseling?
3. What are the most effective family strategies to promote change?

4. What is the relationship between behavior change and life stages?
5. What are the major barriers to implementing community intervention to improve the health of its members?
6. What types of community-based interventions are most effective in improving the health of special populations?

CONSIDERATIONS FOR PRACTICE IN HEALTH PLANNING

Developing a plan to counsel clients about their health behaviors is a major responsibility of nurses in practice. The nurse must possess the skills necessary to guide clients to participate in developing a realistic, positive plan. Nurses who have a working knowledge of current guidelines will ensure that accurate, up-to-date information is incorporated into the plan. An interdisciplinary approach may be more effective in interpreting the assessment data and recommending appropriate goals. Support is critical during the change process, so the nurse also must learn to identify family and other sources of support for the client, and to develop creative strategies to incorporate their support into the plan. The plan must be adapted to life-span issues and gender and cultural differences.

Knowledge of cultural issues that may play a role is important to the design of a culturally sensitive, age- and gender-appropriate plan. Whenever possible, technology should be incorporated in developing the plan. Interactive software that provides feedback on achieving outcomes increases motivation, as immediate results are available. Developing a health promotion-prevention plan is straightforward but complex. The nurse must continually update skills to assist clients in this important process.

Summary

The health promotion-prevention plan provides individuals and families with a systematic approach to improve health practices and lifestyle. All clients should be provided with a paper or electronic health portfolio that contains a summary of their health assessment, their health promotion-prevention plan, and other relevant health records. It is imperative that clients have all the information and planning documents needed to follow through successfully with their desired behavior changes. Focusing on outcomes desired by the client will energize and direct implementation of the plan. Adjusting the plan as needed to ensure client success is vital to effective health-promoting care. In recent years, community-level plans that address broad-based health concerns have been developed. Increasing evidence supports the efficacy and effectiveness of developing health promotion-prevention plans at the community level.

Learning Activities

1. Using the nine-step planning process, select a partner and develop an individual health plan for each other. Evaluate your experiences and outcomes.
2. Using the nine-step planning process, develop a health plan for a family with teenagers. Write a two-page summary of your experiences and outcomes.
3. Write a one-page summary to describe how community factors influence the individual and family planning processes you developed in learning activities 1 and 2.

Selected Web Sites

Agency for Health Research and Quality: Guide to Clinical Preventive Services
http://www.ahrq.gov/clinic/prevenix.htm

Biomedicine and Health in the News
http://library.uchc.edu/bhn/nyt.html

Centers for Disease Control and Prevention
http://www.cdc.gov

National Guideline Clearinghouse
http://www.guideline.gov

Occupational Safety and Health Administration
http://www.osha.gov

Office of Disease Prevention and Health Promotion
http://www.hhs.gov/diseases/index.shtml

Office of the Surgeon General, U.S. Public Health Service
http://www.surgeongeneral.gov

2008 Guide to Clinical Preventive Services
http://www.prevent.org/ncpp

References

Agency for Healthcare Research and Quality (ARHQ). (2007a). *Women: Stay healthy at any age*. AHRQ Pub. No. 07-1P005-A. Rockville, MD: AHRQ.

_____ (2007b). *Men: Stay healthy at any age*. AHRQ Pub. No. 07-1P006-A.Rockville, MD: AHRQ

Allegante, J. P., Peterson, J. C., Boutin-Foster, C., Ogedegbe, G., & Charlson, M. F. (2008). Multiple health-risk behavior in a chronic disease population: What behaviors do people choose to change? *Preventive Medicine, 46*, 247–251.

Allicock, M., Sandelowski, M., DeVellis, B., & Campbell, M. (2008). Variations in meaning of the personal core value: Health. *Patient Education and Counseling, 93*, 347–353.

AMA (1997). *AMA guidelines for adolescent preventive service (GAPS): Recommendations monograph*. Baltimore, MD: Williams & Wilkins.

Aveyard, P., Massey, L., Parsons, P., Manaseki, S., & Griffen, C. (2009). The effect of the transtheoretical model based interventions on smoking cessation. *Social Science & Medicine, 68*, 397–403.

Barnett, E., Anderson, T., Blosnich, J., Halverson, J., & Novak, J. (2005). Promoting cardiovascular health: From individual goals to social environmental change. *American Journal of Preventive Medicine, 29*(5S1), 107–112.

Cameron, K. A. (2009). A practitioner's guide to persuasion: An overview of 15 selected persuasion theories, models and frameworks. *Patient Education and Counseling, 74*, 309–317.

Giles-Corti, B. (2006). People or places: What should be the target? *Journal of Science and Medicine in Sports, 9*, 357–366.

Hall, H. L., & Rossi, J. S. (2008). Meta-analytic examination of the strong and weak principles across 48 health behaviors. *Preventive Medicine, 46*(3), 266–274.

Kennett, D. J., Worth, N. C., & Forbes, C. A. (2009). The contributions of Rosenbaum's model of self-control and the transtheoretical model to the understanding of exercise behavior. *Psychology of Sports and Exercise, 10*(6), 1–7.

Laustria, M. L., Cortese, J., Noar, S. M., & Glueckauf, R. L. (2009). Computer-tailored health interventions delivered over the Web: Review and analysis of key components. *Patient Education and Counseling, 74*, 156–173.

Maciosek, M. V., Coffield, A. B., Edwards, N. M., Goodman, M. J., Flollemesch, T. S., & Solberg, L. I. (2006). Priorities among effective clinical preventive services: Results of a systematic review and analysis. *American Journal of Preventive Medicine, 31*, 52–61.

U.S. Services Preventive Task Force (USPSTF). (2008). *The guide to clinical preventive services*. Rockville, MD: AHRQ.

Williamson, D. A., Champagne, C. M., Harsha, D., Han, H., Martin, C. K., Newton, R., et al. (2008). Louisiana (LA) health: Design and methods for a childhood obesity preventive program in rural schools. *Contemporary Clinical Trials, 29*, 783–795.

PART 3

Interventions for Health Promotion and Prevention

CHAPTER 6

Physical Activity and Health Promotion

OBJECTIVES

1. Describe the benefits and risks of physical activity.
2. Discuss strategies to develop a physically active lifestyle across the life span.
3. Describe the application of theories and models to promote physical activity.
4. Discuss the relationship of built environments with active lifestyles in communities.
5. Discuss the pros and cons of community interventions to promote physical activity.
6. Describe strategies for developing and implementing culturally appropriate physical activity interventions.

Outline

Regular physical activity is essential for healthy, energetic, and productive living. Modern life, with its automobiles, televisions, computers, video games, and low levels of physical activity in school and work environments, necessitates the commitment of significant leisure time to physical activity to gain health benefits. *Physical activity* is defined as any bodily movement produced by skeletal muscles that results in expenditure of energy and includes occupational, leisure-time, and routine daily activities. Lifestyle physical activities are those carried out in the course of everyday life that contribute to energy expenditure, such as climbing the stairs instead of taking the elevator. *Exercise* is a subcategory of physical activity performed during leisure time that is planned, structured, repetitive, and aimed at improving or maintaining physical fitness or health. *Physical fitness* is a measure of a person's ability to perform physical activities that require endurance, strength, or flexibility and is determined by a combination of cardiorespiratory endurance (aerobic power), flexibility, balance, and body composition (U.S. Department of Health and Human Services [USDHHS], 2008a). The term *physical activity* is used in this chapter to encompass a broad range of activities that, if performed regularly, will improve health.

Maintenance of regular physical activity is dependent on personal and social motivation within the day-to-day environment. Family, peers, and the community play a powerful role in encouraging active lifestyles. Many individuals rely on the school or work environments to create programs to help them achieve their physical activity goals. Others cycle through periods of activity and inactivity, never establishing regular physical activity patterns. Obesity is now one of the most serious and prevalent health problems in the United States. The alarming increase in the prevalence of overweight and obesity among both adults and adolescents is thought to be due to genetic influences as well as environmental influences, namely dietary and physical activity behaviors (Sallis, Story, & Lou, 2009c). Despite the evidence that physical inactivity is related to weight gain, a significant proportion of the U.S. population remains sedentary. Because of the central role of physical activity in health, this chapter focuses on strategies to increase physical activity for clients of all ages and racial, ethnic, and socioeconomic groups.

HEALTH BENEFITS OF PHYSICAL ACTIVITY

Regular physical activity contributes to physiologic stability and high-level functioning and assists individuals in actualizing their physical performance potential. Research has demonstrated the health benefits of participating in regular physical activity (USDHHS, 2008a). The USDHHS Physical Activity Guidelines Advisory Committee rated the evidence of health benefits as strong, moderate, or weak for children and adolescents, and adults and older adults. The rating decision was based on the type, number, and quality of published research, as well as consistency of findings across studies. The rated health benefits of physical activity are shown in Table 6–1.

The health benefits of physical activity are seen in all ages and all ethnic and racial groups. Scientific evidence documents the role of physical activity in reducing the risk

---

TABLE 6–1   Health Benefits Associated with Regular Physical Activity

Children and Adolescents

Strong evidence

- Improved cardiorespiratory and muscular fitness
- Improved bone health
- Improved cardiovascular and metabolic health biomarkers
- Favorable body composition

Moderate evidence

- Reduced symptoms of depression

Adults and Older Adults

Strong evidence

- Lower risk of early death
- Lower risk of coronary heart disease
- Lower risk of stroke
- Lower risk of high blood pressure
- Lower risk of adverse blood lipid profile
- Lower risk of type 2 diabetes
- Lower risk of metabolic syndrome
- Lower risk of colon cancer
- Lower risk of breast cancer
- Prevention of weight gain
- Weight loss, particularly when combined with reduced calorie intake
- Improved cardiorespiratory and muscular fitness
- Prevention of falls
- Reduced depression
- Better cognitive function (for older adults)

Moderate to strong evidence

- Better functional health (for older adults)
- Reduced abdominal obesity

Moderate evidence

- Lower risk of hip fracture
- Lower risk of lung cancer
- Lower risk of endometrial cancer
- Weight maintenance after weight loss
- Increased bone density
- Improved sleep quality

Source: U.S. Department of Health and Human Services. (2008). Physical activity guidelines for Americans. Retrieved July 17, 2009, from http://www.health.gov/paguidelines

of premature death, improving cardiorespiratory and metabolic health, decreasing the risks for overweight and obesity, and preserving bone, joint, and muscle health. In addition, regular physical activity improves or maintains physical function, lowers the risk for colon and breast cancer, and lessens the risk for depression and cognitive decline. Millions of Americans are at risk for a wide range of chronic diseases and mental health problems that might well be prevented by active lifestyles. Among children and adolescents, weight-bearing exercise is needed for normal skeletal development and attainment of peak bone mass. Regular physical activity increases strength and agility, prevents falls among older adults, and increases their independence in activities of daily living. It also improves the functional capacity of individuals with disabilities (USDHHS, 2008b).

POTENTIAL RISKS OF PHYSICAL ACTIVITY

Moderate intensity physical activity is associated with very low risk for adverse events (USDHHS, 2008a). An overly aggressive approach to physical activity may exaggerate existing clinical conditions and put individuals, particularly older adults, at risk for untoward effects. If an individual has an undiagnosed heart condition and is habitually sedentary, strenuous physical activity may create arrhythmias or precipitate a cardiac arrest or myocardial infarction, although adverse events are not common. Individuals over 50 years of age or with an existing chronic illness should be evaluated medically before starting regular physical activity. Persons with cardiovascular disease or other chronic conditions should be cautioned to avoid activity at levels that are physiologically untenable or result in untoward symptoms. Overstressing muscles and joints may result in muscle soreness and joint pain. The risk of musculoskeletal injury increases with the total amount of physical activity. A program of gradually increasing physical activity is recommended, with emphasis on moderate activity for older adults. The benefits of appropriate physical activity far outweigh the potential risks.

Proper warm-up and cool-down is important for any physical activity. Warming up is important to increase blood flow to the heart and skeletal muscles, enhance oxygenation of tissues, and increase flexibility of muscles before physical activity. The warm-up period allows the heart rate and body temperature to increase gradually and the joints to become more flexible prior to initiating physical activity. Warming up can include activities such as slow walking, arm circles, leg exercises, or wall push-ups. The warm-up period should last about 7–10 minutes and be followed immediately by moderate or vigorous physical activity. Following physical activity, a cooling down period is essential. Taking time to cool down for 5–10 minutes following physical activity is important because activity raises heart rate, blood pressure, body temperature, and lactic acid in the muscles. Cooling down allows the heart rate to decrease gradually, preventing pooling of blood in muscles and resultant lightheadedness. It helps eliminate lactic acid in muscles and maintains blood flow to and from the muscle. During the cool-down period, it is important to keep the lower extremities moving in activities such as slow walking, jogging, or cycling. At the end of the cooling-down period, the client's heart rate should be lower than 100 beats per minute.

GENETICS, ENVIRONMENT, AND PHYSICAL ACTIVITY

The interaction between genetics and the environment and their contribution to health has become a priority area of research. In a gene–environment interaction, the magnitude and direction of the effect that a genetic variant has on a phenotype varies as the environment changes (Olden, 2009). In other words, the genetic risk can be modified by the environment, or the effect of the environmental exposure depends on the genetic background. It is now established that genes only explain a small number of complex diseases. Geographic differences in the incidence of disease, as well as differences in disease in immigrant populations, support a role for environmental influences, which includes lifestyles.

Gene–environmental interactions have been studied to document the role of genetic factors in physical activity. In spite of the diversity in samples studied and assessment methods, these factors have accounted for 29–62% of the variation in daily exercise at the population level (Bryan, Hutchinson, Seals, & Allen, 2007). Various mechanisms have been proposed, including specific genes for motivation and maintenance of exercise, differential sensitivity to the mental health benefits of exercise, and genetic selection advantage for participating in physical activity (de Geus & de Moor, 2008). As research unfolds, attention will be needed to tailor interventions to promote physical activity, depending on individual genetic variations.

Twin studies and obesity research have also shed light on the gene–environment interaction in physical activity. Although genetic factors are critical, environment is also an important contributor (Bergeman & Ong, 2007; Maia, Thomas, & Beunen, 2002). Shared influences, such as social learning and parent role modeling, may offer potential mechanisms operating in the environment to promote physical activity. Obesity results from genetic factors as well as environmental influences, such as overeating and physical inactivity (Clement, 2006). Multiple genetic markers have been identified that increase susceptibility to weight gain, especially in an environment that promotes overeating and little physical activity.

PRESCRIBING PHYSICAL ACTIVITY TO ACHIEVE HEALTH BENEFITS

To achieve health benefits, medium and high levels of regular physical activity are essential. Baseline activities are the light intensity activities of daily life, such as climbing stairs, standing, or carrying lightweight objects. People who only do baseline activity are considered inactive. Health-enhancing physical activity is activity that produces health benefits. The 2008 Physical Activity Guidelines describe four levels of physical activity: inactive, low, medium, and high (USDHHS, 2008a). Low levels of physical activity amount to activity less than 150 minutes per week. Medium physical activity refers to a range of 150–300 minutes of moderate-intensity physical activity a week or 75–150 minutes of vigorous-intensity physical activity to obtain substantial benefits. A high level of physical activity is defined as more than 300 minutes of moderate-intensity activity a week.

A range of 500–1000 metabolic equivalents (METs) of activity per week has been shown to provide substantial health benefits. The benefits show a dose-response relationship in that 1,000 METs per week produce greater benefits than 500 METs per week. A MET is the ratio of the rate of energy expenditure during an activity to the rate of energy expenditure at rest. One MET is the rate of energy expenditure at rest. Moderate intensity activity is defined as 3–5.9 METs. Walking at three miles per hour is equivalent to 3.3 METs, so this is considered a moderate intensity activity. Moderate intensity activity is also defined as 40–59% of aerobic capacity reserve, where 0% of reserve is resting and 100% of reserve is maximal effort. Vigorous intensity activities are considered 6 METS or greater. Running at ten minutes per mile is classified as vigorous activity, as it is a 10-MET activity. Vigorous activities are 60–74% of aerobic capacity reserve.

The American College of Sports Medicine includes frequency and duration, as well as intensity, in its guidelines and recommends 30 minutes of moderate intensity activity five days a week, or a minimum of 20 minutes of high-intensity activity on three days a week (Haskell et al., 2007). The 30 minutes daily can be accumulated in 10-minute bouts. Intensity (how hard), frequency (how often), and duration (how long) all make up the exercise prescription. However, research has shown that the total amount of activity (minutes of moderate intensity physical activity) is more important than any one component for health benefits (USDHHS, 2008a). Examples of light, moderate, and vigorous intensity activities and MET equivalents are shown in Table 6–2.

Because the public is not familiar with METS and aerobic reserve, activity recommendations should be discussed in number of minutes needed per week and level of intensity. The minimum number and range of minutes per week for activities of moderate intensity needed is straightforward. Adults should participate in at least 30 minutes of moderate-intensity activity on a minimum of five days a week for a total of at least 150 minutes. A moderate intensity activity can be explained as a level of effort of 5–6 on a scale of 0–10, where 0 is the effort level when sitting and 10 is all-out maximal effort. This effort produces noticeable changes in heart rate and breathing. A vigorous intensity activity is 7 or 8 on a 10-point scale. This effort produces large increases in heart rate and breathing. The general rule of thumb is that one minute of vigorous intensity activity is equivalent to two minutes of moderate-intensity activity. A person doing moderate-intensity activity is able to talk but not sing during the activity, and a person who is doing vigorous intensity physical activity is only able to say a few words before pausing for a breath. Another recommendation for daily physical activity in the past has been to walk 10,000 steps per day (Tudor-Locke, 2003). More recent research has indicated that moderate intensity activity is equivalent to walking 3,000 steps in 30 minutes for five days each week or three daily bouts of 1,000 steps in ten minutes for five days each week (Marshall et al., 2009). The authors concluded that moderate intensity activity is equivalent to a minimum of 100 steps per minute. However, due to errors in using step counts as METs, this should be a general guideline only and a minimum number of steps per minute to see health benefits.

PROMOTING PHYSICAL ACTIVITY ACROSS THE LIFE SPAN

Interest in life-span patterns of physical activity has been fueled by the realization that many risk factors for cardiovascular disease including obesity, high blood pressure, and elevated cholesterol are evident in early childhood. Further, of the major modifiable risk factors for coronary heart disease (elevated cholesterol, smoking, hypertension, and inactivity), physical inactivity is most prevalent across the life span. Despite the evidence for the health benefits, more than half of the American population is not active enough to gain physical and mental health benefits.

TABLE 6–2   MET Equivalents of Light, Moderate, and Vigorous Activities

Light <3.0 METs	Moderate 3.0–6.0 METs	Vigorous >6.0 METs
Walking	Walking	Walking, jogging & running
Walking slowly around home, store or office = 2.0	Walking 3.0 mph = 3.3	Walking at very very brisk pace (4.5 mph) = 6.3
	Walking at very brisk pace (4 mph) = 5.0	Walking/hiking at moderate pace and grade with no or light pack (<10 lb) = 7.0
		Hiking at steep grades and pack 10–42 lb = 7.5–9.0
		Jogging at 5 mph = 8.0
		Jogging at 6 mph = 10.0
		Running at 7 mph = 11.5
Household & occupation		
Sitting—using computer, work at desk, using light hand tools = 1.5	Cleaning—heavy: washing windows, car, clean garage = 3.0	Shoveling sand, coal, etc. = 7.0
Standing performing light work such as making bed, washing dishes, ironing, preparing food or store clerk = 2.0–2.5	Sweeping floors or carpet, vacuuming, mopping = 3.0–3.5	Carrying heavy loads such as bricks = 7.5
	Carpentry—general = 3.6	Heavy farming such as baling hay = 8.0
	Carrying and stacking wood = 5.5	Shoveling, digging ditches = 8.5
	Mowing lawn—walk power mower = 5.5	
Leisure time & sports		
Arts & crafts, playing cards = 1.5	Badminton—recreational = 4.5	Basketball game = 8.0
Billiards = 2.5	Basketball—shooting around = 4.5	Bicycling—on flat: moderate effort (12–14 mph) = 8.0; fast (14–16 mph) = 10
Boating—power = 2.5	Bicycling—on flat: light effort (10–12 mph) = 6.0	Skiing cross country—slow (2.5 mph) = 7.0; fast (5.0–7.9 mph) = 9.0
Croquet = 2.5	Dancing—ballroom slow = 3.0; ballroom fast = 4.5	Soccer—casual = 7.0; competitive = 10.0
Darts = 2.5	Fishing from river bank & walking = 4.0	Swimming—moderate/hard = 8–11[†]
Fishing—sitting = 2.5	Golf—walking pulling clubs = 4.3	Tennis singles = 8.0
Playing most musical instruments = 2.0–2.5	Sailing boat, wind surfing = 3.0	Volleyball—competitive at gym or beach = 8.0
	Swimming leisurely = 6.0	
	Table tennis = 4.0	
	Tennis doubles = 5.0	
	Volleyball—noncompetitive = 3.0–4.0	

From Haskell, W. L., Lee, I-M., Pate, R. R., et al. (2007). Physical activity and public health: Updated recommendation for adults. From the American College of Sports Medicine and the American Heart Association. *Circulation, 116*(9), 1081–1093.

Patterns of physical activity that begin early in life are likely to persist over time. It is easier to develop positive physical activity patterns early in life rather than to change unhealthy behaviors after they are established habits. Lifestyle activity provides flexibility for increasing energy expenditure through altering patterns of daily activities such as walking to work or school, taking the stairs, and walking during lunchtime or after school or work. Gender and type of physical activity influence motivation for exercise and should be considered in planning programs during adolescence. The 2008 Physical Activity Guidelines promote physical activity across the life span, beginning with age 6 years and older (USDHHS, 2008a). These guidelines are used in this chapter.

PROMOTING PHYSICAL ACTIVITY IN CHILDREN AND ADOLESCENTS

Regular physical activity has many immediate and long-term health benefits for children and adolescents. It improves cardiovascular fitness, increases bone mass, enhances mental well-being, and is associated with less obesity, hypertension, and cigarette smoking, which prevents the development of cardiovascular disease, diabetes, and other chronic diseases in adulthood (Trost & Loprinzi, 2008). However, a significant number of children and adolescents do not participate in the level of regular activity needed to achieve health benefits. In addition, the rise in childhood and adolescent obesity is alarming. In the past 30 years, the prevalence of obesity has more than doubled among children and more than tripled in adolescents (Bennett & Sothern, 2009). Although evidence indicates the trend is beginning to level, the large number of obese children and adolescents warrants strategies for lifestyle change. Evidence consistently shows that only about a third of high school adolescents achieve the recommended amount of daily physical activity, and about two-thirds of children 9–13 years do. Adolescent males are more physically active than adolescent girls, and white are more physically active than Hispanics or African-Americans.

The long-term goal of physical activity research among youths is to design age-, gender-, and culturally appropriate interventions to promote lifelong physical activity. Pubertal changes (onset of menarche, changing patterns of body fat distribution) and social transitions (moving from elementary school to junior high school to senior high school) correspond to changes in sports participation and patterns of physical activity. Longitudinal studies are needed to identify changing activity patterns and successful strategies to promote physical activity across childhood and adolescence.

Physical Activity and Gender

Physical activity patterns vary by gender across many studies. Gender differences are seen starting in adolescence. Boys report greater physical activity than girls in the preteen years and have been shown to increase their level of physical activity until about 11 years of age, plateau, and then decrease beginning about 13 years of age (Kahn et al., 2008). Girl adolescents increase their activity until 12 or 13 years and then decrease, as in boys. Boys exhibit higher levels of screen time than girls in sedentary time. Gender-specific factors are associated with the decline. For boys, changes in attitude toward physical education, perceived parental attitude about body shape and fitness, and risk behaviors (binge drinking and marijuana use) are associated with the decline. For boys and girls, body mass index (BMI) self-esteem, perceived peer attitudes about physical activity, and parental attitude about physical activity are associated with the decline (Kahn et al., 2008). Research has consistently documented similar determinants and suggests that interventions should be implemented before the anticipated decline. Adolescent interventions also need to address individual, environmental, and parental factors that are modifiable.

Implementing Guidelines for Physical Activity

A minimum of 60 minutes or more of moderate or vigorous physical activity every day is recommended for adolescents and children (USDHSS, 2008a). Children and adolescents should participate in vigorous intensity activities at least three days per week. Three types of activity are important: aerobic, muscle-strengthening, and bone-strengthening activities. Aerobic activities increase cardiorespiratory fitness and include such things as running, hopping, skipping, jumping rope, swimming, dancing, and bicycling. Muscle-strengthening activities in this age group are usually unstructured, such as climbing on playground equipment. Structured muscle strengthening activities for adolescents may include weight lifting. Activities that promote bone growth and strength include running, basketball, hopscotch, and jumping rope. Adolescents are more likely to engage in structured programs or play sports that provide aerobic benefits.

Physical activity should be age appropriate and enjoyable and should include a variety of activities. Sedentary and obese children may have difficulty beginning physically activity for 60 minutes, so it is recommended that exercise begin gradually and increase 10% per week until the recommendation time is achieved (Bennett & Sothern, 2009). Developmentally appropriate activities are those that are suitable for the child's physical and cognitive development. A range of noncompetitive and competitive activities, age and ability appropriate, should be offered. Interventions also should be aimed at decreasing sedentary behavior, such as limiting television and video game time to two hours daily. A review of studies using pedometers to promote physical activity in youth indicates that pedometers can be used successfully to promote physical activity in adolescents when used for self-monitoring (Lubans, Morgan, & Tudor-Locke, 2009). Examples of aerobic, muscle-building, and bone-strengthening activities are shown in Table 6–3.

The national physical activity guidelines do not include preschool children, ages 3–5 years. However, the number of overweight preschoolers has also increased. In a seven-country study of preschoolers, only 54% of the children were sufficiently physically active (Tucker & Gilliland, 2007). The amount of time spent in daycare, increase in screen viewing (e.g., television, video games, computers), and greater parental constraints in play places and safety concerns has resulted in a dramatic increase in sedentary behavior. Physical activity habits begin to develop in preschool years, so this group also needs interventions to increase physical activity. The National Association for Sports and Physical Education (NASPE) recommends 60 minutes of structured physical activity daily and at least 60 minutes of unstructured physical activity for preschoolers (NASPE, 2002). Preschools are an important site to implement interventions because more than half of children in the United States attend. The limited number of studies conducted indicates that when the preschooler, teacher, and parent are involved in the intervention, positive changes result (Williams, Carter, Kibbe, & Dennison, 2009). In addition, activity-friendly playgrounds yield increases in physical activity if accompanied with active supervision and structured physical activity (Cardon, Labarque, Smits, & de Bourdeaudhuij, 2009).

TABLE 6–3 Aerobic and Muscle- and Bone-Strengthening Activities		
Type of Physical Activity	**Age Group**	
	Children	**Adolescents**
Moderate-intensity aerobic	• Active recreation such as hiking, skateboarding, rollerblading • Bicycle riding • Walking to school	• Active recreation, such as canoeing, hiking, cross-country skiing, skateboarding, rollerblading • Brisk walking • Bicycle riding (stationary or road bike) • House and yard work such as sweeping or pushing a lawn mower • Playing games that require catching and throwing, such as baseball, softball, basketball and volleyball
Vigorous–intensity aerobic	• Active games involving running and chasing, such as tag • Bicycle riding • Jumping rope • Martial arts, such as karate • Running • Sports such as ice or field hockey, basketball, swimming, tennis or gymnastics	• Active games involving running and chasing, such as flag football, soccer • Bicycle riding • Jumping rope • Martial arts such as karate • Running • Sports such as tennis, ice or field hockey, basketball, swimming • Vigorous dancing • Aerobics • Cheerleading or gymnastics
Muscle-strengthening	• Games such as tug of war • Modified push-ups (with knees on the floor) • Resistance exercises using body weight or resistance bands • Rope or tree climbing • Sit-ups • Swinging on playground equipment/bars • Gymnastics	• Games such as tug of war • Push-ups • Resistance exercises with exercise bands, weight machines, handheld weights • Rock climbing • Sit-ups • Cheerleading or gymnastics
Bone-strengthening	• Games such as hop-scotch • Hopping, skipping, jumping • Jumping rope • Running • Sports such as gymnastics, basketball, volleyball, tennis	• Hopping, skipping, jumping • Jumping rope • Running • Sports such as gymnastics, basketball, volleyball, tennis

Source: Centers for Disease Control and Prevention. Retrieved July 17, 2009, from http://www.cdc.gov /physicalactivity/everyone/guidelines/what_counts.html

Promoting Physical Activity in Families

Family-based activities are important in promoting a health lifestyle in children and adolescents. Parent's lifestyles influence adolescent's risk of developing active or inactive lifestyles as young adults (Crossman, Sullivan, & Benin, 2006). For example, parental obesity places male and female adolescents at greater risks for being overweight as adults. Parents influence their children's physical behavior as role models, being directly involved in activities with their children, offering encouragement and support, and providing opportunities and resources to engage in recreational sports and programs (Madsen, McCulloch, & Crawford, 2009). Family-based programs encourage parents to change their behaviors and to be active with their children in relationship-building experiences. For example, weekend family bike outings and parent–child aerobic or recreational activities create opportunities for parents to be role models for active lifestyles. Parental support is also needed for children to walk and cycle to school. Although the physical environment is important in the decision to walk to school, research indicates that parental support for walking is associated with increases in physical activity, especially among younger children (Hume, Timperio, Salmon, Carver, & Giles-Corti, 2009). Interventions, including school-based programs, to increase physical activity behaviors in children and adolescents should target the entire family. A review of 14 clinical trials that involved parents in interventions to increase physical activity in youth found that programs need to engage parents directly in training and counseling (O'Connor, Jago, & Baranowski, 2009). Family-based programs are a major challenge, as often parents are difficult to reach and recruit due to their work commitments. Contacting families during organized activities is more effective than sending written materials home with the child. Telephone interventions with family members also show promise. Findings also indicate that the dosage of the intervention needs to be high enough to produce an effect. In other words, more intensive programs may be needed to result in behavior change. Programs that involve the parent in physical activity have been successful in increasing time spent in physical activity by the child as well as the parents. Childhood and adolescence are ideal periods in the life span to cultivate regular physical activity that can reap positive health benefits throughout life. Family involvement increases the health habits of the parents as well as the children.

Promoting Physical Activity in Schools

Schools play a major role in promoting involvement of children in recreational activities that they can enjoy for a lifetime. By promoting physical activity on a daily basis, teaching the personal value of regular activity, and encouraging continuing involvement in moderate and vigorous activities both at school and at home, schools contribute to the goal of an "active" generation. Schools are an ideal setting because they have intense and continuous contact with most children ages 6–16 years, teachers who have an interest in health promotion, appropriate facilities (e.g., gymnasium, sports equipment, playground) to promote activity, a structure with blocks of time available to train children (recess, lunch), and the capacity to interact with the community-based activity providers (Trost & Loprinzi, 2008). Physical activity can be promoted at break times or after school. Results of a meta-analysis that included 14 studies to promote physical activity indicate that after-school programs can improve physical activity levels (Beets, Beighle, Erwin, & Huberry, 2009).

In a review of studies evaluating the effectiveness of programs to increase physical activity in schools, results indicate all increased activity levels (Zaga, Briss, & Harris, 2005). School-based programs are effective in increasing levels of physical activity, physical fitness, aerobic capacity, and time spent in moderate to vigorous activities. Based on the consistency of results, the U.S. Task Force on Community Interventions recommends that these programs should be adapted for all elementary, middle, and high school students. The most widely disseminated school based programs are the Sports Play and Active Recreation for Kids (SPARKS) program and The Child and Adolescent Trial for Cardiovascular Health (CATCH). Both programs target physical activity behaviors as well as behavior change skills and parental involvement. SPARKS has been disseminated in more than 300 schools, and CATCH has been disseminated in more than 1,800 schools in Texas (Trost & Loprinzi, 2008). Key reasons for sustainability of these school-based programs are strong support by the school principal, availability of adequate equipment, teachers who engaged in physical activity themselves, and availability of ongoing training (Owens, Glanz, Sallis, & Kelder, 2006). Barriers to success include lack of resources (large class size, inadequate number of physical education specialists, and inadequate school facilities). Placing physical activity as a low priority in the curriculum was a major barrier to implementation in schools.

PROMOTING PHYSICAL ACTIVITY IN ADULTS AND OLDER ADULTS

Cardiovascular diseases (heart disease and stroke), type 2 diabetes, and cancer are the leading causes of illness, disability, and death among Americans and the most costly and preventable (Centers for Disease Control and Prevention [CDC]; see Web sites at the end of this chapter). Chronic diseases account for 70% of all deaths in the United States, and one-third of the years of potential life lost before age 65. Heart disease and stroke account for almost one-third of all deaths in the United States and are preventable. Physical inactivity has consistently been shown to be associated with the risk of developing the major chronic diseases. Regular physical activity has been shown to prevent or reduce the risk for these diseases, as well as improve quality of life in adults and older adults. Physical activity in older adults protects against loss of mobility and increases functional independence through improved muscle mass, increased bone density, and cardiovascular fitness (Rosenberg et al., 2009).

The individual-focused theories and models discussed in Chapter 2 have been used to guide most of the adult physical activity research. Social cognitive theory, the transtheoretical model, the theory of planned behavior, the health belief model, and the health promotion model have all been used with limited success, along with social support theory, motivational interviewing, and relapse prevention theory. These theoretical models have focused on the cognitive, affective, and social influences on individuals and although they have shown success, the amount of explained variance has remained low. Researchers, practitioners, and policy makers see the value of paying attention to additional factors in the social and physical environment that also influence lifestyle behaviors and have implemented new approaches, such as social ecological theory to guide health promotion interventions and policy initiatives. Social ecological models include intrapersonal, interpersonal, and environmental approaches that are interdependent in their effects on lifestyle behaviors (see Figure 6–1). These models offer

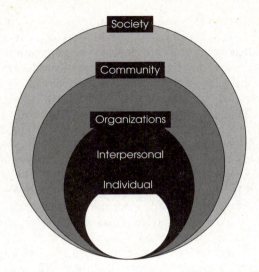

FIGURE 6-1   Socio-Ecological Framework   *Source*: Reprinted from *Journal of Science and Medicine in Sport,* Billie Giles-Corti, "People or places: What should be the target?," pages 357–366, Copyright 2006, with permission from Elsevier.

a greater likelihood of success, as they approach physical activity from the individual's perspective and include the social and physical forces operating in the environment that also influence health behaviors. Several individual models, such as the health promotion model and the health belief model, include concepts such as barriers, facilitating conditions, and contextual factors. These concepts should be considered more broadly to account for environmental factors and their interaction with individual concepts in the models. Socio-ecological and other environmental models that explain individual behavior–environmental interactions are important to guide research and policy to develop, implement, and evaluate effective physical activity interventions.

Gender and Physical Activity

Evidence indicates that physical activity plays a role in the primary prevention of cardiovascular disease, diabetes, and some cancers in women, as in men (Brown, Burton, & Rowan, 2007). However, women report less leisure-time physical activity than do men as they spend more time in paid and unpaid working roles. Multiple family obligations decrease women's time for physical activity. Unmarried women are generally more active than married women with children at home. In addition, leisure-time physical activity is influenced by role changes in women's lives such as parenthood, employment, children leaving home, and retirement. The Baltimore Longitudinal Study of Aging found that a greater decline in total and high-intensity leisure-time physical activity is a predictor of all-cause mortality in men, but not in women (Talbot, Morrell, Fleg, & Metter, 2007). However, men and women did not differ in the inverse dose-response relationship between leisure-time physical activity and the metabolic syndrome (Halldin, Rosell, de Faire, & Hellenius, 2007).

In addition to the time barrier, other obstacles to engaging in physical activity have been consistently reported by women. Lack of social support and encouragement to be physically active from family members or close friends and lack of child care may reinforce sedentary lifestyles (Hoebeke, 2008). Low-income women report that exhaustion from completing the daily demands of child care and family and work responsibilities leave little energy for themselves. In some ethnic groups, cultural barriers exist, as physical activity may not be considered an appropriate activity for women. Neighborhood safety issues and lack of facilities tailored to women's needs further impede adoption of active lifestyles. All of these barriers should be considered in planning programs for women.

Implementing Physical Activity Guidelines

The 2008 Guidelines recommend that adults under age 65 years need to participate in at least 150 minutes each week of moderate-intensity aerobic (endurance) activity, or 75 minutes of vigorous intensity physical activity each week to obtain substantial benefits for lowering one's risk of heart disease and stroke, type 2 diabetes, and depression (USDHSS, 2008a). As stated previously, the benefits are dose-related, so 300 minutes per week results in additional benefits, including lower risk for colon and breast cancer and prevention of weight gain. The activity should be performed on at least three days a week to produce health benefits and can be performed in bouts of 10 minutes. The activity may be either moderate intensity, vigorous intensity, or a combination of both (see Table 6–2 for physical activities and MET equivalents). Muscle-strengthening activities to increase muscle fitness and bone strength are also recommended. Muscle-strengthening activities include weight lifting, resistance bands, calisthenics, carrying heavy loads, and gardening. These activities should be done two days a week and count if they work the major muscle groups and are at moderate-to high-intensity levels.

Inactive adults need to begin slowly and gradually increase the activity over a period of weeks to months. For example, they may begin with five minutes of slow walking several times a day and slowly increase each session. Initially, muscle-strengthening activities can be performed one day a week at a light or moderate intensity effort. Active adults can increase the number of minutes per week to exceed the minimum level or perform higher-level intensity activities and do muscle strengthening activities at least two days per week.

Structured programs have been successful with adults and older adults. The Sedentary Exercise Adherence Trial (SWEAT2) promoted swimming and walking in sedentary women, aged 50 to 70 years (Cox et al., 2008). Adherence and physical fitness was similar in both groups at six months. Increased physical fitness at six months was maintained at 12 months. Comparison of a home-based program support by telephone calls with structured, supervised weekly classes, and a control group resulted in similar improvements in the structured and home-based program at six months (Opdenacker, Boen, Coorevits, & Delecluse, 2008). However, at 12 months, the home-based group maintained their physical activity levels compared with the structured group, providing support for lifestyle home-based programs in older adults.

Sedentary behavior increases with age, and older adults (aged 65 years and older) are the most sedentary group. However, aerobic and strength-building activities are essential for healthy aging, and older adults should be encouraged to develop or continue healthy lifestyle habits (Nelson et al., 2007). The same guidelines for younger adults apply to individuals aged 65 years and older: a minimum of 150 minutes of moderate-intensity physical activity, 75 minutes of vigorous-intensity physical activity each week, or a combination of the two. All types of activities count, including walking the dog and taking an exercise class. Dog walking promotes physical activity, and research shows that dog walkers are less likely to be obese than non–dog walkers (Coleman, Rosenberg, Conway, Sallis, & Saelens, 2008). The activities may be done in 10-minute bouts if performed at a moderate or vigorous intensity level. Supervision may be needed initially for older adults to learn to exercise at a moderate level of effort, especially for adults with low fitness levels.

Muscle-strengthening activities are also recommended for older adults. They should perform 8–10 exercises using resistance, such as weights, at least 10–15 repetitions for each exercise, a minimum of two days a week. These exercises should be done at the same levels of intensity as aerobic activities, 5–6 on a 10 point scale for moderate intensity and 7–8 for vigorous intensity. Vigorous-intensity activities should be performed under supervision or by adults who have continued to be physically fit. Older adults at risk for falls also need to perform balance training three days a week. Examples of exercises in a balance program include walking backward, walking sideways, heel and toe walking, and standing from a sitting position. Tai Chi has been shown to prevent falls, so enrolling in one of these exercise classes is another option to improve balance.

Older adults consist of the young old (65 to 74 years), middle old (75 to 84 years), and very old (over 85 years). Ability to be physically active varies over this age spectrum. Barriers to physical activity are an important consideration for the elderly. Although work and family demands may lessen with age, convenience of facilities, cost, opportunities for physical activity with others, fear of resultant illness or injury, disability, and sensory impairment become more salient. Concern about existing medical conditions may be a further deterrent to an active lifestyle. Environmental barriers, such as weather (extreme temperatures), presence or quality of sidewalks, and lack of places to sit and rest while walking are concerns of older adults (Brawler, Rejeski, & King, 2003). Many older adults also have misconceptions about physical activity, believing that it can be unhealthy. Barriers can be addressed by inclusion of an educational component with physical activity programs. Emphasis should be placed on reducing sedentary activity and increasing moderate activity, leaving vigorous activities for select older adults with appropriate fitness levels (Nelson et al., 2007). A stepwise program is also recommended to decrease the risks of injury and to gain experience and self-confidence performing the activities. Table 6–4 describes strategies for all adults to overcome the major barriers to physical activity.

Inactive adults and adults with chronic conditions should consult with their health care provider, who will assess their ability to participate in physical activity. Inactive adults should begin very slowly and increase activity gradually over a period of months. They should aim for 150 minutes a week. If an older adult who has a chronic condition is unable to meet the target goal of 150 minutes a week, even 60 minutes of moderate-intensity activity will produce some health benefits. Warm-up and cool-down activities are important.

Programs to increase physical activity in adults should be tailored to their interests, preferences, and readiness to change (Zaga et al., 2005). Based on scientific evidence, the Guide to Community Preventive Services (Zaga et al., 2005) recommends that programs teach behavior skills needed to make leisure-time physical activity a daily habit. Other components of successful programs are setting goals for physical

TABLE 6–4   Strategies for Overcoming Barriers to Physical Activity

Barrier	Strategies
Lack of time	Identify available time slots. Monitor your daily activities for one week. Identify at least three 30-minute time slots you could use for physical activity. Add physical activity to your daily routine. For example, walk or ride your bike to work or shopping, organize school activities around physical activity, walk the dog, exercise while you watch TV, park farther away from your destination, etc. Select activities requiring minimal time, such as walking, jogging, or stair climbing.
Social influence	Explain your interest in physical activity to friends and family. Ask them to support your efforts. Invite friends and family members to exercise with you. Plan social activities involving exercise. Develop new friendships with physically active people. Join a group, such as the YMCA or a hiking club.
Lack of energy	Schedule physical activity for times in the day or week when you feel energetic. Convince yourself that if you give it a chance, physical activity will increase your energy level; then, try it.
Lack of motivation	Plan ahead. Make physical activity a regular part of your daily or weekly schedule and write it on your calendar. Invite a friend to exercise with you on a regular basis and write it on both your calendars. Join an exercise group or class.
Fear of injury	Learn how to warm up and cool down to prevent injury. Learn how to exercise appropriately considering your age, fitness level, skill level, and health status. Choose activities involving minimum risk.
Lack of skill	Select activities requiring no new skills, such as walking, climbing stairs, or jogging. Take a class to develop new skills.
Lack of resources	Select activities that require minimal facilities or equipment, such as walking, jogging, jumping rope, or calisthenics. Identify inexpensive, convenient resources available in your community (community education programs, park and recreation programs, worksite programs, etc.).
Weather conditions	Develop a set of regular activities that are always available regardless of weather (indoor cycling, aerobic dance, indoor swimming, calisthenics, stair climbing, rope skipping, mall walking, dancing, gymnasium games, etc.).
Travel	Put a jump rope in your suitcase and jump rope. Walk the halls and climb the stairs in hotels. Stay in places with swimming pools or exercise facilities. Join the YMCA or YWCA (ask about reciprocal membership agreement). Visit the local shopping mall and walk for half an hour or more. Bring your mp3 player with your favorite aerobic exercise music.

(continued)

TABLE 6–4 (Continued)	
Barrier	**Strategies**
Family obligations	Trade babysitting time with a friend, neighbor, or family member who also has small children.
	Exercise with the kids: go for a walk together, play tag or other running games, get an aerobic dance or exercise tape for kids (there are several on the market) and exercise together. You can spend time together and still get your exercise.
	Jump rope, do calisthenics, ride a stationary bicycle, or use other home gymnasium equipment while the kids are busy playing or sleeping.
	Try to exercise when the kids are not around (e.g., during school hours or their nap time).
Retirement years	Look upon your retirement as an opportunity to become more active instead of less. Spend more time gardening, walking the dog, and playing with your grandchildren. Children with short legs and grandparents with slower gaits are often great walking partners.
	Learn a new skill always been interested in, such as ballroom dancing, square dancing, or swimming.
	Now that you have the time, make regular physical activity a part of every day. Go for a walk every morning or every evening before dinner. Treat yourself to an exercycle and ride every day while reading a favorite book or magazine.

Source: Centers for Disease Control and Prevention. Retrieved July 20, 2009, from http://www.cdc.gov /physicalactivity/everyone/getactive/barriers.html

activity, monitoring progress, building social support, incorporating self-rewards for the new behaviors, and learning to problem solve to maintain change and prevent relapse (Zaga et al., 2005). Programs can be delivered individually, in groups, or by telephone, mail, or computer.

Social support interventions have been successful, as they build, strengthen, and maintain social networks to promote physical activity (Zaga et al., 2005). These programs establish buddy systems and contracts or form walking groups. Group members or buddies provide motivational support as well as companionship and encouragement to engage in regular leisure-time physical activities. Group facilitators provide encouragement and formal discussions to address barriers and other issues related to behavior change. Telephone calls to provide encouragement and monitor progress are also useful.

Promoting Physical Activity in the Work Site

An increasingly sedentary workplace, an aging workforce, and a rising rate of preventable chronic diseases make health promotion workplace programs a priority. Work sites are ideal places to promote healthy changes, as large numbers of employees are available for an extended period of time. Employers have multiple tools and resources with which to engage employees, such as department meetings, telephone or computer-based interventions, email communication, signage on bulletin boards, and the ability to make policy and health benefit changes (Pronk & Kottke, 2009). Health promotion programs in work settings are thought to help employees stay healthy, satisfied, and productive. Also important is the projected savings in health care costs and lost productivity.

Scientific evidence supports the need to implement and test programs to promote leisure-time physical activities. Wellness programs that focus on nutrition and physical activity have been associated with a decrease in absenteeism and improvement in cardiovascular risk factors (Aldana, Merrill, Price, Hardy, & Hager, 2005; Muto, Hashimoto, Haruyuma, & Fukuda, 2006). The Worksite Opportunities for Wellness (WOW) promotes wellness through dietary and physical activity programs, pedometers, group exercise classes, weight-loss classes, and rewards. Differences in BMI and fat mass were noted between the intervention and control groups after 12 months (Racette et al., 2009). However, improvements were observed with personalized health assessments and personalized reports without the intervention. The Move to Improve 12-month clinical trial, which was implemented in Home Depot work sites, resulted in physical activity increasing to 51% in the intervention sites, compared with 25% in the control sites (Dishman, DeJoy, Wilson, & Vandenberg, 2009). Participants exceeded the 300 minutes per week of moderate to vigorous activity and 9,000 daily pedometer steps. At year five, a health promotion campaign and rearrangement of the environment to promote walking resulted in an increase in high-density lipoprotein cholesterol levels in middle-age employees (Naito et al., 2008).

In general, positive findings have been reported for physical activity programs; however, the research continues to suffer from numerous barriers in the workplace. The most successful programs incorporate a social-ecological approach, targeting the individual as well as the environment, and engage the organization (Simpson et al., 2000). Currently, employers can deduct the cost of on-site facilities from their taxes if provided to benefit employees. However, if the services are outsourced, employees must pay income tax on this benefit (Wamp, 2009). Policy changes are needed to eliminate tax barriers for employers and employees.

INTERVENTIONS IN THE COMMUNITY TO PROMOTE PHYSICAL ACTIVITY

Interventions in the community to promote physical activity take place in schools, work sites, churches, and other community organizations. These programs reach a larger group than do one-on-one interventions. These community-based programs focus on groups of individuals in the various sites. Community-level interventions focus on the entire population through mass media campaigns or by changing the physical or built environment. Recently the term *whole community* has been used to describe community interventions that are based on social ecological approaches. Whole community interventions use participatory planning to develop strategies to intervene at the individual, social, environmental, and legislative levels (Mummery & Brown, 2009). Although individual factors, such as motivation, are important, it is well documented that community interventions require multiple intervention components, including mass media, community activities to enhance social networks and social support, engagement with community members, participatory planning, and community partnerships (Reger-Nash, Bauman, Cooper, Chey, & Simon, 2006). Whole community approaches include

(1) social marketing through local mass media, (2) other community strategies to raise awareness, (3) individual counseling, (4) engaging voluntary and nongovernment agencies, (5) working in specific settings, such as work sites and schools, and (6) environmental change strategies (Mummery & Brown, 2009).

Community-based approaches have been implemented to promote physical activity at all ages and socioeconomic groups with success. The Keep Minnesota Active clinical trial for adults aged 50–70 years successfully used a telephone- and mail-based activity maintenance intervention to promote maintaining physical activity at six months for participants in a large managed care organization (Martinson et al., 2008). In a clinic-based community-supported lifestyle intervention for women (WISEWOMAN Project), women aged 40–60 years reported greater physical activity, although the findings were not statistically significant (Keyserling et al., 2008). The Hartslag Limburg five-year community intervention program was successful in preventing age- and time-related unfavorable changes in walking and leisure-time activities, particularly among low socioeconomic status women (Wendel-Vos et al., 2009). Two physical activity programs, Active for Life and Active Living Everyday, were successfully translated into a wide range of institutions in community settings (Wilcox et al., 2008). Positive results were consistent across sites. A multilevel walking intervention implemented in a continuing care retirement community for adults over age 65 was successful in increasing walking in the intervention group (Rosenberg et al., 2009). The multilevel intervention components included pedometers for self-monitoring, social support, changing perceptions about the environment, and counseling for goal setting.

The Guide to Community Preventive Services (Zaga et al., 2005) recommends five evidence-based components that should be tailored to individual community needs:

- Community-wide media campaigns
- School-based physical education
- Individual adapted behavior change interventions
- Social support interventions
- Increased access to places for physical activity

Media campaigns should use television, newspapers, radio, and other media as appropriate. Social support interventions include organizing a buddy system, walking groups, or community physical activities, such as dances. Individual evidence-based interventions must be adapted for larger audiences. Interventions to increase access include work site programs and providing access to school playgrounds and gymnasiums (Zaga et al., 2005).

Community-based physical programs must be evaluated to identify programs that are effective and can be recommended for practice. The CDC Physical Activity Evaluation Handbook recommends six steps in the evaluation process (see Web site at the end of the chapter). These include the following:

1. Engage stakeholders in the evaluation process
2. Plan and describe the program
3. Focus the evaluation
4. Justify conclusions
5. Gather credible evidence
6. Disseminate the lessons learned

Four community-wide walking programs were evaluated for program effectiveness (Reger-Nash et al., 2006). The evaluation plan included formative, process, and outcome evaluation strategies. The authors reported six major lessons learned from the evaluation process: (1) participatory planning is an essential first step, (2) it is important to coordinate media approaches and stay focused on the message, (3) knowing the media market is key, (4) organizers must be aware of the resources that will be needed to change, (5) having a community organizer who maintains links with stakeholders is critical, and (6) the sustainability of the program must be monitored (Reger-Nash et al., 2006). Community-based interventions are complex, require financial and human resources, and need time to be implemented and evaluated. Ongoing monitoring and evaluation is important using multiple sources of data.

The cost-effectiveness of community-based interventions also must be evaluated. Seven physical activity interventions were evaluated for costs, health gains, and cost-effectiveness in a simulated cohort of healthy adults (Roux et al., 2008). All of the interventions included individually adapted behavior change, social support interventions, informational outreach activities, and the creation of access to places for physical activity. Cost-effectiveness ratios ranged from $14,000 to $69,000 per quality-adjusted life year (QALY) gained, relative to no intervention. All of the interventions were found to be cost-effective with gains in survival and health-related quality of life, supporting any of the seven programs to promote physical activity.

Changing the Built Environment to Promote Physical Activity

Physical activity is considered the most place-dependent health behavior (Sallis, 2009). Places hinder or facilitate physical activity on the basis of the presence or absence of a supportive infrastructure; in other words, some places are physical activity friendly, and others are considered physical activity unfriendly. Sallis (2009) classifies physical activity environments as a subset of physical environments, which encompass natural and built environments. Built environments include all spaces, buildings, and objects that are created or modified by people, such as homes, schools, workplaces, parks, and transportation systems. The regulations and policies that govern built environments also hinder or facilitate physical activity. For example, policy reform may need to occur to implement and maintain walking paths or recreational parks.

Neighborhood built environments influence physical activity behaviors. In a study comparing two Alabama cities, the low socio-economic status (SES) city had one public recreation area with monthly use fees ranging from $25 to $35 per month, whereas three of the four public facilities in the contrasting city did not charge a fee (Bovell-Benjamin, Hathorn, Ibraim, & Bromfield, 2009). The low SES city also provided limited opportunities for physical activity. Moderate physical activity has also been shown to be higher in high-walkability neighborhoods compared with low-walkability ones (Sallis, et al., 2009b). In addition, overweight/obesity was higher in low-walkability neighborhoods. *Walkability* refers to the ability of individuals to walk to nearby destinations. Walking has been associated with access to an aesthetically pleasing neighborhood, convenient facilities, safe neighborhoods, and limited traffic. Neighborhood environments were compared in 11 countries for their relationship with physical activity (Sallis, Bowles et al., 2009a). The environmental variables included single-family houses or housing type, shops within walking distance, transit stop 10–15 minutes from home, sidewalks on most streets, bicycle facilities in or near neighborhoods, low-cost recreation facilities, and crime rate. Five of the seven variables were significant with having sidewalks on most streets in the neighborhood, the most significant predictor of physical activity. In contrast, unsafe neighborhoods are barriers to physical activity. Research supports the need to design activity-friendly communities to provide opportunities and facilities for families and their children to participate in leisure time physical activity. Additional research is needed to refine the indicators of activity-friendly communities and develop measures that can be used to design friendly physical activity environments. Multiple sectors in the community play a role in promoting physical activity in the community (USDHHS, 2008a). Concerns about crime and safety involve law enforcement. Urban planners play a major role in designing activity friendly communities, and the transportation sector plays a role in building pedestrian and bicycle paths for walking to school or work, or for leisure activities. Parks and recreation departments need to be involved to facilitate access to recreational facilities and playgrounds for all.

Ecological models have proven useful to guide physical activity interventions. Rigorous evaluation of these community-level models across the multiple levels is complex, but it is necessary to begin to understand the usefulness of multilevel interventions. Kelly, Hoechner, Baker, Ramirez, & Brownson (2006) develop an ecological framework with indicators amenable to evaluation (see Figure 6–2). The model encompasses the physical environment (land use, aesthetics, transportation), sociocultural

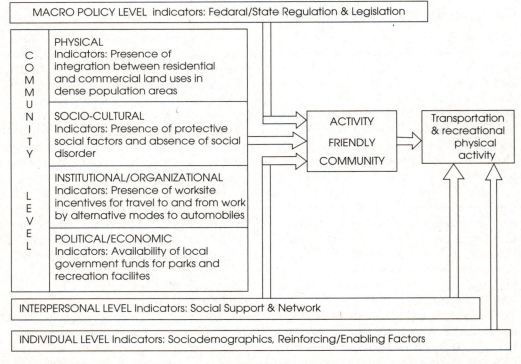

FIGURE 6–2   Ecological Framework for Activity Friendly Communities   *Source:* Reprinted from *Evaluation and Program Planning,* Volume 29(3), Kelly, C. M., Hoehner, C. M., Baker, E. A., Brennan Ramirez, L. K., Brownson, R. C., (2006). "Promoting physical activity in communities: Approaches for successful evaluation of programs and policies," pages 280–292, Copyright 2006, with permission from Elsevier.

environment (protective social factors, disorder), institutional/organizational environment (workplace, schools), and political/economic environment (local and regional
politics). The interpersonal level (social support and social networks), the individual or
intrapersonal level, and the macro or policy level are also included in the model. All of
these factors determine an activity-friendly community. Objective indicators have been
suggested for all of the domains, and measurement approaches have been described
(Kelly et al, 2006). Although the model has undergone limited testing, it is a first step in
evaluating ecological interventions for physical activity, in which multiple levels of
change are implemented.

DESIGNING PHYSICAL ACTIVITY INTERVENTIONS FOR DIVERSE POPULATIONS

People of color and lower socioeconomic status report the lowest levels of regular
physical activity and are most vulnerable to chronic conditions, such as cardiovascular
disease and diabetes. In addition, inequality in environments also influences the ability
to meet physical activity guidelines in these groups. People of color and those with low
SES have less leisure time and energy to exercise, limited access to safe and affordable
places to exercise, less support for regular physical activity, and are exposed to more
stressful living conditions than non-Hispanic whites (Lee & Cubbin, 2009). Living in
impoverished neighborhoods is associated with depression, anxiety, anger, and apathy,
which lead to increased stress and physical inactivity.

The built environment has a negative influence on physical activity in low-income
communities. Low-income neighborhoods also have fewer recreational facilities, and
the available ones may be of lower quality and less likely to be maintained. Less money
is spent on parks and open spaces in low-income communities of color than spending
in affluent areas (Wolch, Wilson, & Fehrenbach, 2005). The amount of commute time is
also a factor in leisure-time physical activity, especially for those who use public transportation. Long commute times leave little time for social interaction and physical
activity after work. Changing environmental conditions in these communities is a
challenge for individuals, local governments, and policy makers.

Cultural factors also must be taken into consideration in promoting physical
activity in diverse populations. Cultures are not homogeneous, and subgroup variations in language, income, education, and acculturation also must be recognized.
Gender socialization and role expectations also differ across cultures. Cultural beliefs
and practices contribute to different patterns of activity across groups. Racial/ethnic
differences include variations in cultural attitudes as well as differences in geographic
residence, degree of urbanization, family size, household composition, neighborhood
characteristics, and degree of segregation (Kumanyika, 2008). Cultural attitudes influence physical activity as well. Cultural values of automobiles and televisions as indicators of sufficient income promote inactivity. Physical activity may be seen as work in
some groups, so leisure time is considered a time for sedentary activities.

Several factors should be considered in designing culturally appropriate
programs for diverse populations across the life span (Gordon, 2004). Nurses first
should become familiar with the community's history, the cultural values, and potential cultural barriers to physical activity. Every cultural group has historical events that
have influenced it. Nurses should learn which cultural values are critical to incorporate
in a physical activity intervention. For example, African-Americans value faith-based

communities. Barriers may be environmental, interpersonal, financial, or legal. For example, transportation may not be available to reach safe walking paths. As mentioned in prior chapters, members of the target community must be engaged beginning with the planning stage. Nurses must integrate the cultural values and strategies to minimize barriers in the activity plan and focus on the community's strengths and resources to maximize their assets. All of these steps must be tailored to the diversity of cultural patterns and practices, including the group's history, beliefs, and preferences.

Examples of differences among underserved groups have been documented (Yancey, Ory, & Davis, 2006). African-Americans value faith-based institutions and the collectivist versus the individualist approach. Physical activity programs may be more successful if faith-based and physical messages need to increase positive ethnic identity, promote physical activity participation as entitlement, and promote prominent African-American athletes as role models. Latino interventions must focus on changing female perceptions of activity and also link group physical activity to traditional celebrations and intergenerational activities. American Indian tribes share several cultural concepts, including the oral tradition, intergenerational activities, and use of ceremonies for health. Native Americans have norms about not telling others what to do, indicating that different strategies to increase physical activity are needed. In addition, many do not think physical activity is normal. Incorporating Indian music and pow-wow dances has been done in one Native American "Celebrate Fitness" program to make activity a source of motivation and pride (Brown & Kraft, 2008). Asians and Pacific Islanders value collectivism, intergenerational living, and respect for elders. Group physical activity participation, such as dance and martial arts, are potential interventions for this population.

In summary, physical activity programs should be built into the cultural practices of the community (Brown & Kraft, 2008). The program should blend into community activities without changing social norms and community values. Intergenerational approaches, which include children as well as elders, are also recommended. The preferences of the community are respected and incorporated into program, and assets are emphasized. Programs should be flexible in accommodating the culture, offering choices to the extent possible. These steps empower diverse communities to take an active role in promoting the health of its members through physical activity.

Recommendations have also been suggested to address the built environment in low-income diverse communities (Floyd, Taylor, & Whitt-Glover, 2009). First, identify the most critical environmental needs and social variables. Second, determine how the environmental factors can be modified through policy, management, or programming changes, taking culture in to consideration. Last, ensure adequate representation of community members using community-based participatory methods. Stakeholders should be community members as well as members of community organizations. Involve stakeholders in all phases of development, implementation, and evaluation. These steps will help to ensure success in changing the built environment to positively influence physical activity in low-income communities.

OPPORTUNITIES IN PHYSICAL ACTIVITY RESEARCH

More research is needed to better understand how to tailor exercise programs to the needs of diverse populations. Particular focus should be placed on developing and testing interventions that assist very young children to adopt physical activity as enjoyable and rewarding. Interventions to prevent the decrease in physical activity during adolescence also needs further study. Focusing on development of healthy behaviors rather than behavior change is critical; after behaviors are established in youth, they are highly resistant to change. Additional suggestions for future research include the following:

1. Describe family and environmental influences during early childhood that promote or inhibit the development of physically active lifestyles.
2. Test multiple levels of socio-ecological model to promote physical activity in low-income communities.
3. Test the effects of changing the built environment in rural communities on physical activity in older adults.
4. Develop and test strategies to promote the adoption and maintenance of physical activity for low-income sedentary women across the life span.
5. Investigate the interaction of genetic makeup, environment, and behavior on the adoption and maintenance of physical activity.
6. Test the long-term effectiveness of family interventions to increase physical activity for children and parents.
7. Test the effectiveness of changing national policies to promote physical activity on the health of the community.
8. Develop and test community level measure to assess socio-ecological concepts and built environments.

CONSIDERATIONS FOR PRACTICE TO PROMOTE PHYSICAL ACTIVITY

This chapter emphasizes approaches for increasing physical activity. This information can guide nurses in counseling persons of all ages to adopt regular physical activity. Within any given age, gender, or cultural group, nurses should start by assessing the client's level of physical activity. For example, when working with children, the nurse should assess patterns of physical activity; preferred activities; perceptions of barriers to being active; availability of active parents, siblings, and friends; access to safe recreational facilities; and time spent outdoors. Counseling should assist children and adolescents to select activities they enjoy and not focus solely on competitive sports. Children should be encouraged to engage in activities that can be carried into adulthood and are easily incorporated into their daily life year-round. Appropriate safety equipment should be used to prevent injuries, and youth should be counseled to avoid use of any anabolic steroids. By offering simple recommendations to children and parents, nurses play a key role in promoting lifelong physical activity.

Adult clients should be asked about their physical activity habits at work, at home, and during leisure time to determine if these activities are sufficient to confer health benefits. Adults should be assisted in planning a program of physical activity that is medically safe, enjoyable, convenient, realistic, and structured to achieve self-selected goals. Routine monitoring, follow-up, and booster sessions are essential to assist clients in maintaining their exercise programs. Home exercise programs may work for some adults, whereas for others structured programs may need to be offered at work sites or convenient community locations. Group activities may be particularly appealing to adults who prefer the social support and comradeship of group programs. For older adults, current health status, existing medical conditions, disabilities, fear of injury, and preferences need to be assessed.

Nurses should consider developing or using existing computer-based tailoring programs to optimize physical activity. Assessment and counseling should be followed up with mail, email, or telephone calls at periodic intervals. These contacts should focus on providing appropriate strategies to increase or maintain activity and overcome barriers to being active that they have encountered.

The nurse should collaborate with the health care team to establish systems that will facilitate regular physical activity counseling for all clients. Physical activity components of health promotion and prevention systems should consist of screening systems to assess patterns of physical activity, agency guidelines for physical activity counseling, chart reminders for counseling at client visits, relevant client education materials, and follow-up protocols to reinforce interventions. When health care agencies systematize counseling protocols, physical activity counseling is much more likely to be an integral part of care by all health professionals.

Summary

Nurses, as key health professionals, must assume responsibility for using evidence-based knowledge to assist clients to develop lifelong habits of physical activity. Physical activity must be an integral part of everyday life to have optimum effects on health. Evidence promotes focusing on multiple levels in the environment as well as individual behaviors to promote leisure-time physical activity. Maintaining physical fitness can be enjoyable and rewarding for persons of all ages and contributes significantly to extending longevity and improving the quality of life.

Learning Activities

1. Review the guidelines for promoting physical activity in children. Develop an exercise plan for a healthy child, 8 years of age. Tailor the plan to a sedentary child and describe steps and activities needed to reach the recommended activity guidelines.
2. Apply the recommended steps for physical activity programs for diverse populations to a low-income cultural group of your choice. Outline how you would ensure that the program is sensitive to gender (females), age (persons aged 65 years and over), and the cultural values of the community.
3. Develop a plan to promote physical activity for workers employed by Wal-Mart. Describe work site and leisure-time strategies to enable them to meet the national physical activity guidelines.
4. Find the percentage and estimated cost of obesity for all racial/ethnic groups in your region on the CDC Web site listed at the end of the chapter.

Selected Web Sites

2008 Physical Activity Guidelines for Americans
http://health.gov/paguidelines

President's Council on Physical Fitness and Sports
http://www.presidentschallenge.org

National Institutes of Health
http://nihseniorhealth.gov/exercise.html

Centers for Disease Control and Prevention, Division of Nutrition and Physical Activity
http://www.cdc.gov/nccdphp/dnpa/physical/index.htm

Centers for Disease Control and Prevention Division of Adolescent and School Health
http://cdc.gov/HealthyYouth/physicalactivity

U.S. Preventive Services Task Force (USPSTF)
http://www.ahrq.gov/clinic/uspstf/uspsphys.htm

American College of Sports Medicine
http://www.acsm.org

American Heart Association
http://www.americanheart.org/catalog/Health_catpage9.html

Mayo Clinic Rochester Aerobic Exercise and Fitness Guidelines
http://www.mayo.edu:80/cv/wwwpg_cv/cv-whc/mc1952/mc1952.htm

National Association for Sports and Physical Education [NASPE]
http://www.aahperd.org/naspe/template.cfm?template=toddlers.html
First Ever Physical Activity Guidelines for Infants & Toddlers

Statistics Related to Overweight and Obesity
www.niddk.nih.gov/health/nutrit/pubs/statobes

References

Aldana, S. G., Merrill, R. M., Price, K., Hardy, A., & Hager, R. (2005). Financial impact of a comprehensive multisite workplace health promotion program. *Preventive Medicine, 40,* 131–137.

Beets, M. W., Beighle, A., Erwin H. E., & Huberry, J. L. (2009). After-school program impact on physical activity: A meta-analysis. *American Journal of Preventive Medicine, 36*(5), 527–537.

Bennett, R., & Sothern, M. S. (2009). Diet, exercise, behavior: The promise and limits of lifestyle change. *Seminars in Pediatric Surgery, 18,* 152–158.

Bergeman, C. S., & Ong, A. D. (2007). Behavioral genetics. In J. E. Birren (Ed.), *Encyclopedia of Gerontology*, (2nd ed., pp. 149–160). New York: Elsevier Science.

Bovell-Benjamin, A. C., Hathorn, C. S., Ibraim, S., & Bromfield, E. M. (2009). Healthy food choices and physical activity opportunities in two contrasting Alabama cities. *Health & Place, 15,* 429–438.

Brawler, L. B., Rejeski, W. J., & King, A. G. (2003). Promoting physical activity for older adults: The challenge of changing behavior. *American Journal of Preventive Medicine, 25*(3Sii), 172–183.

Brown, L. D., & Kraft, M. K. (2008). Active living as an institutional challenge: Lessons from the Robert Wood Johnson Foundation's "Celebrate Fitness" program. *Journal of Health Politics, Policy and Law, 32,* 497–523.

Brown, W. J., Burton, N. W., & Rowan, P. J. (2007). Updating the evidence on physical activity and health in women. *American Journal of Preventive Medicine, 35,* 404–411.

Bryan, A., Hutchinson, K. E., Seals, D. R., & Allen, D. L. (2007). A transdisciplinary model integrating genetics, physiological, and psychological correlates of voluntary exercise. *Health Psychology, 26,* 30–39.

Cardon, G., Labarque, V., Smits, D., & de Bourdeaudhuij, H. (2009). Promoting physical activity at the pre-school playground: The effects of providing markings and play equipment. *Preventive Medicine, 48,* 335–340.

Clement, K. (2006). Genetics and human obesity. *C.R. Biologies, 329,* 608–622.

Coleman, K. J., Rosenberg, D. E., Conway, T. L., Sallis, J. F., & Saelens, B. E. (2008). Physical activity, weight status, and neighborhood characteristics of dog walkers. *Preventive Medicine, 47,* 309–312.

Cox, K. L., Burke, V., Beilin, L. J., Derbyshire, A. J., Grove, J. R., Blanksby, B. A., et al. (2008). Short and long-term adherence to swimming and walking programs in older women: The Sedentary Women Exercise Adherence Trial (SWEAT 2). *Preventive Medicine, 46,* 511–517.

Crossman, A., Sullivan, D. A., & Benin, M. (2006). The family environment and American adolescents' risk of obesity as young adults. *Social Science & Medicine, 63,* 2255–2267.

de Geus, E., & de Moor, M. (2008). A genetic perspective on the association between exercise and mental health. *Mental Health and Physical Activity, 1*, 53–61.

Dishman, R. K., DeJoy, D. M., Wilson, M. G., & Vandenberg, R. J. (2009). Move to improve: A randomized workplace trial to increase physical activity. *American Journal of Preventive Medicine, 36*, 133–141.

Floyd, M. F., Taylor, W. C., & Whitt-Glover, M. (2009). Measurement of park and recreation environments that support physical activity in low-income communities of color: Highlights of challenges and recommendations. *American Journal of Preventive Medicine, 36*(4S), S156–S160.

Giles-Corti, B. (2006). People or places: Which should be the target? *Journal of Science and Medicine in Sports, 9*(5), 357–366.

Gordon, C. (2004). Cultural approaches to promoting physical activity in older adults. *The Journal on Active Aging, 4*(1), 22–28.

Halldin, M., Rosell, M., de Faire, U., & Hellenius, M. L. (2007). The metabolic syndrome: Prevalence and association to leisure time and work related physical activity in 60 year old men and women. *Nutrition, Metabolism, & Cardiovascular Diseases, 17*, 349–357.

Haskell, W. L., Lee, I., Pate, R. R., Powell, K. E., Blair, S. N., Franklin, B. A., et al. (2007). Physical activity and public health: Updated recommendation for adults from the American College of Sports Medicine and the American Heart Association. *Circulation, 117*, 1081–1093.

Hoebeke, R. (2008). Low-income women's perceived barriers to physical activity: Focus groups results. *Applied Nursing Research, 21*, 60–65.

Hume, C., Timperio, A., Salmon, J., Carver, A., & Giles-Corti, B. (2009). Walking and cycling to school: Predictors of increases among children and adolescents. *American Journal of Preventive Medicine, 36*, 195-200.

Kahn, J. A., Huang, B., Gillman, M. W., Field, A. E., Austin, S. B., Colditz, G. A., et al. (2008). Patterns and determinants of physical activity in U.S. adolescents. *Journal of Adolescent Health, 42*, 369–377.

Kelly, C. M., Hoechner, C. M., Baker, E. A., Ramirez, L. K., & Brownson, R. C. (2006). Promoting physical activity in communities: Approaches for successful evaluation of programs and policies. *Evaluation and Program Planning, 29*, 280–292.

Keyserling, T. C., Hodge, C. D., Jilcott, S. B., Johnston, L. F., Garcia, B. A., Gross, M. D., et al. (2008). Randomized trial of clinic-based, community-supported, lifestyle intervention to improve physical activity and diet: The North Carolina enhanced WISEWOMAN project. *Preventive Medicine, 46*, 499–510.

Kumanyika, S. K. (2008). Environmental influences on childhood obesity: Ethnic and cultural influences in context. *Physiology & Behavior, 94*, 61–70.

Lee, R. E., & Cubbin, C. (2009). Striding toward social justice: The ecologic milieu of physical activity. *Exercise and Sports Sciences Reviews, 37*, 10–17.

Lubans, D. R., Morgan, P. J., & Tudor-Locke, C. (2009). A systematic review of studies using pedometers to promote physical activity among youth. *Preventive Medicine, 48*, 307–315.

Madsen, K. A., McCulloch, C. E., & Crawford, P. B. (2009). Parent modeling: Perceptions of parents' physical activity predict girls' activity throughout adolescence. *Journal of Pediatrics, 154*, 278–283.

Maia, J. A., Thomas, M., & Beunen, G. (2002). Genetic factors in physical activity levels: A twin study. *American Journal of Preventive Medicine, 23*(2S), 87–91.

Marshall, S. J., Levy, S. S., Tudor-Locke, C. E., Kolkhorst, F. W., Wooten, K. M., Ji, M., et al. (2009). Translating physical activity recommendations into a pedometer-based step goal: 300 steps in 30 minutes. *American Journal of Preventive Medicine, 36*, 410–415.

Martinson, B. C., Crain, A. L., Sherwood, N. E., Hayes, M., Pronk, N. P., & O'Connor, P. J. (2008). Maintaining physical activity among older adults: Six month outcomes of the Keep Active Minnesota randomized controlled trial. *Preventive Medicine, 46*, 111–119.

Mummery, W. K., & Brown, W. J. (2009). Whole of community physical activity interventions: Easier said than done. *British Journal of Sports Medicine, 43*, 39–43.

Muto, T., Hashimoto, M., Haruyama, Y., & Fukuda, H. (2006). Evaluation of a workplace health promotion program to improve cardiovascular disease risk factors in sales representatives. *International Congress Series, 1294,* 131–134.

Naito, M., Nakayama, T., Okamura, T., Miura, K., Yanagita, M., Fujieda, Y., et al. (2008). Effect of a 4-year workplace-based physical activity intervention program on the blood lipid profiles of participating employees' health promotion (HIPOP-OHP) study. *Atherosclerosis, 197,* 784–790.

National Association for Sport and Physical Education (NASPE). (2002). Active start: A statement of physical activity guidelines for children birth to five years. Retrieved from http://www.NASPE.org

Nelson, M. E., Rejeski, W. J., Blair, S. N., Duncan, P. W., Judge, J. O., King, A. C., et al. (2007) physical activity and public health in older adults: Recommendations from the American College of Sports Medicine and the American Heart Association. *Circulation, 116,* 1094–1105.

O'Connor, T. M., Jago, R., & Baranowski, T. (2009). Engaging parents to increase youth physical activity: A systematic review. *American Journal of Preventive Medicine, 37,* 141–149.

Olden, K. (2009). Human health and disease: Interaction between the genome and the environment. In F. W. Huntington & G. S. Ginsburg (Eds.), *Genomic and Personalized Medicine,* (pp. 47–59). New York: Elsevier.

Opdenacker, J., Boen, P., Coorevits, N., & Delecluse, C. (2008). Effectiveness of a lifestyle intervention and a structured exercise intervention in older adults. *Preventive Medicine, 46,* 518–524.

Owens, N., Glanz, K., Sallis, J. F., & Kelder, S. H. (2006). Evidence-based approaches to dissemination and diffusion of physical activity interventions. *American Journal of Preventive Medicine, 31*(4S), S35–S44.

Pronk, N. P., & Kottke, T. E. (2009). Physical activity promotion as a strategic corporate priority to improve worker health and business performance. *Preventive Medicine 49*(4), 316–321.

Racette, S. B., Deusinger, S. S., Inman, C. L., Burlis, T. L., Highstein, C. R., Buskirk, T. D., et al. (2009). Worksite opportunities for Wellness (WOW): Effects on cardiovascular disease risk factors after 1 year. *Preventive Medicine 49*(2–3), 108–114.

Reger-Nash, B., Bauman, A., Cooper, L., Chey, T., & Simon, K. J. (2006). Evaluating

communitywide walking interventions. *Evaluation and Program Planning, 29,* 251–259.

Rosenberg, D., Kerr, J., Sallis, J. F., Patrick, K., Moore, D. J., & King, A. (2009). Feasibility and outcomes of a multilevel place-based walking intervention for seniors: A pilot study. *Health & Place, 15,* 173–179.

Roux, L., Pratt, M., Tengs, T., Yore, M., Yamagawa, T., Van den Bos, J., et al. (2008). Cost effectiveness of community-based physical activity interventions. *American Journal of Preventive Medicine, 35,* 578–588.

Sallis, J. F. (2009). Measuring physical activity environments: A brief history. *American Journal of Preventive Medicine, 36,* S86–S92.

Sallis, J. F., Bowles, H., Bauman, A., Ainsworth, B., Bull, F., Craig, C., et al. (2009a). Neighborhood environments and physical activity among adults in 11 countries. *American Journal of Preventive Medicine, 36,* 484–490.

Sallis, J. F., Saelens, B. E., Frank, L. D., Conway, T. L., Slymen, D. J., Cain, K. L., et al. (2009b). Neighborhood built environments and income: Examining multiple health outcomes. *Social Science & Medicine, 68,* 1285–1293.

Sallis, J. F., Story, M., & Lou, D. (2009c). Study designs and analytic strategies for environmental and policy research on obesity, physical activity, and diet: Recommendations from a meeting of experts. *American Journal of Preventive Medicine, 36*(2 Suppl. 2), S72–S77.

Simpson, J. M., Oldenburg, B., Owen, N., Harris, D., Dobbins, T., Salmon, A., et.al. (2000). The Australian National Workplace Health Project: design and baseline findings. *Preventive Medicine, 31*(3), 249–260.

Talbot, L. A., Morrell, C. H., Fleg, J. L., & Metter, E. J. (2007). Changes in leisure time physical activity and risk of all-cause mortality in men and women: The Baltimore Longitudinal Study of Aging. *Preventive Medicine, 45,* 169–176.

Trost, S. G., & Loprinzi, P. D. (2008). Exercise-Promoting health lifestyles in children and adolescents. *Journal of Clinical Lipidology, 2,* 162–168.

Tucker, P., & Gilliland, J. (2007). The effect of season and weather on physical activity: A systematic review, *Public Health, 121,* 909–922.

Tudor-Locke, C. (2003). *Manpo-Kei: The art and science of step counting: How to be naturally active and lose weight!* New Bern, NC: Trafford.

U.S. Department of Health and Human Services [USDHHS]. (2008a). 2008 Physical activity guidelines for Americans, Retrieved from http://www.health.gov/paguidelines

USDHHS National Center for Chronic Disease Prevention and Health Promotion. (2008b). Chronic disease overview. Retrieved from http://www.cdc.gov/needphp/overview .htm

Wamp, Z. (2009). Creating a culture of movement: The benefits of promoting physical activity in schools and the workplace. *American Journal of Preventive Medicine, 36*(2S), S56–S57.

Wendel-Vos, W., Dutman, A. E., Verschuren, M., Ronickers, E. T., Ament, A., van Assema, P., et al. (2009). Lifestyle factors of a five-year community intervention program: The Hartslag Limburg intervention. *American Journal of Preventive Medicine, 37*, 50–56.

Wilcox, S., Dowda, M., Leviton, L. C., Bartlett-Prescott, J., Bazzarre, T., Campbell-Voytal, K., et al. (2008). Active for Life: Final results from the translation of two physical activity programs. *American Journal of Preventive Medicine, 35*, 340–351.

Williams, C. L., Carter, B. J., Kibbe, D. L., & Dennison, D. (2009). Increasing physical activity in preschool: A pilot study to evaluate animal trackers. *Journal of Nutrition Education and Behavior, 41*, 47–52.

Wolch, J., Wilson, J. P., & Fehrenbach, J. (2005). Parks and parks funding in Los Angeles: An equity mapping analysis. *Urban Geography, 26*, 4–35.

Yancey, A. K., Ory, M. G., & Davis, S. M. (2006). Dissemination of physical activity promotion interventions in underserved populations. *American Journal of Preventive Medicine, 31*(4S), S82–S91.

Zaga, S., Briss, P. A., & Harris, K. W. (Eds.) (2005). *The community guide to preventive services: What works to promote health?* New York: Oxford University Press.

CHAPTER 7

Nutrition and Health Promotion

OBJECTIVES

1. Review the U.S. federal dietary guidelines for healthy eating.
2. Describe MyPyramid and its role in implementing guidelines for healthy eating.
3. Examine evidenced-based factors that influence eating behaviors.
4. Describe the nutritional needs of infants and children, adolescents, and older adults.
5. Examine factors related to overweight/obesity and intervention goals in weight loss.

Outline

- **Promoting Healthy Diets and Nutrition**
  A. Nutritional Health of Americans
  B. Dietary Guidelines for Americans
  C. MyPyramid: A Personalized Approach to Healthy Eating
  D. Issues in Under-Nutrition
- **Factors Influencing Eating Behavior**
  A. Genetic–Biologic Factors
  B. Psychological Factors
  C. Socioeconomic and Cultural Factors
  D. Environmental Factors
  E. Health Policy Factors
- **Nutritional Needs of Special Populations**
  A. Infants and Children
  B. Adolescents
  C. Older Adults
- **Promotion of Dietary Change**
- **Interventions to Promote Dietary Change**
- **Research-Tested Intervention Programs (RTIPs)**
  A. Promoting Healthy Living: Assessing More Effects (PHLAME)
  B. Body and Soul

Good nutrition is one of the primary determinants of good health. An unhealthy diet and lack of activity are two major risk factors responsible for the global increase in obesity and other noncommunicable disease. The role of nutrition has expanded from a focus on nutrients needed to feed populations to its role in promoting health and preventing disease. The emphasis on healthy nutrition for children and adolescents is critical, as diet and eating behaviors that develop during these years tend to persist throughout life. Good nutrition is influenced by multiple factors, making successful promotion of optimal diets a challenge. Policy makers and health promotion experts acknowledge the need for multilevel changes, including programs that target individuals and communities, and policies that are aimed at changing the environment and food industry.

PROMOTING HEALTHY DIETS AND NUTRITION

Chronic diseases, such as coronary artery disease, cardiovascular disease, cancer, diabetes, and obesity, account for about 60% of deaths and almost half of the burden of disease worldwide (World Health Organization [WHO], 2002). However, a large percentage of these diseases could be avoided, as they are either initiated or accelerated by unhealthy nutrition in addition to other etiologies. Food and activity choices are influenced by food preferences, portion sizes, and inactivity, as well as culture, socioeconomic status, advertising, the built (human-made) environment, and other "obesogenic" (unhealthy eating) factors (McKinnon, Reedy, Handy, & Rodgers, 2009). Successful dietary change first requires an understanding of the national dietary guidelines and the MyPyramid approach to healthy eating.

Nutritional Health of Americans

The obesity epidemic is responsible for many of the health problems of Americans and for the increasing cost of health care in America. The incidence of chronic disease in young people is increasing, as the obesity rate in this population rises (Centers for Disease Control and Prevention, 2009). In *F as in Fat: How Obesity Policies Are Failing in America* (Robert Wood Johnson Foundation, 2009), 8 of the 10 states with the highest percentage of obese people are in the South. In addition, 30 or more percent of children in 30 states are overweight or obese.

Americans rank prevention as the most important health reform priority. The shift of Americans' support of prevention over the past two decades is impressive, increasing from 45% in 1986 to 59% in 2009 (Trust for America's Health, 2009). Yet obesity rates in adults and children have doubled and tripled respectively over the past 30 years. Overweight and obesity levels in America and the majority of developed countries are major health concerns (Kaila & Raman, 2008; Robert Wood Johnson Foundation, 2009).

Current evidence suggests that distribution of body fat may be more significant that quantity of fat, represented by the body mass index (BMI) (Kragelund & Omland, 2005). Specifically, increased abdominal fat, measured by waist circumference and waist–hip ratio, has been associated with metabolic risk factors, even in high-risk individuals with a BMI below 30 (BMI greater than 30 is considered obese). Individuals with a large muscle mass, such as body builders, may have a higher BMI, but less fat. Both BMI and waist circumference have been shown to be clinically useful in identifying adolescents at risk for later cardiovascular disease onset (Messiah, Arheart, Lipschultz, & Miller, 2008). However, in older adults, waist circumference is a more relevant measure, due to age-related changes in body size and composition that limit the usefulness of BMI in this population (Srikanthan, Seeman, & Karlamangla, 2009). This finding is consistent with white and black adult men and women younger than 65 years, in which waist-to-hip ratio had the strongest association with cardiovascular disease and mortality (Gelber et al., 2008; Reis et al., 2008).

Findings consistently indicate that waist circumference and waist-to-hip ratios are better predictors of risk than BMI. Knowing one's waist circumference is a primary step in knowing one's risk of disease. However, BMI remains an important screening tool for excess body weight. It is important to keep in mind that BMI and waist measurements are indirect measures and should be used to get a better picture of the individual's health risk, along with an assessment of lifestyle, the presence of other chronic diseases, other risk factors, and family history.

Dietary Guidelines for Americans

The *Dietary Guidelines for Americans* are published every five years, by the U.S. Department of Agriculture and U.S. Health and Human Services, and form the basis for the federal nutrition policy. The guidelines focus on dietary advice for Americans aged 2 years and older and provide information about how to reduce risk for chronic disease with good dietary habits. The *Dietary Guidelines for Americans 2005* remain the current guidelines until the updated guidelines are published in fall 2010 (http://www.cnpp .usda.gov/DGAsMeeting3.htm).

An important component of each five-year review of the dietary guidelines is the analysis of new scientific information. The latest research is summarized and synthesized into recommendations for a pattern of eating that can be adopted by the public. A premise of the *Guidelines for Americans* is that food should provide all of the nutrients that an individual needs to be healthy. Although dietary supplements and fortified foods may be useful sources for one or two nutrients, they cannot replace a healthy diet. The 2005 guidelines place greater emphasis on decreased calorie consumption and increased physical activity to maintain a healthy body weight. The dietary guidelines Web site is consumer friendly and offers important information and downloadable materials (see http://www.DietaryGuidelines.gov).

Two examples of eating patterns that are used to model the *Dietary Guidelines for Americans* are the U.S. Department of Agriculture Food Guide (http://usda .gov/cnpp/pyramid.html) and the Dietary Approaches to Stop Hypertension (DASH) (http://www.nhlbi.nih.gov/). Originally developed to study eating patterns to prevent and treat hypertension, the DASH eating plan is a balanced plan consistent with the dietary guidelines. Both of these eating plans illustrate healthy ways to eat.

The *Guidelines for Americans* are used by policy makers, health care providers, nutritionists, and educators to develop educational materials, and design and implement nutrition-related programs. Modifications are necessary to integrate the food preferences of different ethnic and racial groups, vegetarians, and other special groups. The guidelines are based on a 2000-calorie level, but the recommended intake will vary according to age, gender, and activity level. The recommendations are interrelated and all of them should be followed. However, following just some of the recommendations will have positive health outcomes. The guideline's basic principles for healthy eating are shown in Table 7–1 and Table 7–2 compares the saturated fat of foods.

The American Diabetic Association also has published nutrition recommendations and interventions for the primary prevention of diabetes (American Diabetes Association, 2008). Lifestyle changes for moderate weight loss—which include reduction of calories and intake of dietary fats, regular physical activity, encouragement of at least 14 g of dietary fiber/100 kcal and foods containing whole grains daily, and a greater intake of low-glycemic index foods rich in fiber—are recommended for adults and adolescents at risk for type 2 diabetes. Monitoring carbohydrates is a key recommendation for achieving glycemic control in persons with diabetes as well. Dietary fat should be limited to less than 7% of total calories. Although there is insufficient evident to suggest modifying usual protein intake, high-protein diets are not recommended. These guidelines are applicable to all who wish to follow a healthy diet (see http://www.diabetes.org).

Some scientists suggest that dietary guidelines share some responsibility for the obesity epidemic in America. When dietary guidelines recommended that people eat less dietary saturated fat, sugar consumption increased, people doubled their caloric intake, and obesity increased. According to some scientists, the message should have been formulated to promote less caloric intake, reduce portion size, and increase physical activity (Marantz, Bird, & Alderman, 2008). However, other scientists counter that as science has progressed, it is now evident that both saturated fat and calorie intake are important, so a change has been made to address both fat intake and calories

---

TABLE 7–1   Nutrition and Your Health: Dietary Guidelines for Americans

1. Consume a variety of foods within and among the basic food groups while staying within energy needs.
2. Control calorie intake to manage body weight.
3. Be physically active every day.
4. Increase daily intake of fruits and vegetables, whole grains, and nonfat or low-fat milk and milk products.
5. Choose fats wisely for good health.
6. Choose carbohydrates wisely for good health.
7. Choose and prepare foods with little salt.
8. If you drink alcoholic beverages, do so in moderation.
9. Keep food safe to eat.

Source: U.S. Department of Health and Human Services, U.S. Department of Agriculture. Dietary guidelines for Americans 2005. Retrieved from http://www.healthierus.gov/dietaryguidelines/dga2005/report/HTML/A_ExecSummary.htm

TABLE 7–2   A Comparison of Saturated Fat in Some Foods

Food Category	Portion	Saturated Fat Content in Grams	Calories
Cheese			
Regular cheddar cheese	1 oz.	6.0	114
Low-fat cheddar cheese	1 oz.	1.2	49
Ground beef			
Regular ground beef (25% fat)	3 oz. (cooked)	6.1	236
Extra lean ground beef (5% fat)	3 oz. (cooked)	2.6	148
Milk			
Whole milk (3.24%)	1 cup	4.6	146
Low-fat (1%) milk	1 cup	1.5	102
Breads			
Croissant (med)	1 medium	6.6	231
Bagel, oat bran (4")	1 medium	0.2	227
Frozen desserts			
Regular ice cream	½ cup	4.9	145
Frozen yogurt	½ cup	2.0	110
Table spreads			
Butter	1 tsp.	2.4	34
Trans-free soft margarine	1 tsp.	0.7	25
Chicken			
Fried chicken (leg)	3 oz. (cooked)	3.3	212
Chicken breast	3 oz. (cooked)	0.9	140
Fish			
Fried fish	3 oz.	2.8	195
Baked fish	3 oz.	1.5	129

Source: U.S. Department of Health and Human Services, U.S. Department of Agriculture. Dietary guidelines for Americans 2005. Retrieved from http://www.health.gov/dietaryguidelines/dga2005/report/HTML/table_e2.htm

(Woolf & Nestle, 2008). Dietary guidelines are one important strategy to provide the best science-based information available to improve nutrition and diet.

MyPyramid: A Personalized Approach to Healthy Eating

MyPyramid translates the *Dietary Guidelines for Americans 2005* into messages that consumers can more easily understand and practice. MyPyramid, shown in Figure 7–1, replaced the widely recognized nutrition education tool *Food Guide Pyramid* in 2005. MyPyramid moves away from the one-size-fits-all approach of the *Food Guide Pyramid.* Interactive tools and personalized recommendations are offered to help individuals make changes (Britten, Haven, & Davis, 2006; Britten, Marcoe, Yamini, & Davis, 2006). The MyPyramid Web site is an excellent teaching resource for nurses and health care professionals as well as the lay public, as it offers information for preschoolers (2–5 years), children (6–11 years), mothers, and the general population; information to develop a personalized plan; weight loss information; dietary analysis; and a tip-of-the-day section. Information can be downloaded on MP3 players, and

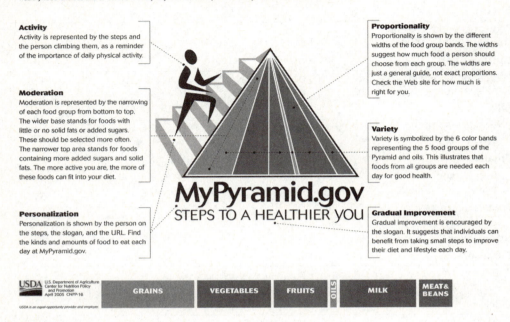

Anatomy of MyPyramid

One size doesn't fit all
USDA's new MyPyramid symbolizes a personalized approach to healthy eating and physical activity. The symbol has been designed to be simple. It has been developed to remind consumers to make healthy food choices and to be active every day. The different parts of the symbol are described below.

Activity
Activity is represented by the steps and the person climbing them, as a reminder of the importance of daily physical activity.

Moderation
Moderation is represented by the narrowing of each food group from bottom to top. The wider base stands for foods with little or no solid fats or added sugars. These should be selected more often. The narrower top area stands for foods containing more added sugars and solid fats. The more active you are, the more of these foods can fit into your diet.

Personalization
Personalization is shown by the person on the steps, the slogan, and the URL. Find the kinds and amounts of food to eat each day at MyPyramid.gov.

Proportionality
Proportionality is shown by the different widths of the food group bands. The widths suggest how much food a person should choose from each group. The widths are just a general guide, not exact proportions. Check the Web site for how much is right for you.

Variety
Variety is symbolized by the 6 color bands representing the 5 food groups of the Pyramid and oils. This illustrates that foods from all groups are needed each day for good health.

Gradual Improvement
Gradual improvement is encouraged by the slogan. It suggests that individuals can benefit from taking small steps to improve their diet and lifestyle each day.

MyPyramid.gov
STEPS TO A HEALTHIER YOU

USDA
U.S. Department of Agriculture
Center for Nutrition Policy and Promotion
April 2005 CNPP-16

USDA is an equal opportunity provider and employer.

GRAINS   VEGETABLES   FRUITS   OILS   MILK   MEAT & BEANS

FIGURE 7–1   Anatomy of MyPyramid: Steps to a Healthier You

MyPyramid can be followed on Twitter (http://www.twitter.com/MyPyramid). The interactive Web site is also available (see http://www.mypyramid.gov/tips _resources/index.html).

Issues in Under-Nutrition

Although the major problem in American is over nutrition, under-nutrition is a problem in some segments of the population. Under-nutrition has been documented in persons living below the poverty line, as well as children, adolescents, and the elderly.

Iron deficiency, the world's most common nutritional deficiency, is associated with multiple health problems. Chronic iron deficiency in childhood has an adverse effect on growth and development. Iron deficiency anemia is commonly caused by a decrease iron intake due to a diet insufficient in iron. The correction of iron deficiency that is accompanied with anemia is important to correct developmental delays, impaired behavior, diminished intellectual functioning, and decreased resistance to infection (Trost, Bergfield, & Calogeras, 2006).

Inadequate calcium intake in youth, another health problem caused by under-nutrition, may result in failure to attain peak bone mass during the years of bone mineralization (up to age 20 years). This is thought to be a later predisposition for osteoporosis (Gao, Wilde, Lichtenstein, & Tucker, 2006).

Eating disorders such as anorexia nervosa and bulimia are nutritional threats to the health of youth, particularly young white females. These diagnoses are rare in black females. The incidence of anorexia and bulimia stabilized during the 1990s, and the occurrence of bulimia continues to decrease. Anorexia nervosa affects about 1 in 100 adolescents between 12 and 18 years of age (U.S. Department of Health and Human Services [DHHS], Centers for Disease Control and Prevention, National Center for Health Statistics, 2008). Many of the physical complications of eating disorders are secondary to malnutrition with osteoporosis and cardiac changes being significant problems (Hoek, 2006; Winston, 2008). Promising prevention programs are reducing risk factors and eating pathologies, resulting in better outcomes (Stice, Shaw, & Marti, 2007).

Under-nutrition is also a major problem in the elderly. In nursing home settings, the elderly may experience weight loss due to multiple issues, including loss of appetite and decreased ability to feed themselves. Undernourished nursing home patients (defined by BMI, weight loss, and anthropometric measurements) require increased nutritional supplements to prevent recurring infections and premature death (Baker, 2007; Furman, 2006). The assessment of the nutritional status of the elderly is critical to intervene to restore nutritional adequacy and healthy aging.

FACTORS INFLUENCING EATING BEHAVIOR

Making wise food choices is a cornerstone of good health. However, the multi-causal nature of eating behaviors makes change a challenge. Eating behaviors are an integral part of individual, family, and community lifestyles. A strong cultural component adds to the difficulty of making modifications. Effective changes require consideration of all factors that influence eating behavior, the use of appropriate behavior-change strategies, and environmental and policy changes. Eating behaviors are influenced by multiple factors, including genetic–biologic, psychologic, socioeconomic, cultural, environmental, and health policy factors.

Genetic–Biologic Factors

Food intake and energy expenditure are controlled and kept in balance by complex neural systems. Humans have the ability to store a tremendous energy supply (fat) for later use. This ability has resulted in one of the major health risks for many human populations—obesity. The effectiveness of our neural system is seen in the body's ability to defend the lower limits of body weight by initiating external and internal nutrient-depletion signals, such as increased appetite, foraging, and stimulating the autonomic and endocrine systems to go into an internal energy saving mode.

The extra-hypothalamic brain structures that are responsible for reward, emotions, decision making, and choice (i.e., type of food intake) appear to assist the hypothalamus regulators in managing inadequate nutrition, but not over-nutrition. The challenge is to understand why the neural system does not respond to over-nutrition as it does to under-nutrition (Morrison & Berthoud, 2007; Wells, 2006). The predisposition to overeat may be due to inability of the complex neural system to adapt to environmental changes (Morrison & Berthoud, 2007).

Heredity explains more than half of the variation in weight among individuals, indicating why some individuals gain weight and others do not (Bloom, 2007). There are numerous regulatory mechanisms in the body and their redundancy speaks to the biological importance of body weight regulation and to the futility of managing obesity without considering the neuro-regulatory determinants of energy balance.

The exposure to the food environment—such as the availability of fast food, take away meals, and convenience foods—makes people with genetic risk more susceptible to eating unhealthy foods. Obese individuals may have an inappropriately high set point in the brain that allows them to overeat without receiving the "full" message. Along with reduced energy expenditure, overweight or obesity develops (Kelly, Yang, Chen, Reynolds, & He, 2008).

Considerable research is underway to understand the physiological and cellular mechanisms that regulate energy balance and the events that converge to result in obesity. Multiple factors regulate eating behaviors include recently discovered hormones and genes. In the mid-1990s, the "ob" (obesity) gene was isolated from adipose tissue and its protein product, Leptin, was also identified. Leptin, an adipocyte-derived protein hormone that circulates in the blood in proportion to whole body adipose tissue mass, is thought to serve as the signal to the brain to regulate the balance of food intake and energy expenditure (Morrison, 2008). The neurobiology of leptin is being investigated through two possible mechanisms to explain metabolic and neural disorders: leptin resistance versus central leptin insufficiency (Kalra, 2008). Both hypotheses are under investigation to clarify the role of leptin and its contribution to energy balance. Evidence shows that increased leptin sensitivity protects against obesity, whereas loss of leptin sensitivity predisposes obesity, opening the doors for potential pharmacological interventions (Morrison, 2008). In addition, leptin is undergoing investigations as a potential biomarker for childhood obesity (Venner, Lyon, & Doyle-Baker, 2006).

How genetic disposition relates to energy regulation is poorly understood, as more than 400 genes have been associated with weight regulation (Knecht, Ellger, & Levine, 2008). However, it is acknowledged that genetic disposition as well as behavior and environment all play a role in eating behaviors.

Epigenetics is study of factors that can change the way genes respond without changing the genetic code itself. Single nutrients, toxins, behaviors, or environmental changes can stimulate a chemical that mobilizes a group of molecules—called a methyl group—that attaches to the control segment of a gene. The gene is either silenced or activated, altering its intended course of activity. Scientists describe methylation "as putting gum on a light switch. The switch isn't broken, but the gum blocks its function." Methylated genes can be demethylated through nutrients, drugs, and positive life experiences (Ptak & Petronis, 2008). However, an environmental toxin, a single nutrient deficient, or a negative behavioral experience can stay dormant and cause cancer, asthma or other diseases decades later.

The link between the environment and epigenetics is largely unexplored. However, evidence has begun to show that the environment and nutrition can perturb the way genes are controlled by DNA methylation (Feil, 2006). The "nature or nurture" debate is no longer valid as the environment and genes are inextricably linked.

The biologic changes of aging have a marked effect on eating behavior. A progressive loss of taste buds on the anterior tongue occurs with age, resulting in decreased sensitivity to sweet and salty tastes. In contrast, taste buds sensitive to bitter and sour increase with age. This taste distortion may result in decreased enjoyment of food and decreased intake nutrients.

Gastric secretions may result in limited absorption of iron, calcium, and vitamin B_{12} in the elderly. Decreased gastric motility augments the need for foods high in fiber (fresh fruits, raw vegetables, whole-grain breads, and cereals) and increases the importance of water consumption to promote regularity in bowel evacuation. A decrease in basal metabolic rate with aging has also been associated with a decrease in caloric intake.

Psychological Factors

Eating, drinking, and food choices are the most commonly performed human behaviors. Although simple behaviors, they are determined by many factors, including individual, psychologic determinants. Individual factors must be addressed among persons of all ages if healthy nutritional practices are to become a reality.

Affective processes (e.g., depression, low self-esteem, and lack of personal control over one's life) influence nutritional practices. Negative emotions (e.g., anger, frustration, fear, and insecurity) may also effect the motivation to eat. Stress-related eating has been associated with weight gain. Emotions can decrease food intake in some individuals and increase food intake in others (Macht, 2008). Eating driven by emotional states provides comfort. The emotion that is producing the change in food intake must be addressed before the behavior can be modified.

Habits constitute another important determinant of eating behavior. A habit is a behavior that occurs often and is performed automatically or with little conscious awareness. Habits are performed so frequently that many cues within the environment serve as signals for the behavior. They often result in a psychological addiction to certain behaviors because they become a pervasive part of lifestyle. Such behaviors are known as *consummatory* because the response itself (eating) provides the reinforcement. People may also become psychologically addicted to the consequences of habitual behaviors such as the "energy spurt" experienced after the ingestion of highly refined sugars (e.g., doughnuts, sweet rolls, snack foods) or caffeine (e.g., sodas, coffee, energy drinks).

The public has expressed varying beliefs about the causes of obesity. The majority of 1,139 adults surveyed believed that individuals were responsible for overeating resulting in overweight and obesity (Fuemmeler, Baffi, Mâsse, Atienza, & Evans, 2007). Most respondents (66%) did not believe that obesity was caused by genes or due to a lack of knowledge of what constituted a healthy diet. Gender differences were evident, with women less likely to endorse the concept of "lack of willpower" as a contributing factor to overeating. Also, more women than men believed that the cost of healthy food was a factor in maintaining a healthy diet. The socialization processes of men and women may influence gender differences, as men often believe that they have more personal control over factors that affect their lives than women (Chipperfield & Perry, 2006). Also, women are more likely to grocery shop for the family and experience the cost of healthy food. Half of the respondents, regardless of gender, believed that society made it difficult for individuals to maintain a healthy weight; although individual responsibility is important, the opportunity to make healthy choices is not equality distributed among people. Sociological, economic, and cultural factors play dominant roles in eating behaviors and nutrition.

Socioeconomic and Cultural Factors

People exist within a social and cultural context that shapes their eating behaviors and their access to healthy foods. Many lower socioeconomic status individuals and racial/ethnic minorities believe that overeating and obesity are due to societal influences (Fuemmeler et al., 2007). Other groups who support society's major role in obesity are unemployed and nonmarried individuals, and older, retired persons who are overweight or obese.

The relationship between socioeconomic position and consumption of fast foods has been suggested as a possible reason for higher levels of obesity among individuals of low socioeconomic status (Shahar, Shai, Vardi, Shahar, & Fraser, 2005). The regular consumption of fast food (high fat, salt, and sugar; low fiber) has been associated with higher levels of overweight and obesity. Within these groups, the likelihood exists that these individuals have been exposed to situations that make it difficult to manage their weight.

Ethnic minority populations are also more likely to experience higher exposures to environmental and psychological stressors associated with discrimination, economic security, and personal safety. Food may be used for coping with the day-to-day stressors. This type of unhealthy eating may result in the disposition of abdominal fat and risks for chronic diseases, as described previously in the chapter.

Ethnicity and culture also serve as important influences on eating behavior. Attitudes toward body size and shape are culturally defined, as well as traditional uses and meanings of foods. In addition, cultural traditions exist about which foods are harmful and protective as well as how food relates to health (Kumanyika et al., 2008). Food creates social interactions and conveys symbolic meanings across cultures. Ethnic foods are a source of pride and identity for many groups and may have deep emotional meaning for individuals because of their association with their country of origin or because of fond childhood memories of holidays on which particular foods were served.

Cultural factors may contribute to patterns of obesity in childhood and youth in many U.S. minority populations (Kumanyika et al., 2008). Cultural wisdom may be strongly ingrained due to past economic deprivation, which led to a need to feast whenever food was available. High status and highly valued foods associated with survival are often red meats, sugars, and fatty foods. Larger body sizes have been associated with beauty, fertility, wealth, and power. In some cultures, overweight may be considered neutral or positive unless it is linked with a health problem, especially for women.

Suggestions for promoting healthy nutrition in diverse cultural communities include the following as well as those described in Chapter 12:

- Understand cultural beliefs about the interrelationships between food and health.
- Recognize how food consumption practices contribute to cultural identity.
- Assess the extent of acculturation to dominant-group nutritional behaviors.
- Offer nutrition or nurse consultants of similar ethnic backgrounds to clients.
- Recognize nutritional attributes of ethnic foods.
- Reinforce ethnic nutritional practices that are positive.
- Provide information on nutrient values of ethnic foods to clients.
- Work with ethnic restaurants to offer healthy choices that are acceptable.
- Incorporate healthy ethnic food choices into work site and school site cafeterias.

Sensitivity to the difficulties that ethnic groups may have in identifying the contents of foods packaged in the United States and in understanding nutrition labeling is imperative. Inability to obtain familiar foods and trying to eat unfamiliar foods may be a source of frustration and distress. Language barriers and confusing mass media messages about nutritious foods often serve as barriers to good nutrition among members of varying ethnic groups.

Environmental Factors

A population's preference for an unhealthy diet and large portions is influenced by advertising, the food environment, and other obesogenic influences. Food and nutrition environments are believed to be major contributors to obesity and chronic diseases (Glanz, 2009). Food environments include home, school, work site, and neighborhoods. The macro level food environment consists of food and agriculture policy, economics and pricing, and food marketing and advertising.

Obesogenic environments are all of the surroundings, opportunities, or conditions that promote obesity in individuals and populations (Ulijaszek, 2007). Exposure to obesogenic environments is mediated by social, political, and economic factors. Obesogenic food environments include the production, distribution, and affordability of foods that contribute to obesity. The availability of fast foods, 24-hour take-away, and home delivery has resulted in the consumption of fewer whole grains and greater high fat, high sugar foods.

The importance of the neighborhood environment as a promoter of obesity has been documented (Harrington & Elliott, 2009). Neighborhoods that discourage physical activity and have few parks and walking paths as well as a high concentration of fast food places to eat are obesogenic. Walking trails, well-maintained sidewalks, and affordable recreational facilities, as well as access to supermarkets and health-related stores, promote healthy lifestyles, compared with a neighborhood with only convenience stores and fast food restaurants. Neighborhood disparities in access to food are of concern because of the potential influence on obesity. Neighborhood socioeconomic disadvantage may also play a role in an obesogenic environment as previously described. All of these factors reinforce the complexity of geography and eating behaviors.

For individuals to make healthy food choices, healthy food resources must be *accessible*, *available*, and *affordable* (Sharkey, 2009). The complexities of modern life make it difficult for many individuals to consistently maintain access to foods rich in important nutrients.

Cost of food is a critical consideration for many families, given the increasing numbers of families living at or below the poverty level. Sources of complex carbohydrates (fruits, vegetables, and grains) may exceed the cost of highly refined sugar products. Proteins also vary greatly in per-unit cost. Assisting families in identifying low-cost, high-nutrition options within their "choice" environments is an important responsibility of the nurse providing nutritional guidance to diverse populations.

Seasonal variation in availability of foods such as raw vegetables and fresh fruits determines both accessibility and affordability. Seasonal patterns in the types of fruits and vegetables can be followed to maximize nutrient quality and lower cost. Use of frozen fruits and vegetables in their natural juices rather than those canned during off-season is recommended to decrease the intake of sugar and salt. Home-frozen products are an important source of nutrients at reasonable cost.

Ease of preparation also plays an important role in food selection. Quick and effortless preparation techniques appeal to many families because of busy work schedules. In addition, attractiveness of prepared foods is an important consideration. Assisting the client in selecting nutritious foods that are quickly prepared and aesthetically appealing increases the likelihood of sustaining positive eating behavior.

Health Policy Factors

As science advances, new regulations are implemented. For example, beginning in 2006, the Food and Drug Administration (FDA) required the labeling of the amount of "trans fat" per serving. The new regulations were added to the Dietary Guidelines for Americans to reflect the change. However there was no coordinated effort to publicize the change, and the public learned of the change through the mass media. Based on the sales immediately following the news coverage, the recommendations were heeded as fewer products containing trans fats were purchased. However, this trend was short-lived, and after one week, sales of trans fats products reached pre-news levels (Niederdeppe & Frosch, 2009). Sustained change needs a well-planned and ongoing public awareness campaign.

In modern society, food additives are used to retard spoilage and prevent deterioration of quality, improve nutritional value, enhance consumer acceptability, and facilitate preparation. By law, labels of many products must list the manufacturer, packer, and distributor, and the amount of each ingredient. Even when ingredients are listed, information on the products is often by itself insufficient to guide knowledgeable food selection. Not only are potentially carcinogenic additives used in the preparation of foods (e.g., nitrosamines in bacon), but unintentional food additives such as pesticides and other agricultural chemicals may appear in foods. Unfortunately, some of the synergistic, cumulative, and long-term effects of many additives will be determined only after years of use and exposure within human populations (Finucane & Holup, 2005).

NUTRITIONAL NEEDS OF SPECIAL POPULATIONS

Infants and Children

The caloric and nutrient intakes of children are critical for supporting growth and development. Infants whose diet is primarily mother's milk or infant formula consume 40% or more of their calories from fat, which is appropriate during infancy. When children reach 2 years of age, however, they should be encouraged to consume a diet lower in total fat, saturated fat, and cholesterol than the usual American diet (36–40%) as a basis for lowering the risk for chronic diseases in later years (U.S. DHHS, Office of Disease Prevention and Health Promotion, and U.S. Department of Agriculture, 2005). It is recommended that total fats and cholesterol be restricted in the diets of children 2 years of age and older with saturated fats to 10% of calories, total fats to 30% of calories, and dietary cholesterol to less than 300 mg/d (U.S. DHHS et al., 2005).

African-American children and children from low-income families have diets least consistent with the national recommendations (Shahar et al., 2005). When the diets of African-American children were examined separately, their major sources of total dietary fat were franks, sausages, luncheon meats, and bacon, with whole milk a close second (U.S. DHHS et al., 2005).

A healthy start for infants also means encouraging mothers to breast-feed or use iron-rich formulas for formula-fed infants. During pregnancy and lactation, mothers must maintain sufficient iron intake through iron-rich foods or supplements, as this increases the likelihood that their children will not be iron deficient during the early years of life (Centers for Disease Control and Prevention, Pediatric and Pregnancy Nutrition Surveillance System, 2007).

The dietary habits of young children are profoundly affected by family food prepa-ration and eating behaviors. Parental beliefs about good nutrition for children may not match healthy recommendations and thus may actually contribute to an unhealthy diet. Substituting 1% milk for whole milk consumed, skim-milk cheese for whole-milk cheese, and skim milk for low-fat milk consumed would markedly decrease total fat intake. Not all children find the substitutes acceptable, and not all are willing to consume them all the time. However, moderate changes in food consumption patterns results in favorable changes in dietary intake for most children.

The nutrition beliefs and practices of day care providers, other relatives, and preschool personnel have a significant influence on children in their care. Organized day care is an important setting for teaching nutrition and healthy behaviors. Cost consciousness on the part of caretakers should not interfere with the provision of good nutrition. It is important that parents monitor the food provided in child care facilities until they are assured that healthy nutrition guidelines are followed (Ward et al., 2008).

Adolescents

Adolescence is a period of biologic and social change. Body size, composition, func-tions, and physical abilities are changing rapidly. Under-nutrition slows height and weight growth and may delay puberty. Among adolescents, minimal dietary require-ments are those that maintain an optimal rate of pubertal development and growth. Adolescents who are vigorously active have increased energy needs. Thus, adolescents should consume diets providing more total nutrients than they consumed as young children.

Moderation is a good rule, as adolescents whose caloric intake is too high will gain weight, potentially leading to obesity. A caloric intake that is too low will result in loss of energy, weight loss, and, in the extreme, eating disorders that can lead to health problems and even premature death (Boschi et al., 2003). Adolescents with chronic diseases such as type 1 diabetes have special nutrition needs, because absorption, me-tabolism, or excretion of particular nutrients may change both as a result of adolescent biologic changes and as a result of the disease.

In terms of fat intake, adolescents should be given dietary counseling to reduce total fat to less than 30% of calories per day with less animal fat, and cholesterol to less than 300 mg/d to lower risk factors for chronic disease. Because many adolescents con-sume fast foods at lunchtime or during the evening hours, selecting low-animal-fat fast foods is a significant challenge.

An example of a high-fat, fast food meal is a double burger with sauce, milkshake, and French fries. The fat calories are 46% of the total calories in this meal. Because the goal should be less than 30% calories from fats, it is easy to see why consumption of such meals day after day increases the risk for cardiovascular disease and type 2 diabetes as early as adolescence. There is accumulating evidence that this "risk" carries over into adulthood (U.S. Task Force on Preventive Services, 2007).

Adolescent girls in the United States typically begin menstruating at 12½ years of age. Menstrual losses and increased physical activity increase the need for iron. Particular attention should be given to adequate intake of iron in the diet for women in general and, in particular, for very active young women. The mineral calcium helps to build strong bones. An adequate intake of calcium throughout childhood to age 25 years may reduce the risk of osteoporosis in later life. Young girls should learn to select foods that ensure adequate calcium, iron intake, and vitamin D (U.S. Task Force on Preventive Services, 2007).

Heightening awareness of the importance of good nutrition is important for overall adolescent health and performance. The challenge is to make nutritious food options appealing to adolescents who may eat primarily for taste rather than for good nutrition or health reasons. Peer support for healthy eating practices is also critical, as the desire to be accepted by peers is extremely high during the adolescent years. Meal skipping contributes to poor nutrition and should be discouraged. Eating fast food, yet selecting lower-fat options, creates opportunities for adolescents to be with their peers. Adolescents who model good eating habits may also influence their peers to make better choices.

Pressure on fast food establishments to offer healthier options will help create a supportive environment for healthy nutrition practices among adolescents. Schools are a vehicle for early health promotion activities. School lunch programs are more carefully monitored than in the past, and because at-risk children are eligible for reduced or free breakfast and/or lunch, these children's nutritional statuses have improved.

Efforts should continue to implement nutrition education beginning in preschool through grade 12. Efforts also should be made to integrate nutrition concepts throughout the entire curriculum, including courses in which it is not traditionally taught, such as math, chemistry, and history. Parents and guardians must be included in efforts to improve the nutrition of all students.

Older Adults

Research on the nutritional needs of older adults is expanding rapidly as the American population ages. Aging is thought to alter nutrient requirements for calories, protein, and other nutrients as a result of changes in lean body mass, physical activity, and intestinal absorption. Although many older Americans maintain healthy eating patterns, for some, changing nutritional needs may be accompanied by deterioration in diet quality and quantity, jeopardizing nutritional status, quality of life, and functional independence.

Many elderly people skip meals and exclude whole categories of food from their diet because of reduced appetites, infrequent grocery shopping, lack of interest in cooking, and difficulties in chewing and swallowing. For these individuals, supplementation may be required but should be initiated after consultation with health professionals. Self-medication may result in toxic levels of some vitamin and mineral supplements.

Polypharmacy is common in older adults so the interaction of food and drugs must be considered. Medications can affect the absorption of nutrients, foods, and other medicines. For example, crackers, dates, jelly, and other carbohydrates may slow down the rate of absorption of analgesics and limit their effectiveness in reducing pain.

Milk, eggs, cereals, and dairy products may inhibit the absorption of iron. Antibiotics such as tetracycline are less readily absorbed when milk, dairy products, or iron supplements are taken. Prune juice, bran cereal, and high-fiber foods may increase intestinal emptying time to the point where some drugs cannot be adequately absorbed. There is a need for further exploration of food–drug interactions that commonly occur among the elderly (Mallet, Spinewine, & Huang, 2007).

For individuals aged 65 years and older, recommended eating patterns lower in saturated fatty acids, total fat and saturated fats, and cholesterol help maintain desired body weight and lower the risk of cardiovascular heart disease (CHD). All of the risk factors for CHD, except cigarette smoking, are influenced by diet in some way. CHD is linked to nutritional patterns throughout life, with the damage manifest most frequently in middle-aged and older adults. Daily physical activity, along with a healthy diet to maintain adequate weight, can prevent premature mortality from heart disease and maintain vigor into old age (Hays & Roberts, 2006).

Essential components of the diets of older Americans generally are complex carbohydrates and fiber. Many elderly people have chewing and swallowing disorders that make eating fruits and vegetables difficult. Average daily fiber intake among the elderly is less than half of the recommended 20–35 g. Health benefits attributed to fiber include proper bowel function, reduced risk of colon cancer, reduction of serum cholesterol, and improved glucose response. Six daily servings of whole grains are the recommended minimum for the elderly.

Energy requirements decline with reductions in body size, lean body mass, basal metabolism rate, and decreased physical activity. Because physical activity maintains muscle mass, it is highly desirable to keep physically active in later years. Diets of the elderly may also be deficient in protein along with calories as the result of an inability to chew meat or afford the cost of protein-rich foods. Infections, trauma, and other metabolic stresses may increase protein needs. Inadequate protein in the diet may lower resistance to disease and delay recovery from illness (Hays & Roberts, 2006). See Chapter 4 for recommendations on assessing an elderly client's nutritional status.

Older adults with limited economic means should be assisted in selecting low-cost foods that meet recommended nutritional requirements. They may need guidance to learn to read label information to select and prepare foods so that they are easier to chew and swallow. Nutrition is integral to quality of life for the elderly. Thus, it is a primary area of focus for nurses providing care to the elderly in primary care and long-term care settings.

PROMOTION OF DIETARY CHANGE

Altering nutrition education, the food environment, and food consumption patterns contributes to better nutrition and healthier lives. To alter nutrition patterns, all ages must be exposed to nutrition education through mass media and Internet sources, education at schools and work sites, tailored self-help nutrition education packages, and nutrition counseling in primary health care services. Information technology plays an increasingly larger role, so nutrition education approaches must be assessed to see if they are evidenced based and user friendly. Interactive computer nutrition programs, nutrition videos, and healthy nutrition instant messaging are all important in broad-based nutrition education (Park et al., 2008).

Dietary information must evolve as scientific discoveries are published (Kumanyika et al., 2008; Woolf & Nestle, 2008). Research is also needed to establish the effectiveness of interventions for low-income and ethnic minorities and the efficacy of policy and environmental interventions (Fuemmeler et al., 2007). Despite the gaps in current knowledge, cumulative research findings support the basic advice: Take in fewer calories, eat less fat, move more, and eat more vegetables, fruits, and grains.

The food industry must be challenged to recognize its role in moving Americans toward a healthier society. Current legislation and regulation about the production and availability of food options influence cost and product development. Populations at school and work sites are captive and rely primarily on others to provide and prepare their food for a considerable part of the day, so the availability of healthy options from cafeterias and vending machines greatly affect nutrition behaviors. Furthermore, healthy food choices must have appeal in terms of taste and texture. Widespread research in the food production industry continues to create food options that are both consistent with dietary recommendations and acceptable to the public (Fuemmeler et al., 2007; Turrell & Giskes, 2008).

INTERVENTIONS TO PROMOTE DIETARY CHANGE

Interventions are evidenced-based strategies implemented to change unhealthy behavior(s). Most interventions target the individual and may occur in the home, school, organized child care centers, and work sites. Interventions also target populations such as churches, schools, and communities. Individual intervention formats include one on one, group, technology driven (telephone, Internet, and/or video), or combinations of these formats.

Individual targeted interventions to reduce obesity have had little long-term success. Preventing obesity in the population (population intervention) and helping overweight individuals prevent further weight gain (individual intervention) require new and different approaches (Franz et al., 2007). Interventions strategies for addressing change in dietary and eating patterns include the following:

- Increasing accessibility to nutrition information, education, counseling, and healthy foods in all settings and for all subpopulations.
- Preventing chronic diseases associated with diet and weight, beginning in early childhood.
- Strengthening the link between nutrition and physical activity in health promotion.

Evidenced-based interventions are necessary to continue to build the body of knowledge about nutrition and how to change eating behaviors. The U.S. Task Force on Preventive Services (2007) provides a valuable service to health care professionals, policy makers, researchers, and others through its *Community Guide*.

The *Community Guide* conducts multiple systematic reviews of types of interventions that have been tested and evaluates their effectiveness. The Task Force's findings are used to make recommendations for practice, policy changes, and future research. It has conducted systematic reviews of the evidence on nutrition and physical activity to determine the effectiveness of work site– and school-based interventions to prevent overweight and obesity.

School- and work site–based interventions are the most potentially effective intervention sites because children and adults spend most of their time in these respective sites. School sites offer intensive contact with the majority of children and adolescents in America and are generally supportive of programs offered to improve students' health. Work sites provide access to approximately 65% of the population aged 16 years and older. Workers are accessible in a controlled environment with communication networks that facilitate employee participation. Facilities are also available to support interventions such as cafeterias, vending machines, and meeting space. A substantial proportion of calories are consumed at schools and work sites on a daily basis, making them ideal sites for dietary changes.

The Task Force on Preventive Services recommends four strategies for school-based interventions aimed at weight control: (1) include both nutrition and physical activity, (2) incorporate additional time for activity during the school day, (3) include noncompetitive sports such as dance, and (4) reduce sedentary activities. Recommendations for work site interventions include combining instruction in better nutrition and eating habits with a structured physical activity program.

Comprehensive population-based interventions that address the interaction of multiple individual and social and physical environmental factors are needed to bring about effective dietary change (Kumanyika et al., 2008). However, the challenge is to develop interventions that are powerful enough to counteract the higher intake of calories and obesogenic factors in the environment for at-risk populations. Kumanyika et al. (2008) conclude that the difficulty lies in the identity of the set of interventions that would be effective in shifting the BMI distribution for a whole community.

Population-based interventions must be complementary to individual-focused interventions. Population-based interventions address the health of the larger community, whereas individual interventions are tailored to the needs to specific individuals within the community. Population-based health interventions should promote healthy living for all, yet recognize and value the differences that exist in subpopulations. Individuals are responsibility for their lifestyles; however, society has the ultimate responsibility for providing population-based interventions to improve the health of all.

RESEARCH-TESTED INTERVENTION PROGRAMS (RTIPs)

Research tested intervention programs (RTIPs) move science into programs for people. These interventions have been reviewed and determined to have positive outcomes. Two RTIPs are presented as examples of strategies to promote better eating behaviors and improve health: The Promoting Health Living: Assessing More Effects (PHLAME) (Elliot et al., 2007) and Body and Soul activities (Resnicow et al., 2004).

Promoting Healthy Living: Assessing More Effects (PHLAME)

The PHLAME intervention promotes healthy eating, regular exercise, and appropriate weight among firefighters. Healthy eating is defined as five or more servings of fruits and vegetables each day and less than 30% of calories from fat. Peer-led team-centered scripted lesson plans are used in 11 (45 minutes per session) team sessions scheduled over one year. Sessions include nutrition, physical activity, and energy balance. The curriculum incorporates aspects of social-cognitive theory. The intervention is intended for professional firefighters and implemented in fire stations. Team materials cost approximately $25 per participant.

Body and Soul

The Body and Soul intervention offers a unique opportunity to increase fruit and vegetables intake among African-Americans. The program includes three church-wide nutrition activities, one event with the church pastor, and one policy change, such as establishing guidelines for the type of food served at church functions. Lay counselors, who make at least two 15-minute calls to five participants, are given 12–16 hours of training. The program is suitable for implementation in home and church settings for African-American church members, aged 17–89 years. Implementation time varies based on length of church involvement.

STRATEGIES FOR MAINTAINING RECOMMENDED WEIGHT

Weight maintenance is a lifelong health goal to reduce the multiple health problems that result from obesity. The physical basis for excessive weight gain is relatively simple and straightforward, as overweight and obesity result from an imbalance in energy as a result of too many calories and not enough physical activity. Weight management means balancing the number of calories consumed with the number of calories burned. Despite the multiple factors involved, diet and exercise are the cornerstones to prevention of overweight and obesity. Homes, schools, work sites, and the community must all work together to promote healthy eating and physical activity. Strategies to promote healthy eating habits and physical activity can be accessed at the National Institute of Diabetes, Digestive and Kidney Diseases weight control information network Web site. Strategies include the following.

- Choose sensible portions of foods lower in fat. Watch portion sizes.
- Learn healthier ways to make favorite foods.
- Learn to recognize and control environmental cues that make you want to eat.
- Have a healthy snack an hour before a social gathering.
- Engage in moderate-intensity physical activity for 30 minutes every day.
- Take a walk instead of watching television.
- Do not eat meals in front of the television.
- Keep records of your food intake and physical activity. Weigh yourself weekly.
- Pay attention to why you are eating.

STRATEGIES FOR INITIATING A WEIGHT-REDUCTION PROGRAM

Obesity is a global epidemic and continues to increase in the United States. It is estimated that two-thirds of adults are either overweight or obese (Brown, Fujioka, Wilson, & Woodworth, 2009). As mentioned in previous chapters, overweight is defined as a BMI in the range of 25–29.9, and obesity as a BMI 30 or greater. Location of excess body fat is also important, as intra-abdominal fat is a risk factor for diabetes and cardiovascular disease. Obesity increases the risk of cardiovascular disease, type 2 diabetes, and other chronic diseases. The epidemic represents a public health crisis that requires primary and secondary prevention efforts to stop the escalating costs of managing chronic diseases associated with obesity as well as detrimental effects on quality of life. Weight management is difficult and requires a lifelong commitment, making it a challenge for the individual and the health care provider. Individuals who are overweight and obese and desire to lose weight should consult a health care provider before starting an aggressive weight loss program. Consultation will assist with the type of dietary program to select. In addition, the health care provider will perform a health and family history, physical examination, BMI and waist circumference or hip–waist ratio measures, blood lipid and glucose analysis, and electrocardiogram or exercise stress test before beginning a weight-loss program. Careful assessment of current dietary habits is essential to develop an individualized, effective program. Other questions to assist in the assessment include the following:

- Is the person strongly motivated to lose weight?
- Is the person willing or able to commit the time and financial resources needed?
- Does the person believe he or she can be successful in a weight loss program?
- Does the person understand the possible risks of weight loss interventions?
- Are weight loss goals realistic?
- What is the person's attitude toward physical activity?
- Does the person have a support system to facilitate weight loss?
- What are the potential barriers to successful weight loss?
- Has the person had past successes in weight loss? If so, what worked? What did not work?
- What factors caused the person to relapse in the past?

Caloric reduction with attention to portion size, while maintaining adequate nutrient levels, adequate vitamins and minerals, and adequate fiber is the best way to achieve and maintain desired weight, in conjunction with a regular physical activity program. Radical changes in food consumption patterns are not recommended. It is important for clients to understand that even modest weight loss is beneficial.

Dietary preferences and the individual's ability to incorporate a particular diet into his or her daily routine should be taken into consideration when planning the type of dietary intervention (Aronne, Wadden, Isoldi, & Woodworth, 2009). Dietary interventions include low carbohydrate, low fat, high protein, high fiber, and meal replacements. Meal replacement diets have become increasingly popular for those who do not have time to prepare meals and have difficulty controlling portion size. The meal substitutes are considered nutritionally well-balanced diets, and the result has been favorable with sustained weight loss for as long as four years. Very low calorie diets should be avoided or undertaken under the close supervision.

Behavioral management techniques refer to principles used to change an individual's behavior and lifestyle. The client must develop new skills to facilitate long-term change. These techniques have been shown to be an important component of weight loss programs (Hainer, Toplak, & Mitrakou, 2008). Behavioral modification techniques include self-monitoring, stress management, stimulus control, problem solving, rewarding behavior changes, cognitive restructuring, social support, and relapse prevention training. Learning to control daily food choices and physical activity is crucial to long-term success. Learning to plan and self-monitor are considered two of the most useful behavioral management strategies (Lang & Froelichler, 2006). Planning meals for healthy dietary intake and time for physical activity, and keeping records to assess one's progress give insight into personal behavior.

Although short-term change has been documented, it is much more difficult to maintain weight loss long term. A supportive approach with extended contacts has been shown to be effective in maintaining behavior change. Other strategies for long-term weight loss maintenance that have been successful include the following:

- Relapse prevention training to teach specific skills,
- Telephone prompts to provide frequent contacts,
- Peer/social support, and
- Extended behavioral therapy.

Effective weight-loss programs for children suffer from many barriers, including lack of family motivation, financial costs, and lack of time. A meta-analysis of research interventions for children aged 6–16 years reported that the use of structured dietary and exercise regimens are effective in promoting weight loss (Snethen, Broome, & Cashin, 2006). Diet, exercise, behavioral techniques, and parental involvement are all important in promoting the effectiveness of weight loss programs in this group. Parents should be included in the intervention, as they have control over the food purchased, meal planning and preparation, as well as modeling healthy eating.

Obesity in older persons is beginning to receive attention due to the increased prevalence of obesity in this population. A systematic review was undertaken to investigate the evidence of weight loss interventions in older adults (Bales & Buhr, 2008). Loss of lean body mass was noted in several studies. In general, the findings show benefits for osteoarthritis, physical function, and possibly type 2 diabetes and coronary heart disease. Results suggest that in persons aged 65 years and older, weight loss interventions should be considered on an individual basis with attention to the weight history and the medical conditions of the client. Resistance exercises should be part of all weight loss interventions for older adults.

OPPORTUNITIES FOR RESEARCH IN NUTRITION AND HEALTH

The health consequences of overweight and obesity in America make research a priority to identify and test new strategies and treatments to reverse the trend. Research results indicate that the benefits of dieting interventions have had limited success for sustained weight loss (Mann, Tomiyama, Lew, Samuels, & Chatman, 2007). The role of physical activity warrants careful study as a treatment for obesity. Clinical trials that compare activity-only groups with diet-only and diet and exercise groups will help researchers to better understand the role of physical activity in weight loss. Strategies to sustain weight loss also should be identified and tested. In addition, preschool interventions to promote physical activity and make healthy food choices need development, testing, and follow-up of long-term health outcomes. Measures of obesogenic environments and food environments should be developed that can be used to assess neighborhoods and communities. Multilevel approaches are needed to take into consideration the context of the individual. Community level interventions must be carefully planned, implemented, and evaluated. Interventions that target ethnic and low-income communities and build on the existing community strengths and assets to bring about social change should be investigated. Interventions to increase the long-term effectiveness for family–child dietary pattern changes are also needed. It is no longer sufficient to focus solely on the individual to promote health food choices. The complexity of the multiple factors involved necessitates a multidisciplinary approach and the involvement of government officials and health policy makers.

CONSIDERATIONS FOR PRACTICE IN NUTRITION AND HEALTH

Health professionals are important role models for healthy eating patterns. Nurses and other health professionals should not only advocate healthy diets for others, but also put the dietary guidelines into practice as a part of their own lifestyles. Modeling recommended eating behaviors, as well as managing issues that surround maintenance of positive nutritional practices, will indicate sincerity and commitment to good health practices that speak louder than words to clients.

The responsibility for monitoring the nutritional health of individuals, families, and the community is shared among all members of the health promotion team. Lack of facilitation of positive dietary habits and good nutrition has resulted in a sizable population of children, adolescents, and adults who are overweight and/or obese. The chronic health problems that follow are costly in terms of resources and life quality. Dietary counseling and education should be an integral part of nursing practice in all settings. Counseling and follow-up of clients who are at risk for or who are overweight or obese is a priority. Health teaching should begin with preschoolers, so that they learn healthy eating habits early that can be sustained.

Opportunities should be created to engage clients and others in dialogue about their dietary practices and changes to improve their health. School nurses and occupational health nurses must work with schools, work places, industry, and policy makers to improve the food choices in cafeterias and vending machines. Internet Web sites that focus on nutrition are a quick way to keep current on the latest research findings and practice guidelines. The nurse can help clients understand and select accurate information.

Summary

Lifelong patterns of health eating are needed to avoid the chronic health problems of overweight and obesity. Individual, social, and physical environmental barriers to changing eating behaviors must be addressed to facilitate lifestyles that promote healthy eating behaviors. Promoting good nutrition is a critical concern in prevention and health promotion and an important dimension of competent self-care. Cultural and ethnic backgrounds influence eating behavior and must be accounted for in changing eating patterns. The individual, family, and community must all be part of nutritional interventions. Research has substantiated the complexity of factors that determine eating behaviors, and all of these determinants must be part of a strategy for successful change to occur.

Learning Activities

1. Using the *Dietary Guidelines for Americans*, compare your diet with the recommendations, and identify two modifications you are willing to make in your diet.
2. Use MyPyramid to assist you in making the modifications you identified in #1.
3. Select, explore, and evaluate the nutritional information on two Web sites from the list at the end of the chapter.
4. Engage an adolescent and older adult in discussions to assess their knowledge and understanding of their nutritional needs. Assist them to develop a plan to overcome identified barriers to healthy eating.

Selected Web Sites

Department of Health and Human Services
http://www.dhhs.gov
The Department of Health and Human Services (DHHS) is the principal agency for protecting the health of all Americans and providing essential human services, especially for those who are least able to help themselves.

Weight-Control Information Network (WIN)
http://win.niddk.nih.gov/
The weight-control information network is an information service of the National Institute of Diabetes and Digestive and Kidney Diseases (NIDDK) and provides useful information on understanding obesity.

American Cancer Society Great American Health Challenge
http://www.cancer.org/docroot/subsite/greatamericans/Eat&_Right.asp
The American Cancer Society Great American Health Challenge site offers nutritional information as well as videos and a virtual dietitian.

Centers for Disease Control (CDC)
http://www.cdc.gov/needphp/publications/AAG/obesity.htm
The CDC provide useful information on chronic disease prevention and health promotion and has a targeted Web site on obesity.

Food and Fitness Site
http://www.foodfit.com
Founded by a former Undersecretary of Agriculture, this site offers budget-friendly healthy recipes.

Food and Nutrition Information Center
http://www.nal.usda.gov/fnic
The Center provides accurate and practical resources for nutrition and health professionals, educators, and consumers.

Healthy People 2020
http://www.health.gov/healthypeople
This site allows one to explore Healthy People 2010, the mid-course review, and keep up to date on the progress of the 2020 objectives. Physical Activity Guidelines for Americans can be accessed from this site as well.

National Center for Health Statistics
http://www.cdc.gov/nchs
The National Center compiles statistical information to guide actions and policies to improve the health of Americans.

National Heart, Lung and Blood Institution Food Portion Size Quiz
http://www.hin.nhlbi.nih.gov/portion

National Institute of Diabetes, Digestive and Kidney Diseases
http://win.niddk.nih.gov/publications/understanding.htm

Nutrition and Your Health: Dietary Guidelines
http://www.health.gov/dietaryguidelines
The Guidelines provide authoritative advice for people aged 2 years and older about how good dietary habits can promote health and reduce risk for major chronic diseases.

MyPyramid Steps to a Healthier You
http://www.mypyramid.gov
MyPyramid offers personalized eating plans and interactive tools to help plan and assess food choices based on the Dietary Guidelines for Americans.

Office of Disease Prevention and Health Promotion
http://www.odphp.osophs.dhhs.gov
The Office of Disease Prevention and Health Promotion Web site provides links to projects focusing on health and electronic health tools.

References

American Diabetic Association. (2008). Nutritional recommendations and interventions for diabetes. *Diabetes Care, 31*, S61–S75.

Aronne, L. S., Wadden, T., Isolde, K. K., & Woodworth K. A. (2009). When prevention fails: Obesity treatment strategies. *American Journal of Medicine, 122*, S24–S32.

Baker, H. (2007, October). Nutrition in the elderly: Diet pitfalls and nutrition advice. *Geriatrics, 62*(10), 24–26.

Bales, C. W., & Buhr, G. (2008). Is obesity bad for older persons? A systematic review of the pros and cons of weight reduction in later life. *Journal of the American Medical Directors Association, 9,* 302–312.

Bloom, S. (2007, March). Hormonal regulation of appetite. *Obesity Reviews, 8,* 63–65.

Boschi, V., Siervo, M., D'Orsi, P., Margiotta, N., Trapenese, E., Basile, F., et al. (2003). Body composition, eating behavior, food-body concerns and eating disorders in adolescent girls. *Annals of Nutrition and Metabolism, 47*(6), 284–293.

Britten, P., Haven, J., & Davis, C. (2006). Consumer research for development of educational messages for the MyPyramid food guidance system. *Journal of Nutrition Education and Behavior, 38,* S108–S123.

Britten, P., Marcoe, K., Yamini, S., & Davis, C. (2006). Development of food intake patterns for the MyPyramid food guidance system. *Journal of Nutrition Education and Behavior, 38,* S78–S92.

Brown, V. W., Fujioka, K., Wilson, P. W., & Woodworth, K. A. (2009). Obesity: Why be concerned? *Journal of Nutrition Education and Behavior, 38,* S4–S11.

Centers for Disease Control and Prevention. (2009). *Obesity prevalence 25 percent or higher in 32 states.* Retrieved July 9, 2009, from http://www.cdc.gov/media/pressrel/2009/r090708.htm

Centers for Disease Control and Prevention, Pediatric and Pregnancy Nutrition Surveillance System. (2007). Pediatric Nutrition Surveillance, 2007 Report. Retrieved from http://www.cdc.gov/PEDNSS/ pdfs/ PedNSS&_2007.pdf

Chipperfield, J. G., & Perry, R. P. (2006). Primary- and secondary-control strategies in later life: Predicting hospital outcomes in men and women. *Health Psychology, 25,* 226–236.

Elliot, D. L., Goldberg, L., Kuchl, K. S., Moe, E. L., Breger, R. K., DeFrancesco, C. L., et al. (2007). The PHLAME firefighters' study: Feasibility and findings. *American Journal of Health Behavior, 28*(1), 13–23.

Feil, R. (2006). Environment and nutritional effects on the epigenetic regulation of genes. *Mutation Research, 600,* 46–57.

Finucane, M. L., & Holup, J. L. (2005, April). Psychosocial and cultural factors affecting the perceived risk of genetically modified food: An overview of the literature. *Social Science & Medicine, 60*(7), 1603–1612.

Franz, M. J., VanWormer, J. J., Crain, A. L., Boucher, J. L., Histon, T., Caplan, W., et al. (2007, October). Weight-loss outcomes: A systematic review and meta-analysis of weight-loss clinical trials with a minimum 1-year follow-up. *Journal of American Dietetic Association, 107,* 1755–1767.

Fuemmeler, B. F., Baffi, C., Mâsse, L. C., Atienza, A. A., & Evans, W. D. (2007, January). Employer and healthcare policy interventions aimed at adult obesity. *American Journal of Preventive Medicine, 32*(1), 44–51.

Furman, E. F. (2006, January). Under-nutrition in older adults across the continuum of care: Nutritional assessment, barriers, and interventions. *Journal of Gerontological Nursing, 32*(1), 22–27.

Gao, S., Wilde, P. E., Lichtenstein, A. H., & Tucker, K. L. (2006, November). Meeting adequate intake for dietary calcium without dairy foods in adolescents aged 9 to 18 years (National Health and Nutrition Examination Survey 2001–2002). *Journal of the American Dietetic Association, 106*(11), 1759–1765.

Gelber, R. P., Gaziano, J. M., Orav, J., Manson, J. E., Buring, J. E., & Kurth, T. (2008). Measures of obesity and cardiovascular risk among men and women. *Journal of the American College of Cardiology, 52,* 605–615.

Glanz, K. (2009). Measuring food environments: A historical perspective. *American Journal of preventive Medicine, 36*(4S), S93–S98.

Hainer, V., Toplak, H., & Mitrakou, A. (2008). Treatment modalities of obesity. *Diabetes Care, 31*(S2), S269–S277.

Harrington, D. A., & Elliot, S. J. (2009). Weighing the importance of neighborhood: A multi-level exploration of the determinants of overweight and obesity. *Social Science & Medicine, 68,* 593–600.

Hays, N. P., & Roberts, S. B. (2006, June). The anorexia of aging in humans. *Physiology & Behavior, 88*(3), 257–266.

Hoek, H. W. (2006). Incidence, prevalence and mortality of anorexia nervosa and other eating disorders. *Current Opinions in Psychiatry, 19,* 389–394.

Kaila, B., & Raman, M. (2008, January). Obesity: A review of pathogenesis and management strategies. *Canadian Journal of Gastroenterology, 22*(1), 61–68.

Kalra, S. P. (2008). Central leptin insufficiency syndrome: An interactive etiology for obesity, metabolic and neural diseases and for designing new therapeutic interventions. *Peptides, 29,* 127–138.

Kelly, T., Yang, W., Chen, C. S., Reynolds, K., & He, J. (2008, September). Global burden of obesity in 2005 and projections to 2030. *International Journal of Obesity, 32,* 1431–1437.

Knecht, S., Ellger, T., & Levine, J. A. (2008). Obesity in neurobiology. *Progress in Neurobiology, 84* (1), 85–103.

Kragelund, C., & Omland, T. (2005). A farewell to body mass index? *Lancet, 306,* 79–86.

Kumanyika, S. K., Obarzanek, E., Stettler, N., Bell, R., Field, A. E., Fortmann, S. P., et al. (2008, July). Population-based prevention of obesity: The need for comprehensive promotion of healthful eating, physical activity, and energy balance: A scientific statement from American Heart Association Council on Epidemiology and Prevention, Interdisciplinary Committee for Prevention (formerly the expert panel on population and prevention science). *Circulation, 118,* 428–464.

Lang, A., & Froelichler, E. S. (2006). Management of overweight and obesity in adults: Behavioral intervention for long-term weight loss and maintenance. *European Journal of Cardiovascular Nursing, 5,* 102–114.

Macht, M. (2008). How emotions affect eating: A five-way model. *Appetite, 50,* 1–11.

Mallet, L., Spinewine, A., & Huang, A. (2007, July). The challenge of managing drug interactions in elderly people. *The Lancet, 370*(9582), 185–191.

Malterud, K., & Tonstad, S. (2009). Preventing obesity: Challenges and pitfalls for health promotion. *Patient Education and Counseling,* doi:10.1016/j.pec.2008.12.021. Accessed from http://www.elsevier.com/locate/pateducou

Mann, T., Tomiyama, J., Lew, A., Samuels, B., & Chatman, J. (2007). Medicine's search for effective obesity treatments: Diets are not the answer. *American Psychologist, 62,* 220–232.

Marantz, P. R., Bird, E., & Alderman, M. H. (2008). A call for higher standards of evidence for dietary guidelines. *American Journal of Preventive Medicine, 34,* 234–240.

McKinnon, R. A., Tracy Orleans, C., Kumanyika, S. K., Haire-Joshu, D., Krebs-Smith, S. M., Finkelstein, E. A., et al. (2009, April). Considerations for an obesity policy research agenda. *American Journal of Preventive Medicine, 36*(4), 351–357.

McKinnon, R. A., Reedy, J., Handy, S. L., & Rodgers, A. B. (2009, April). Measuring the food and physical activity environments: Shaping the research agenda. *American Journal of Preventive Medicine, 36*(4, Suppl 1), S81–S85.

Messiah, S. E., Arheart, K. L., Lipschultz, S. E., & Miller, T. L. (2008). Body mass index, waist circumference and cardiovascular risk factors in adolescents. *Journal of Pediatrics, 153,* 845–850.

Morrison, C. D. (2008). Leptin resistance and the response to positive energy balance. *Physiology and Behavior, 94,* 660–663.

Morrison, C. D., & Berthoud, H. R. (2007, December). Neurobiology of nutrition and obesity. *Nutrition Reviews, 65*(12 Pt 1), 517–534.

Niederdeppe, J., & Frosch, D. L. (2009, May). News coverage and sales of products with trans fat: Effects before and after changes in federal labeling policy. *American Journal of Preventive Medicine, 36*(5), 395–401.

Park, A., Nitzke, S., Dritsch, K., Kattelmann, K., White, A., Boeckner, L., et al. (2008, September–October). Internet-based interventions have potential to affect short-term mediators and indicators of dietary behavior of young adults. *Journal of Nutrition Education and Behavior, 40*(5), 288–297.

Ptak, C., & Petronis, A. (2008, February). Epigenetics and complex disease: From etiology to new therapeutics. *Annual Review of Pharmacology and Toxicology, 48,* 257–276.

Reis, J. P., Araneta, M. R., Wingard, D. L., Macera, C. A., Lindsay, S. P., & Marshal, S. J. (2008). Overall obesity and abdominal adiposity as predictors of mortality in U.S. white and black adults. *Annals of Epidemiology, 19,* 134–142.

Resnicow, K., Kramish Campbell, M., Carr, C., McCarty, F., Want, T., Periasamy, S., et al. (2004). Body and soul. A dietary intervention conducted through African-American churches. *American Journal of Preventive Medicine, 27*(2), 97–105.

Robert Wood Johnson Foundation. (2009, July). Issue Report: *F as in Fat: How obesity policies are failing in America,* 2009. Retrieved July 3, 2009 from http://www.healthyamericans.org

Shahar, D., Shai, L., Vardi, H., Shahar, A., & Fraser, D. (2005). Diet and eating habits in high and low socioeconomic groups. *Nutrition, 21*, 559–566.

Sharkey, J. R. (2009, April). Measuring potential access to food stores and food-service places in rural areas in the U.S. *American Journal of Preventive Medicine, 36*(4, Suppl 1), S151–S155.

Snethen, J. A., Broome, M. E., & Cashin, S. E. (2006). Effective weight loss for overweight children: A meta-analysis of intervention studies. *Journal of Pediatric Nursing, 21*, 45–54.

Srikanthan, P., Seeman, T. E., & Karlamangla, S. K. (2009). Waist-hip ratio as a predictor of all-cause mortality in high functioning older adults. *Annals of Epidemiology 19*(10), 724–731.

Stice, E., Shaw, H., & Marti, C. N. (2007, April). A meta-analytic review of eating disorder prevention programs: Encouraging findings. *Annual Review of Clinical Psychology, 3*, 207–231.

Trost, L. B., Bergfield, W. F., & Calogeras, E. (2006). The diagnosis and treatment of iron deficiency and its potential relationship to hair loss. *Journal of the Academy of Dermatology, 54*, 824–844.

Trust for America's Health. (2009). Americans rank prevention as most important health reform priority. Retrieved from http://www.healthyamericans.org/report/70/prevention-survey-Il

Turrell, G., & Giskes, K. (2008, July). Socioeconomic disadvantage and the purchase of takeaway food: A multilevel analysis. *Appetite, 51*(1), 69–81.

Ulijaszek, S. J. (2007). Frameworks of population obesity and the use of cultural consensus modeling in the study of environments contributing to obesity. *Economics and Human Biology, 5*, 443–457.

U.S. DHHS, Centers for Disease Control and Prevention, National Center for Health Statistics. (2008). Information sheet: *NCHS data on eating behaviors.* Retrieved July 12, 2009 from http://www.cdc.gov/nchs/data/infosheets/infosheet&_eatingbehaviors.htm

U.S. DHHS, Office of Disease Prevention and Health Promotion, U.S. Department of Agriculture. (2005). *Dietary Guidelines for Americans 2005.* Retrieved July 18, 2009 from http://www.healthierus.gov/dietaryguidelines/

U.S. Task Force on Preventive Services. (2007, July). *Screening for lipid disorders in children, topic page.* Retrieved July 18, 2009 from http://www.ahrq.gov/clinic/uspstf/uspschlip.htm

Venner, A. A., Lyon, M. E., & Doyle-Baker, P. K. (2006). Leptin: A potential biomarker for childhood obesity? *Clinical Biochemistry, 39*, 1047–1056.

Ward, D. S., Benjamin, S. E., Ammerman, A. S., Ball, S. C., Neelon, B. H., & Bangdiwala, S. I. (2008, October). Nutrition and physical activity in child care: Results from an environmental intervention. *American Journal of Preventive Medicine, 35*(4), 352–356.

Wells, J. C. (2006, May). The evolution of human fatness and susceptibility to obesity: An ethological approach. *Biological Reviews of the Cambridge Philosophical Society, 81*(2), 183–205.

Winston, A. P. (2008, April). Management of physical aspects and complications of eating disorders. *Psychiatry, 7*(4), 174–178.

Woolf, S. H., & Nestle, M. (2008) Do dietary guidelines explain the obesity epidemic? *American Journal of Preventive Medicine, 34*(3), 263–265.

World Health Organization. (WHO). (2002). The world health report 2002. Reducing risks, promising healthy life. Geneva, Switzerland: WHO.

CHAPTER 8

Stress Management and Health Promotion

OBJECTIVES

1. Discuss the relationship between stress and health.
2. Describe four approaches to assist patients to reduce stressful situations.
3. Discuss five psychological conditioning strategies to increase resistance to stress.
4. Discuss the pros and cons of three interventions to manage stress in individuals and groups.

Outline

- Stress and Health
- Stress Across the Life Span
- Approaches to Stress Management
  A. Minimizing the Frequency of Stress-Inducing Situations
  B. Increasing Resistance to Stress
- Complementary Therapies to Manage Stress
  A. Mindfulness-Based Stress Reduction (MBSR)
  B. Progressive Relaxation Through Tension-Relaxation
- Opportunities for Research on Stress Management
- Considerations for Practice in Stress Management
- Summary
- Learning Activities
- Selected Web Sites
- References

Stress is of theoretical and practical interest to nurses. Various aspects of stress have been studied in attempts to understand the stress–illness relationship, as well as how to intervene and promote health through fostering stress resistance and overall resilience among individuals and families. More than three-fourths of visits to health care professionals have been attributed to or made worse by stress (Hogan, 2003). With this high incidence of stress-related health problems, strategies and interventions for promoting stress reduction among clients are critically important to minimize insults to well-being and maximize realization of personal potential.

Stress is an inevitable, unavoidable, human experience in any society and more so in a society characterized by rapid and accelerating change. Selye (1936), a pioneer in stress research, defined stress as "the nonspecific response of the body to any demand made on it." Internal and external manifestations of stress were referred to as the General Adaptation Syndrome (GAS) or the "fight-or-flight" response. Specific physiologic or behavioral changes that occur in response to stressors include the following:

- Dilation of pupils
- Increased respiratory rate
- Increased heart rate
- Peripheral vasoconstriction
- Increased perspiration
- Increased blood pressure
- Increased muscle tension
- Increased gastric motility
- Release of adrenalin
- Increased blood glucose level
- Cold, clammy skin

Although Selye made major contributions to the general adaptation theory of stress and supported the idea of a relationship between prolonged stress and disease, the theory was not without limitations. The role of emotional or cognitive factors in the stress response was not accounted for in his model. All individuals experience stress; however people interpret and react to it differently, resulting in differing vulnerabilities to the deleterious effects of stress. In addition, research has clarified the homeostasis concept by distinguishing between the conditions that are necessary to maintain the internal body systems for survival (*homeostasis*) and those that maintain the system in balance (*allostasis*). The goal of homeostasis and allostasis is to maintain internal stability. The differing reactions of individuals to stress led to a re-evaluation of homeostasis in the face of challenge, bringing about the terms *allostasis* and *allostatic load* (McEwen, 2007).

Allostasis refers to the process of achieving stability through change and is a continuous process of adapting in the face of potentially stressful events. When exposed to a stressor, the body responds by turning on a complex pathway for adapting and coping with physiologic and behavioral responses. The stressful event leads to the release of catecholamines (adrenalin), glucocorticoids (cortisol), and other hormones. When the stressful event has ended or is under control, the response returns to baseline, unless exposure to elevated level of stress continues over weeks and months. A continued elevated stress response results in *allostatic load* and overload, with resultant vulnerability and dysfunction. *Allostatic load* reflects the cumulative negative effects of prolonged environmental and psychosocial stressors. One of the major factors leading to allostatic load is frequently encountered stress (McEwen, 2007). Allostatic load is also affected by health-damaging behaviors, such as excess calorie intake, smoking, and alcohol, as well as by health promoting behaviors. In other words, how individuals cope with challenges over a lifetime influences allostasis, allostatic load, and resulting disease. Allostatic load represents cumulative stress and has the potential to predict risk for a variety of diseases, such as diabetes, cardiovascular disease, and cancer (Loucks, Juster, & Pruessner, 2008).

Because the allostasis stress framework is fairly new, the research base is limited due to many methodological challenges, including measurement of allostatic load. Much work must be done to describe the role of allostatic load as a risk for disease and to identify interventions to decrease allostatic load (Gersten, 2008).

Stressors, or the causes of stress, are defined as "environmental and internal demands and conflicts among them, which tax or exceed a person's resources" (Lazarus & Folkman, 1984). Stress, the body's response to stressors, involves the nervous, endocrine, and immunologic systems, which in turn affect all organ systems. Some stressors are viewed as challenges, creating stimulation and excitement. Other stressors are viewed negatively, perhaps because they are considered undesirable, uncontrollable, or emotionally distressing. There is much scientific interest in the "resistance resources" that enable some individuals to successfully manage stressors and flourish whereas others find the same stressors debilitating.

Coping strategies assist individuals in managing stress and are described as learned and purposeful cognitive, emotional, and behavioral responses to stressors used to adapt to the environment or to change it (Lazarus, 1999). In the coping process, the ability to regulate emotions, behavior, and the environment is critical to successful adjustment. Cognitive appraisal and coping constitute the stress-coping process. Cognitive appraisal consists of two phases. In *primary appraisal*, the person evaluates whether anything is at stake in the encounter: Is there potential harm or benefit to cherished commitments, values, goals, or self-esteem, or to one's health and well-being? If an encounter is threatening, primary appraisal serves to reduce its significance for the person experiencing it. For example, if a person receives notice that the results of a laboratory test are "abnormal," the person may discount the validity of the test (Wenzel, Glanz, & Lerman, 2002). In *secondary appraisal*, the person evaluates what, if anything may be done to overcome or prevent harm, or to improve the prospects of benefit. Various coping options are evaluated, such as altering the situation, accepting it, seeking more information, or holding back from acting in an impulsive way. Primary and secondary appraisals converge to determine if the person–environment transaction is primarily threatening or challenging.

Coping regulates stressful emotions (emotion-focused coping) and alters the person–environment relationship that is causing the distress (problem-focused coping). Both forms of coping occur in stressful encounters. The success of problem-focused coping may in large part depend on the success of emotion-focused coping, because heightened emotions are likely to interfere with the cognitive activity necessary to effectively manage the stressors. Problem-focused coping is likely to be dominant in encounters viewed as changeable, whereas emotion-focused coping often dominates in encounters viewed as unchangeable, with acceptance as the only recourse (Wenzel et al., 2002). Encounters involving threats to self-esteem are often the most difficult to resolve. These threats include the possibility of losing the affection of someone one cares about, losing self-respect or the respect of others, and appearing to be unethical or incompetent.

The World Health Organization (WHO) Global Burden of Disease Survey estimated that stress-related disorders and mental illness will be the second leading cause of disabilities by 2020 (Kalia, 2002). There are many ongoing unmet needs in providing care for the mentally ill and individuals with stress-related illnesses. Disability, absenteeism, decreased productivity, and health-damaging effects of stress and mental illnesses are very costly for businesses and industry. Financial incentives to businesses and health care organizations are needed to help individuals manage stress and avoid its costly, health-impairing effects.

Adults who seek mental health care in primary care settings have fewer visits per year than adults who are seen by specialists. Only about 6% of adults in the United States use their primary care provider for mental health care, so it is imperative that nurses and other primary care providers ensure that all adults and children are screened and treated for stress-related problems and mental health disorders. The mid-course review of the 2010 objectives conducted in 2005 showed that the objective to increase the number of primary care facilities providing treatment and/or referral for mental illness exceeded its goal by moving from a baseline of 62% to 74%. However, mental illness often still goes undiagnosed in primary care settings (Healthy People 2010 Midcourse Review). Nurses in primary care settings including schools, clinics, and work sites have a responsibility to promote and conduct early screening and intervention for mental illness and stress-related problems.

STRESS AND HEALTH

Decreased life satisfaction, the development of mental disorders, the occurrence of stress-related illnesses (e.g., cardiovascular disease, gastrointestinal disorders, low back pain, headaches), and decreased immunologic functioning result from stress. In heart disease, long-term stress is thought to sensitize arterioles to catecholamines, with even short-term stress responses causing overconstriction of the vessels and endothelial damage. Repetitive overconstriction may lead to hypertension, decreased myocardial perfusion, and arrhythmias (Epel, 2009). Social factors are intimately related to the experience of stress and subsequently to health and disease (Vimont, 2008). There is evidence that providing social support may be more beneficial than receiving it. Mortality was significantly reduced for individuals who reported giving support, whereas no change was noted in mortality for those receiving support (Bacon, Milne, Sheikh, & Freeston, 2009). In other instances, the nature of interpersonal relationships may be detrimental to health. A meta-analysis of cohort studies showed a robust estimate of the positive effect of marriage on mortality that did not vary by gender, or between North America and Europe (Manzoli, Villari, Pirone, & Boccia, 2007). Both the absence of social relations and certain characteristics of social relations serve as stressors that may have an impact on health.

Psychoneuroimmunology examines the effects of social and psychological phenomena on the immune system as mediated by the nervous and endocrine systems. This arena of science is particularly important because both acute and chronic infections as well as cancer have been linked to compromised immune functioning. In a series of studies, male undergraduate college students with high heart-rate reactivity to stressors (mental arithmetic test with noise superimposed) were compared with low heart-rate reactors on neuroendocrine and immune responses to stressors. High reactors showed higher stress-related levels of plasma cortisol and increased natural killer (NK) cell lysis than did low reactors. The finding that cortisol was elevated in high reactors is particularly interesting in view of the extensive literature linking cortisol with down-regulation of multiple aspects of cellular immune function. These findings suggest that individual variation in activation of the hypothalamic–pituitary–adrenocortical axis by brief psychological stressors may explain why daily stressors have greater health consequences for some individuals than for others. Different mediating roles may be played by the hypothalamic–pituitary–adrenocortical axis and the sympathetic adrenomedullary systems (Epel, 2009).

Results of a meta-analysis conducted to evaluate evidence that psychological interventions affect the immune system indicate only modest changes in the immune system. The authors suggest that conceptual and methodological issues must be addressed in research before it can be concluded that psychological interventions do not cause changes in immune responses (Pace et al., 2009). Clinical evidence suggests that the immune system is influenced by central nervous system processes that are shaped by psychological factors (Brydon, Walker, Wawrzyniak, Chart, & Steptoe, 2009). A number of physiologic systems are highly responsive to life experiences and the psychological states that accompany them. Further studies of varying human responses to stress are important as a basis for developing effective stress-management techniques, supporting healthy coping mechanisms, and restructuring faulty psychological defenses (Chrousos, 2009). Understanding the mechanisms that integrate our experiences into our biology rely on the emerging field of epigenetics.

Epigenetics, the study of how environmental influences regulate gene expression, is an attempt to describe how experiences such as stress—though not altering the DNA sequence—may modify DNA proteins, leading to enhanced or silenced expression of a specific gene. A total of 21 animal and human studies were reviewed that tested the relationship between psychological factors (stress, coping) and DNA damage. The studies demonstrated causal relations between acute stress and DNA damage in animals and significant correlations between psychological factors and DNA damage in adults (Gidron, Russ, Tissarchondou, & Warner, 2006). These limited findings indicate that psychological factors may influence DNA integrity. The results are further evidence of the person–environment connection. The challenge is to test whether stress management interventions can block stress-induced damage. Investigations are needed to study stress and other environmental and experiential exposures such as infections, toxins, and social interactions that may affect the genome throughout life (Bird, 2007).

A holistic approach that integrates the mind and body has long characterized nursing. Nurses understand the relationships between stress and health and stress and illness as a basis for assessment and nursing care. Nurses are in a key position to identify individuals and families who are coping ineffectively. Coping strategies for stress reduction; perceived controllability, intensity, and duration of stressors; emotional and behavioral regulation skills; and perceived availability of social support should be assessed. Findings will direct the nurse to structure appropriate interventions or make referrals to assist clients in managing stressors before they exert health-damaging effects.

STRESS ACROSS THE LIFE SPAN

Childhood and adolescence are critical periods characterized by increased vulnerability to stressors. Most of the knowledge about stress has been gained from studies of adults, and this information may or may not be directly applicable to children and adolescents.

Children experience stress and develop coping patterns early in life. Some factors known to be related to stress in children are self-esteem, personality characteristics (temperament), gender, social support, parental child-rearing patterns, previous stressful experiences, and illness. Children are mostly concerned about daily events that relate to school, peers, parents, and self. Stressors frequently identified by children include feeling sick, having nothing to do, not having enough money to spend, being pressured to get good grades, and feeling left out of the group.

Children's stress-coping processes must be assessed because of the hazards imposed by prolonged stress. Children with chronic illnesses, compared with well children, are less confident of their ability to handle problems and more often use ineffective coping skills (Walker, Smith, Garber, & Claar, 2007). Environmental and social stressors that place children at high risk include the following:

- Personal safety concerns
- Community violence
- Prolonged poverty
- Increased availability of drugs
- Homelessness

The majority of children, regardless of their environment, have a resiliency that enables them to function well in spite of major stressors. Some children are more affected by stressful situations than others and need intervention (Skybo & Buck, 2007). Competency develops over time (Hood, Power, & Hill, 2009). Children's well-being and health can be enhanced through constructive stress management. Personal resilience and environmental protective factors that mediate the relationship between risk factors and healthy development should be identified and incorporated into family, community, and school interventions. Instruments are available to measure stressors and physiologic and behavioral indicators of acute and chronic stress in children (Ryan-Wenger, Sharrer, & Wynd, 2000).

Adolescents' most common stressors are family-related, such as quarrels in mid-adolescence, peer stressors across early and mid-adolescence, and academic concerns in high school- aged youths. Higher stress in early adolescence is associated with a range of risk-taking behaviors such as smoking, alcohol use, and sexual sensation experiences (Bermudez, Teva, & Buela-Casal, 2009). Nurses and other health professionals may find that the best approach to avoiding substance abuse and other risky behaviors is to assist adolescents in learning effective stress-coping processes to apply across a variety of life circumstances. These processes include the following:

- Behavioral coping (information gathering)
- Decision making (problem solving)
- Cognitive coping (minimizing distress, focusing on the positive)
- Adult social support (talking with an adult)
- Relaxation (Hampel & Petermann, 2006)

How an individual copes with stress does not change from childhood to adolescence to adulthood. Individuals use the same types of coping skills to manage the stressors identified with each developmental stage. However, as individuals age, they increase their use of problem-solving coping and decrease the use avoidance coping, compared with the preteen and adolescence years (Amirkhan & Auyeung, 2007).

The stresses often experienced in young and middle-age adulthood relate to establishing oneself in a productive career, nourishing enduring relationships in a dyadic unit, childbearing and child rearing. Young adults desire to create a sense of self-identity as an independent yet interdependent adult.

The Double ABCX Model of Family Stress and Adaptation (McCubbin & Patterson, 1983) describes how families manage stressful events over a period of time. The model was founded in family stress theory in the 1940s and expanded by McCubbin and Patterson (1983). The initial stressor and accumulation of family demands are referred to as the A factor. Family changes and transitions as well as daily hassles among family members may cause stress. These demands on the family may produce internal tension that requires management. The B factor represents all the adaptive resources that a family can draw on in a time of stress. These include strengths of individual members, strengths of the family unit (open communication, cohesion), and strengths of the community (helpful agencies, supportive social networks). The C factor includes the family's definition and appraisal of all the demands (stressors), and the family's stress-meeting resources. Coping (BC factor) is seen as the family's resources, perceptions, and responses interacting to restore balance in the family. The outcome of the interaction between a family's demands and capabilities is family adaptation (X factor). McCubbin (1999) expanded the model to include family resiliency. Family responses to stressors occur in two stages: adjustment during minor events that do not require major family changes and adaptation during major crisis events to restore balance and harmony in the family. This model has been applied to assist nurses in primary care settings in conceptualizing stressors and coping capabilities of families as a basis for assessment and intervention (McLain & Dashiff, 2008) and understanding adjustment of mothers of children.

Constrained finances or arguments between spouses about how to spend limited income may markedly increase tension in the home. Single parents are particularly vulnerable to stress, as they may lack social support and also find that job demands leave them little time for parenting responsibilities. In the absence of authoritative parenting, children may get into difficulties that further stretch limited psychological resources of parents. Stress-management programs that address how to change the work and home environments to minimize stress and develop effective coping strategies best meet the needs of young and middle-age adults.

Work is often cited as a source of stress. Support at home can buffer work-related stressors, or the existence of additional stressors at home may have a cumulative effect with those at work. Many employers increasingly are offering work-site stress-management programs. Sources of work stress include the following:

- Lack of control over job environment or production demands
- Being "caught in the middle" between supervisors and customers
- Being under-prepared for the job
- Lack of clarity about job expectations
- Unexpected transfers across departments or company locations
- Feeling trapped in a particular job
- Lack of positive relationships with coworkers

Stress often causes deterioration in performance, which can further escalate already existing causes of stress and tension (Couser, 2008).

An analysis of client-centered stress management interventions in the workplace by the Centre for Stress Management is available (at http://managingstress.com/articles /webpage2). A systemic review of job-stress interventions, 1990–2005, found that interventions that are both organizationally and individually focused produce more favorable outcomes than intervention that focus on either alone (Lamontagne, Keegel, Louie, Ostry, & Landsbergis, 2007).

Although some sources of stress may abate in older adulthood, other stressors, particularly those resulting from loss, are more prevalent. The elderly are particularly vulnerable to negative life events such as the death of a spouse, death of a close family member, personal injury or illness, change in one's financial status, and retirement. Hassles of daily living may increase as a result of diminished sensory acuity, decreased dexterity and strength, and loss of flexibility. Cumulative stress, along with depression can compromise immune function, leaving the elderly more vulnerable to acute and chronic disease (Trouillet, Gana, Lourel, & Fort, 2009).

In old age we begin to see the increased morbidity and mortality associated with years of daily hassles and cumulative major life events, particularly when coping strategies have been ineffective. Systemic effects on the cardiovascular, gastrointestinal, neurologic, endocrine, and immune systems are increasingly apparent (Charmandari, Tsigos, & Chrousos, 2005). Decreased resistance to disease means that elderly adults need to learn to use productive coping strategies. Nurses familiar with the issues of aging and the capabilities of older adults can equip them to manage the stressors that they encounter more effectively and efficiently, thus conserving valuable personal resources.

APPROACHES TO STRESS MANAGEMENT

A number of nursing diagnoses specific to problems in stress management (e.g., defensive coping, ineffective family coping) are described by Gordon (2007) in the functional health pattern category of Coping–Stress Tolerance Pattern. The nurse and client must assess the level of existing stress as well as the sources of stress and then determine the appropriate interventions to reduce stress. Many techniques for stress management are reported in the literature. However, the overall effectiveness of some stress management interventions has not been sufficiently studied, so the evidence for the effectiveness and safety of interventions should be closely examined prior to using in one's practice.

Interventions for stress management should aim to achieve the following:

- Minimize the frequency of stress-inducing situations
- Increase resistance to stress
- Avoid physiologic arousal resulting from stress

In general, changing the environment to decrease the incidence of stressors is the "first line of defense." When that is not possible, individual and family coping resources must come into play to reinterpret stress as a challenge and increase resilience against it.

Minimizing the Frequency of Stress-Inducing Situations

The need to adapt to externally imposed change is continuous. Approaches to assisting clients in preventing stressful situations include (1) changing the environment, (2) avoiding excessive change, (3) time control, and (4) time management.

CHANGING THE ENVIRONMENT.   Widely held values and beliefs shape the environment in any society. Changing the environment, when it is possible, is the most proactive approach to minimizing the frequency of stress-inducing situations. Major changes in societal beliefs, values, and actions are necessary if stress is to be reduced for some vulnerable populations. Sexism, racism, and ageism create stress for selected groups as a result of devaluation of their status and lack of acknowledgment of their contributions to society. Discrimination directed at any group can result in decreased educational and employment opportunities, poverty, and personal devaluation. Racial disparities in disease rates are rooted in differences between races in exposure or vulnerability to pathogenic factors in the physical, social, economic, and cultural environment. Perceived discrimination is a stressor that does not vary on the basis of the minority person's social status (Brondolo, Brady Ver Halen, Pencille, Beatty, & Contrada, 2009).

The work environment is frequently identified as a major source of stress. Changes in the work environment itself can reduce the incidence of stressful events. For example, instituting policies that provide flextime, job sharing, or child-care benefits or facilities can ease the stress on parents who must both maintain a job and care for young children. Protecting workers from job-related hazards, redesigning work assignments, creating pleasant work stations, instituting quality circles, and implementing participatory management styles also can foster lower levels of stress at work. Job-related stresses may also be avoided by becoming more aware of persons or experiences that create personal stress and minimizing contact to the extent possible. A study by Lamontagne and colleagues (2007) suggests that the best outcomes for reduction of stress in the workplace occur when a comprehensive framework guides the chosen interventions.

If a job change is required to decrease stress, new employment possibilities should be analyzed to make sure that stress phenomena similar to those already encountered are not an inherent part of the new employment setting. Protective factors in the broader environment that can further decrease stress include a family characterized by warmth and cohesion, cultural events and customs that promote identity, supportive relationships with others outside the family, and involvement in community structures such as churches and neighborhood organizations that promote competence and support.

AVOIDING EXCESSIVE CHANGE.   During periods of significant life change and resulting negative tension states, any additional unnecessary changes should be avoided. For example, if a family is experiencing the illness of one of its family members and a subsequent job loss, this may not be the time to consider geographic relocation, pregnancy, or any other change in lifestyle. Negative tension created by multiple changes is synergistic. Each time a distressing change occurs, the potency of previous change for upsetting stability is increased. Deliberately postponing changes that result in negative tension can assist clients to constructively manage unavoidable change, and postponement prevents the need for multiple adjustments at one point in time.

Any changes that are made in lifestyle during periods of high or moderate stress should be self-initiated and challenge, rather than threaten, the client. Increasing positive sources of tension that promote growth and self-actualization can offset the deleterious effects of negative tension. For example, learning to play tennis, to swim, or to dance may provide a distracting challenge to counterbalance potentially debilitating stress.

TIME CONTROL.   Time control is a technique to set aside specific time to adapt to various stressors. This period of personal time may be daily, weekly, or monthly. It offers clients time to focus on a specific change and develop strategies for adjustment. The major advantage of time control is that it ensures that important goals or concerns are addressed and critical tasks are accomplished. Individuals are encouraged to focus on managing time more effectively to prevent the stress that time shortages produce. This strategy reduces a sense of urgency, a high level of anxiety, and feelings of frustration and failure.

TIME MANAGEMENT.   The time management approach to stress management suggests organizing oneself to accomplish those goals most important in life within the time available. Lack of time is a frequent reason for not participating in health-promoting activities. Teaching clients time management makes a major contribution to their health and fitness. Time-pressured, high-anxiety clients are particularly in need of time-management skills.

Identifying and prioritizing goals serve as a framework for time management. When clients identify time wasted on activities unrelated to personal goals, they can restructure how they spend their time. Overcommitment to others or unrealistic expectations of one-self is a frequent source of stress. Time overload may be avoided by learning to say "no" to demands of others that are unrealistic or of low personal or family priority. Overload results in frustration and loss of satisfaction from the work accomplished, because one seldom expends one's best efforts under strain and pressure.

An important approach to time management is to reduce a task into smaller parts. A task may appear overwhelming; however, if it is broken down into smaller segments, accomplishment becomes feasible. An example may be to learn several effective conditioning exercises before learning a complete conditioning routine, or developing skill with a conditioning routine before beginning a walk-jog activity. Breaking it down into component parts allows mastery and feelings of competence.

Feelings of overload can be avoided by delegating responsibilities to others and enlisting their assistance. Making use of others' skills provides freedom from the expectation of having to be "all things to all people." Another important aspect of time management is to reduce the perception of time pressure and urgency. Not all perceptions of time urgency are warranted; some are needlessly self-imposed. The client should differentiate between time urgencies that are valid and others that are needlessly created. One may avoid time urgencies by minimizing procrastination, as leaving tasks that must be completed until the last minute often results in needless pressure and stress (Davis & Rob, 2008).

Increasing Resistance to Stress

Resistance to stress is achieved through either physical or psychologic conditioning. Physical conditioning for stress resistance focuses on exercise. Psychologic conditioning to increase resistance resources focuses on (1) enhancing self-esteem, (2) enhancing self-efficacy, (3) increasing assertiveness, (4) setting realistic goals, and (5) building coping resources.

PROMOTING EXERCISE.   Exercise is discussed at length in Chapter 6. However, the relationship between exercise and stress is addressed here briefly. Four processes have been suggested that may account for the positive effects of exercise on responses to mental stress. The first is that psychologic changes are the by-product of cardiorespiratory fitness. However, this explanation is weakened by the fact that psychologic responses and fitness are frequently not correlated. A second possibility is that changes in exercise-related self-efficacy and mastery generalize to other situations, resulting in improvements in self-concept and coping ability. A third process that may underlie decreased stress responses following periods of exercise is a blunting of the psychophysiology responsiveness to stressors. Epidemiologic research suggests that physical activity is positively related to good mental health. In general, people who are inactive are twice as likely to be depressed, whereas people who exercise regularly report feelings of well-being. Although increased fatigue, anxiety, and decreased vigor can occur with overtraining, in general, regular physical exercise contributes to good mental health (Ament & Verkerke, 2009).

ENHANCING SELF-ESTEEM.   Self-esteem is the value attributed to self or how one feels about oneself. This valuation is based on a person's concept of his or her desirable and undesirable attributes, strengths and weaknesses, achievements, and success in interpersonal relationships. Hein and Hagger (2007) find that physical activity interventions that target self-identified activities enhance young people's general self-esteem.

Although self-esteem is developed over time, studies have shown that the level of self-esteem may be changed. One approach is positive verbalization. In using this technique, clients identify positive aspects of self or personal characteristics that they value highly. They should also ask significant others to comment on their positive attributes. Each characteristic, one per day, is placed on a 3 × 5 index card, and the cards are placed in a conspicuous place. Each card should be read several times a day. This technique helps clients to spend more time thinking positively about themselves, and it decreases the amount of time spent in self-devaluation. Increased self-awareness of positive characteristics and their presence in conscious thought result in more frequent behavior that reflects these attributes and more positive responses from significant others. Nurse practitioners and school nurses have excellent opportunities to promote positive self-concepts and healthy levels of self-esteem for adolescents as a basis for healthy functioning throughout life.

ENHANCING SELF-EFFICACY.   Mastery experiences help to create a sense of competence to perform effectively and overcome obstacles. Experiencing successful performance of a particular, valued behavior provides positive messages regarding personal skills and abilities. Counseling clients to undertake tasks that are challenging but from which they experience success rather than failure can build a sense of efficacy in a particular domain. Self-beliefs about personal efficacy have wide-ranging ramifications affecting level of motivation, affect, thought, and action. Perceiving oneself to be efficacious has been shown to predict performance better than actual ability. In other words, if people's beliefs in their efficacy are strengthened, they approach situations with more assurance and make better use of the skills that they have.

High self-efficacy has been documented to be beneficial in managing a specific stressor (Folkman, 2009). Persons with high levels of efficacy mentally rehearse success rather than failures at a task, set high goals and make a firm commitment to attain them, perceive more control over personal threats, and are less anxious in the face of day-to-day challenges. Highly efficacious persons also tend to be more assertive in accessing the support they need to optimize their chances of success. The nurse should help clients identify skills most important to them and then assist them in increasing their efficacy in the highly valued areas.

INCREASING ASSERTIVENESS.   Substituting positive, assertive behaviors for negative, passive ones increases personal capacity for psychological resistance to stress. Assertiveness is the appropriate expression of oneself and one's thoughts and feelings, and results in greater personal satisfaction in living. Assertiveness is more constructive than aggression and is more effective than aggression in managing problems. Many books and articles on assertiveness training are available. Assertiveness enables individuals to share their perceptions and feelings with others in a way that facilitates rather than inhibits personal or group productivity. Clients should be encouraged to use the following strategies to become more assertive:

- Make a deliberate effort to greet others and call them by name.
- Maintain eye contact during conversations.
- Comment on the positive characteristics of others.
- Initiate conversation.
- Express opinions.
- Express feelings.
- Disagree with others when holding opposing viewpoints.
- Take initiative to engage in a new behavior or learn a new activity.

Although it is possible for clients to become more assertive through the use of simple techniques, very passive and reserved clients might well benefit from more comprehensive assertiveness training provided by a competent instructor or counselor. The nurse may assist clients in locating such resources for personal development.

SETTING REALISTIC GOALS.   Clients must not only set goals but understand that accomplishment of goals is rewarding. Long- and short-term goals help the client stay on course. Long-term goals set the direction for change, and short-term goals allow for immediate successes. Goals should be set that can be attained within a reasonable time frame. If goals are met, it may reinforce the client's desire to continue to set health-promoting goals. Another useful rule is to plan to change only one behavior at a time. Flexibility on the part of the client permits achievement of desired outcomes through several approaches. Reward or reinforcement is possible through accomplishment of alternative goals. As a result, lack of success in initial attempts to reach goals becomes much less ominous because of the probability of success in achieving alternative goals that bring similar rewards.

BUILDING COPING RESOURCES.   Stress results when there is an imbalance between appraised demands and appraised coping capabilities. More attention should be directed to the resource side of the equation rather than the demand side. Coping resources are more predictive of reactions to stressors than the actual demands. General coping resources that have been identified to enhance stress resistance include the following:

- *Self-disclosure*: Predisposition to share one's feelings, troubles, thoughts, and opinions with others.
- *Self-directedness*: Degree to which a person respects his or her own judgment for decision making.

- *Confidence*: Ability to gain mastery over one's environment and to control one's emotions in the interest of reaching personal goals.
- *Acceptance*: Degree to which persons accept their shortcomings and imperfections and maintain a positive and tolerant attitude toward others.
- *Social Support*: Availability and use of a network of caring others.
- *Financial freedom*: Extent to which persons are free of financial constraints on their lifestyles.
- *Physical health*: Overall health condition, including absence of chronic disease and disabilities.
- *Physical fitness*: Conditioning resulting from personal exercise practices.
- *Stress monitoring*: Awareness of tension buildup and situations that are likely to prove stressful.
- *Tension control*: Ability to lower arousal through relaxation and thought control.
- *Structuring*: Ability to organize and manage resources such as time and energy.
- *Problem solving*: Ability to resolve personal problems.

A commonly used measure of coping is the Ways of Coping Questionnaire (Folkman & Lazarus, 1988). The scale contains eight subscales that measure both emotion-focused and problem-focused coping strategies an individual uses when responding to a stressful situation. After assessing the extent to which the various coping resources are present, nurses should assist clients in maximizing existing strengths and developing additional resistance resources.

COMPLEMENTARY THERAPIES TO MANAGE STRESS

Complementary therapies are used by more than two-thirds of the world population, and Americans have dramatically increased their use of such therapies in recent years: Most older Americans report use of complementary and alternative medicine (Ness, Cirillo, Weir, Nisly, & Wallace, 2005). Complementary therapies are used together with traditional medicine to manage stress and stress-related illnesses. Complementary therapies used to manage stress include self-regulation techniques such as mindfulness, progressive muscle relaxation, imagery, acupuncture, yoga, and self-hypnosis. The goal of these therapies is to achieve a balance of physical, emotional, and spiritual factors in one's life. Mindfulness, progressive relaxation, and imagery are three interventions used to assist clients in managing stress.

Mindfulness-Based Stress Reduction (MBSR)

Mindfulness-Based Stress Reduction (MBSR), developed by John Kabat-Zinn (2005) at the Massachusetts School of Medicine in 1979, is based on an early Buddhist teaching of being aware of everything in the present moment, without judgment. Participants are taught various types of meditation in the psycho-educational stress-reduction program. Mindfulness is about gaining awareness of your body, actions, feelings, and surroundings, deliberately giving your full attention to everything you are involved in from one moment to the next.

A meta-analysis of published and unpublished health-related studies using MBSR was conducted to determine the effectiveness of the intervention. Of the 60 research studies identified, only 20 met the criteria for inclusion in the meta-analysis. The results support the findings that MBSR helped participants cope with a wide range of clinical and nonclinical problems (Grossman, Niemann, Schmidt, & Walach, 2004). A subsequent review substantiates the beneficial results for physical and mental health (Irving, Dobkin, & Park, 2009). A systematic review of the effects of MBSR on sleep disturbances showed positive effects on sleep quality and duration, indicating a decrease in sleep-interfering cognitive processes (Winbush, Gross, & Kreitzer, 2007). Mindfulness training for older people with anxiety and depression has shown very positive results that were maintained a year later (Smith, 2006). Evidence supports the use of MBSR for decreasing mood disturbance and stress symptoms in people of all ages and diagnoses (Carmody, Reed, Kristeller, & Merriam, 2008; Reibel, Greeson, Brainard, & Rosenzweig, 2001; Winbush et al., 2007).

MBSR is a nonreligious, systematic procedure to develop enhanced awareness of moment-to-moment experiences of perceptual processes. Elements of the eight-week (2.5 hours per week) program include an emphasis on a non-goal orientation and a variety of meditation techniques, including body scan meditation, sitting and walking meditation, and Hatha yoga (Kabat-Zinn, 2005). Daily practice and home study are essential program components.

One way to experience a mindful exercise to try is to become mindful while walking. Be aware of the inner chatter of the mind. Listen for the sound of your foot touching the ground and feel the sensation while just being aware of what you are doing. Being mindful is active yet passive, as it can be done anytime or anywhere by simply focusing on what is happening in the present moment.

Progressive Relaxation Through Tension-Relaxation

Progressive Muscle Relaxation (PMR), developed by Edmund Jacobson in 1938, involves decreasing voluntary muscle and sympathetic nervous system activity while increasing parasympathetic functioning. Increasing evidence supports Jacobson's findings that tension levels may be reduced through use of relaxation skills. Relaxation seems to be a way of turning off the body's response to the sympathetic nervous system and decreasing neuro-hormonal changes that take place in reaction to the experience of negative tension states (Kwekkeboom & Gretarsdottir, 2006; Kwekkeboom, Hau, Wanta, & Bumpus, 2008).

The overreaction or underreaction of the immune system to stress may result in disease or illness. Research is mixed on whether PMR has positive effects on the body's immune system (Kwekkeboom & Gretarsdottir, 2006; Snyder & Lindquist, 2007). Positive outcomes have been documented when PMR is used for stress reduction either as the prescribed therapy or as an adjunct therapy. Improvement in pain intensity and pain control has been seen in patients with cancer pain unrelieved by medications (Kwekkeboom et al., 2008). Changes in blood pressure and anxiety levels after PMR have also been reported (Snyder & Lindquist, 2007; Tang, Harms, & Vezeau, 2008). A review of randomized relaxation interventions for pain relief was conducted to determine their effectiveness (Kwekkeboom et al., 2008). There was support for PMR in 8 of 15 studies. Most often, PMR was used to reduce arthritis pain. In a randomized trial of 55 healthy college men and women, after a 25-minute PMR intervention, participants had a significant increase in the nociceptive flexion reflex (NFR) threshold, which allows withdrawal from noxious stimuli, whereas participants in the no-treatment group experienced no change in NFR threshold (Emery, France, Harris, Norman, & Van Arsdalen, 2008). Research comparing PMR with mindfulness skills found both equally effective in reducing psychological distress (Agee, Danoff-Burg, & Grant, 2009). See *Complementary Alternative Therapies in Nursing* (Snyder & Lindquist, 2007) for further information and precautions in the use of PMR. Continued conduct of well-designed research is necessary to determine effective interventions and protocols.

Relaxation is suggested to result in the following changes (Snyder & Lindquist, 2007):

- Decreased oxygen consumption
- Lowered metabolism
- Decreased respiration rate
- Decreased heart rate
- Decreased muscle tension
- Decreased premature ventricular contractions
- Decreased systolic and diastolic blood pressures
- Increased alpha brain waves
- Enhanced immune function

To conduct relaxation training, a very pleasant, quiet, soundproof room in which lighting may be dimmed, with reclining lawn or lounge chairs for clients, provides an optimum setting. Tight clothing should be loosened, glasses and shoes removed, and a comfortable position assumed in the chair. Relaxation should not be taught with clients lying flat. Although this is a common position assumed for rest and sleep, it often results in muscle strain in the upper back and neck along with drowsiness, which interferes with training. A reclining position or sitting position is most appropriate.

At the beginning of each session, clients are encouraged to focus on their own breathing as the air moves gently in and out. The purpose of this focusing activity is to increase awareness of self. Following the focusing activity, clients are moved slowly through tension and relaxation cycles for each of the major muscle groups listed in Table 8–1, maintaining tension for 8–10 seconds and releasing tension instantaneously

TABLE 8–1   Muscle Group Sequence for Tension–Relaxation Cycle

Muscle Group	Abbreviated Instructions
1. Right hand and forearm	Make a fist.
2. Right upper arm	Pull elbow tightly into side.
3. Left hand and forearm	Make a fist.
4. Left upper arm	Pull elbow tightly into side.
5. Forehead	Wrinkle brow.
6. Upper cheeks and nose	Squint eyes and wrinkle nose.
7. Lower cheeks and jaws	Place teeth together and make a "forced" smile.
8. Neck and throat	Pull chin toward chest.
9. Chest, shoulders, and upper back	Take a deep breath. Push shoulder blades toward each other.
10. Upper abdomen	Pull stomach in and hold
11. Lower abdomen	Bear down against the seat of the chair.
12. Right upper leg	Push down against the foot of the chair.
13. Right lower leg and foot	Point toes toward head and body.
14. Left upper leg	Push down against the foot of the chair.
15. Left lower leg and foot	Point toes toward head and body.

on cue. The entire tension–relaxation cycle should be repeated twice during the first session to increase clients' awareness of the differences in body sensations during tensed and relaxed periods. The tension–relaxation instructions should be given very slowly, allowing clients to enjoy the feelings of relaxation they are experiencing. The guidance provided by the nurse is critical for successful relaxation.

To facilitate daily practice of relaxation techniques, clients at home may use training tapes. Clients are asked to keep a schedule of the frequency and length of time that relaxation is practiced, and are encouraged to "think through" the relaxation procedure and do their own coaching. A "prompt sheet" on the sequence of the muscle groups should be provided for easy reference. This is intended to move clients toward independent practice of relaxation rather than encouraging reliance on the nurse or the coaching tape to obtain relaxation cues.

Common problems reported when learning relaxation techniques include the following:

- Overly rapid self-pacing through the relaxation sequence
- Distraction by environmental noise
- Difficulty keeping attention on own monologue
- Distracting thoughts during relaxation
- Residual tension in some muscles after tension–relaxation

Encouraging clients to slow down internal speech or coaching pace usually solves the problem of overly rapid self-pacing. Autogenic phrases such as "I feel calm," "I feel very relaxed," and "my arms and legs feel heavy" may be interspersed throughout self-instruction. Encouraging family members to join in the relaxation practice sessions often fosters stress-management skills among the entire family unit.

PROGRESSIVE RELAXATION WITHOUT TENSION.   Clients may be taught how to relax without first tensing muscles. Relaxation through counting down and relaxation through imagery are frequently used strategies. The major advantage of these techniques is that tension is no longer required. This is particularly important when elevations in blood pressure caused by prolonged or extensive muscle tensing are contraindicated. Deep relaxation without tension is the goal. Phrases that might be repeated to facilitate relaxation include the following:

- "I feel quiet."
- "I am beginning to feel quite relaxed."
- "My feet feel heavy and relaxed."
- "My ankles, my knees, and my hips feel heavy."
- "My solar plexus and the whole central portion of my body feel relaxed and quiet."
- "My hands, my arms, and my shoulders feel heavy, relaxed, and comfortable."
- "My neck, my jaw, and my forehead feel relaxed. They feel comfortable and smooth."
- "My whole body feels quite heavy, comfortable, and relaxed.
- "I am quite relaxed."
- "My mind is quiet."
- "My thoughts are turned inward, and I am at ease."
- "I can visualize and experience myself relaxed, comfortable, and still."

These phrases were suggested as a result of work in biofeedback at the Menninger Foundation (see Web site listed at the end of the chapter). Such phrases result in physiologic imagery that decreases both sympathetic nervous system activity and tension in voluntary muscles.

Relaxation through the countdown procedure initially focuses on each muscle group used previously. The client is encouraged to relax each muscle group progressively as the count proceeds from 10 down to 1. When the client becomes skilled with this procedure, total body countdown is used, relaxing the entire body while silently counting down from 10 to 1. This procedure is particularly useful when facing stressful social situations. In 2–3 minutes, the skilled client can achieve total body relaxation while in a sitting position with eyes open and focused on a specific object. Mini-relaxation sessions several times throughout the day promote generalization of relaxation training to everyday life.

RELAXATION THROUGH IMAGERY. *Guided imagery* is a stress reduction intervention in which the interrelationship of the body and mind is used to influence physiological responses. This cognitive process uses the imagination to bring about positive mind/body responses. It uses many senses, including sight, smell, taste, and touch. The benefits of imagery include its influence on physiological responses of the autonomic nervous system that result in stress reduction. Research supports imagery as an effective intervention for pain management and depressive disorders, and for changing health behaviors (Apostolo & Kolcaba, 2009; Haase, Schwenk, Hermann, & Müller, 2005; Weydert et al., 2006). However, additional research is needed to determine its association with neuro-immunomodulatory effects (Telles et al., 2007). Imagery plus progressive muscle relaxation is thought to be more effective than imagery alone (Morone, Greco, & Weiner, 2008). See *Complementary alternative therapies in nursing* (Snyder & Lindquist, 2007) for further information and precautions in the use of guided imagery.

Using imagery to relax requires passive concentration on pleasant scenes or experiences from the past to facilitate relaxation. Recalling the warmth of the sun, the feeling of warm sand, the sensations of a gentle breeze, the vision of palm trees swaying, or the sounds of ocean waves may be comfortable and pleasant for clients. Clients vary in scenes or images that result in actual changes in muscle tension. For some clients, visualizing specific colors, shapes, or patterns are as effective as visualizing landscapes or scenes. If clients initially have difficulty using imagery or visualization for relaxation, the nurse may use one of the following techniques:

- Have the client, with eyes closed, visualize a particular room of his or her house (living room, bedroom, kitchen), focusing on colors, shapes, and specific objects. The client's mind should wander about the room, describing verbally what is seen in as much detail as possible.
- Have the client focus on a particular piece of clothing that is a personal favorite. The client should describe the color, texture, design, and trim of the piece of clothing and how it feels when worn (e.g., soft, loose, fitted, light, warm).

Individuals will become more vivid in descriptions of concrete objects, and their ability to use less concrete imagery for purposes of relaxation will increase. Imagery is a highly useful relaxation technique in many settings in which muscle tension or biofeedback equipment would be obtrusive.

The opportunity to assist clients to manage stress and pain through science-based interventions is well within the nurse's scope of practice. However, consultation with and/or referral to other professionals who specialize in complementary therapies is an opportunity for nurses to develop collaborative interdisciplinary relationships and referral networks.

OPPORTUNITIES FOR RESEARCH ON STRESS MANAGEMENT

Major advances in understanding the effects of stressors on the neuroendocrine and immune systems have offered new possibilities for managing the brain–body interface to promote health. However, more research is needed to test stress-reducing interventions and their effect on these systems. The profile of stressors most likely to occur at different developmental stages and the best way to match stressors with targeted coping processes are research priorities. A challenge is to discover how to build coping resources, resilience, and personal competence in the early childhood years so that patterns of successful adaptation manifest themselves throughout adolescence and adulthood.

Interventions that decrease environmental and family stressors for vulnerable populations are priorities. Human tolerance for stress is finite, as people can manage only so much stress. The efforts of scientists from multiple disciplines are needed to learn more about the phenomenon of stress.

CONSIDERATONS FOR PRACTICE IN STRESS MANAGEMENT

Individuals who experience the same stressors often respond differently. Stress-related illnesses are very common and require appropriate interventions or referrals to assist the client to manage stress before negative outcomes present. The promotion and conduct of early screenings and developmentally specific interventions are necessary because children, adolescents, young adults, and older adults develop and use different coping strategies. Awareness of these differences ensures that the nurse intervenes at the appropriate time and with the appropriate strategy to achieve stress reduction. Although the stress management interventions discussed in this chapter are within the nurse's scope of practice, he or she should gain expertise in the use of them by working with an experienced provider and through study and practice. The rapidly growing field of stress research mandates that each practitioner stay updated on the latest evidence for practice.

Summary

This chapter presents a number of different approaches for assisting individuals and families in managing stress. Some of the interventions that are suggested are relatively unstructured, whereas others are more defined and complex. The client and the nurse should make collaborative decisions about the most appropriate interventions to use, taking the client's mental and physical health status into account. This decision should also be based on the sources of stress experienced by the client and his or her general patterns of response to stressful events. The nurse must be aware of his or her own comfort level and expertise with stress-reducing interventions and refer clients to other health care providers when appropriate.

Learning Activities

1. Discuss the management of stress in children, young and middle adults, and the elderly.
2. Select one intervention to manage stress and develop a modified protocol for a client of a specific age.
3. Practice mindful walking and describe your feelings, experiences, and sensations.
4. Practice progressive relaxation without tension using some of the suggested phrases until you feel comfortable saying them and you identify a difference in your relaxation state.

Selected Web Sites

American Psychological Association
http://www.apa.org
The American Psychological Association is a scientific and professional organization whose mission is to advance the creation, communication, and application of psychology to improve people's lives. This site provides information and research publications on topics such as stress and mental health.

The Center for Stress Management
http://managingstress.com/articles/webpage2
An analysis of client-centered stress management interventions in the workplace.

The Center for Mindfulness in Medicine, Health Care, and Society
http://www.umassmed.edu/content.aspx?id=41252
Established in 1995, the Center houses the Stress Reduction Clinic. The Center provides information and research on topics related to MBSR.

Healthy People 2020
http://www.healthypeople.gov/hp2020/
Healthy People 2020 focuses on realistic and achievable goals. This site is updated frequently, so it is available to the public to follow the development and implementation of the plan.

National Institute of Mental Health
http://www.nimh.nih.gov/index.shtml
One of the institutes of the National Institutes of Health, this institute provides health and outreach information and research funding to address mental health/illness issues.

The Menninger Foundation
http://www.menningerclinic.org/
Menninger is a leading psychiatric center dedicated to treating individuals with mood, personality, anxiety, and addictive disorders; teaching mental health professionals; and advancing mental health care through research.

The National Center for Complementary and Alternative Medicine
http://www.nccam.nih.gov
The National Center for Complementary and Alternative Medicine is the Federal Government's lead agency for scientific research on diverse medical and health care systems, practices, and products that are not considered part of conventional medicine.

The World Health Organization Global Burden of Disease Survey
http://www.who.int/healthinfo/global_burden_disease/GBD_report_2004update_part2.pdf

References

Agee, J. D., Danoff-Burg, S., & Grant, C. A. (2009). Comparing brief stress management courses in a community sample: Mindfulness skills and progressive muscle relaxation. *Explore*, 5, 104–109.

Ament, W., & Verkerke, G. J. (2009). Exercise and fatigue. *Sports Medicine*, 39(5), 389–422.

Amirkhan, J., & Auyeung, B. (2007, July–August). Coping with stress across the lifespan: Absolute vs. relative changes in strategy. *Journal of Applied Developmental Psychology*, 28(4), 298–317.

Apostolo, J. L., & Kolcaba, K. (2009). The effects of guided imagery on comfort, depression, anxiety, and stress of psychiatric inpatients with depressive disorders. *Archives of Psychiatric Nursing, 23*(6), 402–411.

Bacon, E., Milne, D. L., Sheikh, A. I., & Freeston, M. H. (2009, January). Positive experiences in caregivers: An exploratory case series. *Behavioural and Cognitive Psychotherapy, 37*(1), 95–114.

Bermudez, M. D., Teva, I., & Buela-Casal, G. (2009, May). Influence of sociodemographic variables on coping styles, social stress, and sexual sensation seeking in adolescents. *Psicothema, 21*(2), 220–226.

Bird, A. (2007, May). Perceptions of epigenetics. *Nature, 447*, 396–398.

Brondolo, E., Brady Ver Halen, N., Pencille, M., Beatty, D., & Contrada, R. J. (2009, February). Coping with racism: A selective review of the literature and a theoretical and methodological critique. *Journal of Behavioral Medicine, 32*(1), 64–88.

Brydon, L., Walker, C., Wawrzyniak, A. J., Chart, H., & Steptoe, A. (2009). Dispositional optimism and stress-induced changes in immunity and negative mood. *Brain, Behavior, and Immunity, 23*(6), 810–816.

Carmody, J., Reed, G., Kristeller, J., & Merriam, P. (2008, April). Mindfulness, spirituality, and health-related symptoms. *Journal of Psychosomatic Research, 64*(4), 393–403.

Charmandari, E., Tsigos, C., & Chrousos, G. (2005). Endocrinology of the stress response. *Annual Review of Physiology, 67*, 259–284.

Chrousos, G. P. (2009, July). Stress and disorders of the stress system. *Nature Review Endocrinology, 5*(7), 374–381.

Couser, G. P. (2008, April). Challenges and opportunities for preventing depression in the workplace: A review of the evidence supporting workplace factors and interventions. *Journal of Occupational and Environmental Medicine, 50*(4), 411–427.

Davis, M., & Rob, E. (2008). *The relaxation and stress reduction workbook* (6th ed.). Oakland, CA: New Harbinger Publications.

Emery, C. F., France, C. R., Harris, J., Norman, G., & Van Arsdalen, C. (2008). Effects of progressive muscle relaxation training on nociceptive flexion reflex threshold in healthy young adults: A randomized trial. *Pain, 138*, 375–379.

Epel, E. S. (2009). Psychological and metabolic stress: A recipe for accelerated cellular aging? *Hormones (Athens), 8*(1), 7–22.

Folkman, S. (2009). Questions, answers, issues and next steps in stress and coping research. *European Psychologist, 14*, 72–77.

Folkman, S., & Lazarus, R. S. (1988). Coping as a mediator of emotion. *Journal of Personality and Social Psychology, 54*(3), 466–475.

Gersten, O. (2008). The path traveled and the path ahead for the allostatic framework: A rejoinder on the framework's importance and the need for further work related to theory, data, and measurement. *Social Science & Medicine, 66*, 531–535.

Gidron, T., Russ, K., Tissarchondou, H., & Warner, J. (2006). The relation between psychological factors and DNA-damage: A critical review. *Biological Psychology, 72*, 291–304.

Gordon, M. (2007). *Manual of nursing diagnosis: Including all diagnostic categories approved by the North American nursing diagnosis association* (11th ed.). St Louis, MO: Mosby.

Grossman, P., Niemann, L., Schmidt, S., & Walach, H. (2004, July). Mindfulness-based stress reduction and health benefits: A meta-analysis. *Journal of Psychosomatic Research, 57*(1), 35–43.

Haase, O., Schwenk, W., Hermann, C., & Müller, J. M. (2005, October). Guided imagery and relaxation in conventional colorectal resections: A randomized, controlled, partially blinded trial. *Diseases of the Colon & Rectum, 48*(10), 1955–1963.

Hampel, P., & Petermann, F. (2006, April). Perceived stress, coping, and adjustment in adolescents. *Journal of Adolescent Health, 38*(4), 409–415.

Hein, V., & Hagger, M. S. (2007, January). Global self-esteem, goal achievement orientations, and self-determined behavioural regulations in a physical education setting. *Journal of Sports Science, 25*(2), 149–159.

Hogan, M. F. (2003). The President's New Freedom Commission: Recommendations to transform mental health care in America. *Psychiatric Services, 54*(11), 1467–1474.

Hood, B., Power, T., & Hill, L. (2009, March). Children's appraisal of moderately stressful situations. *International Journal of Behavioral Development, 33*(2), 167–177.

Irving, J. A., Dobkin, P. L., & Park, J. (2009). Cultivating mindfulness in health care professionals: A review of empirical studies of mindfulness-based stress reduction (MBSR). *Complementary Therapies in Clinical Practice, 15*, 61–66.

Kabat-Zinn, J. (2005). *Coming to our senses: Healing ourselves and the world through mindfulness.* New York: Hyperion.

Kalia, M. (2002, June). Assessing the economic impact of stress: The modern day hidden epidemic. *Metabolism, 51*(6 Part 2), 49–53.

Kwekkeboom, K. L., & Gretarsdottir, E. (2006). Systematic review of relaxation interventions for pain. *Journal of Nursing Scholarship, 38*(3), 269–277.

Kwekkeboom, K. L., Hau, H., Wanta, B., & Bumpus, M. (2008, August). Patients' perceptions of the effectiveness of guided imagery and progressive muscle relaxation interventions used for cancer pain. *Complementary Therapies in Clinical Practice, 14*(3), 185–194.

Lamontagne, A. D., Keegel, T., Louie, A. M., Ostry, A., & Landsbergis, P. A. (2007, January–March). A systematic review of the job-stress intervention evaluation literature, 1990–2005. *International Journal of Occupational and Environmental Health, 13*(3), 268–280.

Lazarus, R. S. (1999). *Stress and emotion: A new synthesis.* New York: Springer Publishing Co.

Lazarus, R. S., & Folkman, S. (1984). *Stress, appraisal and coping.* New York: Springer.

Loucks, E. B., Juster, R. P., & Pruessner, J. C. (2008). Neuroendocrine biomarkers, allostatic load, and the challenges of measurement: A commentary on Gerstein. *Social Science & Medicine, 66*, 525–530.

Manzoli, L., Villari, P., Pirone, G., & Boccia, A. (2007, January). Marital status and mortality in the elderly: A systematic review and meta-analysis. *Social Science & Medicine, 64*(1), 77–94.

McCubbin, H. I., & Patterson, J. M. (1983). The family stress process: The Double ABCX Model of adjustment and adaptation. *Marriage and Family Review, 6*(1/2), 7–37.

McCubbin, M. (1999). Normative family transitions and family outcomes. In A. S. Hinshaw, S. L. Feetham, & J. L. Shaver (Eds.), *Handbook of clinical nursing research* (pp. 201–230). Thousands Oaks, CA: Sage Publications.

McEwen, B. S. (2007). Stress, homeostasis, rheostasis, allostasis and allostatic load. In G. Fink (Ed.), *The Encyclopedia of Stress,* (2nd ed., pp. 557–561). San Diego, CA: Academic Press.

McLain, R. M., & Dashiff, C. (2008, May–June). Family stress, family adaptation and psychological well-being of elderly coronary artery bypass grafting patients. *Dimensions of Critical Care Nursing, 27*(3), 125–131.

Morone, N. E., Greco, C. M., & Weiner, D. K. (2008). Mindfulness meditation for the treatment of chronic low back pain in older adults: A randomized controlled pilot study. *Pain, 134*, 310–319.

Ness, J., Cirillo, D. J., Weir, D. R., Nisly, N. L., & Wallace, R. B. (2005). Use of complementary medicine in older Americans: Results from the health and retirement study. *The Gerontologist, 45*, 516–524.

Pace, T. W. W., Negi, L. T., Adame, D. D., Cole, S. P., Sivilli, T. I., Brown, T. D., et al. (2009, January). Effect of compassion meditation on neuroendocrine, innate immune and behavioral responses to psychosocial stress. *Psychoneuroendocrinology, 34*(1), 87–98.

Reibel, D., Greeson, J., Brainard, G., & Rosenzweig, S. (2001). Mindfulness based stress reduction and health related quality of life in a heterogeneous patient population. *General Hospital Psychiatry, 23*, 183–192.

Ryan-Wenger, N. A., Sharrer, V. W., & Wynd, C. A. (2000). Stress, coping and health in children. In V. H. Rice (Ed.), *Handbook of stress, coping, health: Implications of nursing research theory and practice* (pp. 295–333). Thousand Oaks, CA: Sage Publications.

Selye, H. (1936, July). A syndrome produced by diverse nocuous agents. *Nature, 138*, 32.

Skybo, T., & Buck, J. (2007, September–October). Stress and coping responses to proficiency testing in school-age children. *Pediatric Nursing, 33*(5), 413–418.

Smith, A. (2006). "Like waking up from a dream": Mindfulness training for older people with anxiety and depression. In R. A. Baur (Ed.), *Mindfulness-Based Treatment Approaches, Clinician's Guide to Evidence Base and*

Applications (pp. 191–215). Boston, MA: Elsevier Academic Press.

Snyder, M., & Lindquist, R. (2007). *Complementary alternative therapies in nursing* (5th ed.). New York: Springer.

Tang, J-Y, Harms, V., & Vezeau, T. (2008, November). An audio relaxation tool for blood pressure reduction in older adults. *Geriatric Nursing, 29*(6), 392–401.

Telles Nunes, D. F., Rodriguez, A. L., da Silva Hoffmann, F., Luz, C., Filho, A. P. F. B., Muller, M. C., et al. (2007, December). Relaxation and guided imagery program in patients with breast cancer undergoing radiotherapy is not associated with neuroimmunomodulatory effects. *Journal of Psychosomatic Research, 63*(6), 647–655.

Trouillet, R., Gana, K., Lourel, M., & Fort, I. (2009, May). Predictive value of age for coping: The role of self-efficacy, social support satisfaction and perceived stress. *Aging & Mental Health, 13*(3), 357–366.

Vimont, C. (2008, Winter). How to fight stress and ward off illness. *Medline Plus, 3*(1), 5–6.

Walker, L. S., Smith, C. A., Garber, J., & Claar, R. L. (2007, March). Appraisal and coping with daily stressors by pediatric patients with chronic abdominal pain. *Journal of Pediatric Psychology, 32*(2), 206–216.

Wenzel, L., Glanz, K., & Lerman, C. (2002). Stress, coping and health behavior. In K. Glanz, B. K. Rimer, & F. M. Lewis (Eds.), *Health behavior and health education* (3rd ed., pp. 210–240). San Francisco: Jossey-Bass.

Weydert, J. A., Shapiro, D. R., Acra, S. A., Monheim, C. J., Chambers, A. S., & Ball, T. M. (2006, November). Evaluation of guided imagery as treatment for recurrent abdominal pain in children: A randomized controlled trial. *BMC Pediatrics, 6,* 29.

Winbush, N. Y., Gross, C. R., & Kreitzer, M. J. (2007). The effects of mindfulness-based stress reduction on sleep disturbance: A systematic review. *Explore, 3*(6), 585–591.

CHAPTER 9

Social Support and Health

OBJECTIVES

1. Differentiate between social networks, social integration, and social support.
2. Describe the components of an individual's network system that should be assessed in a social systems review.
3. Discuss the major types of social support that should be assessed in a social systems review.
4. Discuss the role of virtual communities in social support.
5. Describe the role of social networks and social support in the promotion of health.
6. Discuss strategies to enhance social support.

Outline

- Social Networks
- Social Integration
- Social Support
  - A. Functions of Social Support Groups
  - B. Family as the Primary Support Group
  - C. Community Organizations as Support Groups
  - D. Peers as a Source of Support
  - E. Virtual Communities as a Source of Support
- Assessing Social Support Systems
- Social Support and Health
  - A. Social Support and Health Behavior
- Enhancing Social Support Systems
  - A. Facilitating Social Interactions
  - B. Enhancing Coping
  - C. Preventing Loss of Support and Loneliness
- Opportunities for Research in Social Support

- Considerations for Practice in Social Support
- Summary
- Learning Activities
- Selected Web Sites
- References

Understanding the social context in which individuals live and work is critically important in health promotion. In human interactions, individuals and groups both give and receive social support, a reciprocal process and interactive resource that provide comfort, assistance, encouragement, and information. Social support fosters successful coping and promotes satisfying and effective living. The amount and type(s) of social support needed fluctuate across the life span and across situations. Individuals and families usually call on personal resources first to cope with unanticipated, difficult, or threatening circumstances. Contacts with others in the support system may then be initiated only when self-reliance fails. All individuals need a system of sustaining support to realize their full potential. However, it is important to note that some may choose not to ask for or accept support. Given that social support is a basic human need, its multiple dimensions have been explored, defined, and measured in various ways. In addition, the relationship between social support and health has been studied extensively. Social support is considered a person–environment interaction that decreases the occurrence of stressors, buffers the impact of stress, and decreases physiologic reactivity to stress.

Much of our understanding of the relationship between social support and health has come from multiple disciplines, including sociology, anthropology, psychology, medicine, and nursing. Continued advances in our understanding of the pathways by which social support affects mental and physical health are essential to be able to design interventions to promote mental, social, and physical well-being. Relationships among social support, health behaviors, and health are addressed in this chapter. In addition, the role of the nurse in assisting clients to assess, modify, and develop effective social support systems that meet their needs is described.

SOCIAL NETWORKS

Although the terms *social networks*, *social integration*, and *social support* are used interchangeably, they are not the same (Moren-Cross & Lin, 2006). *Social networks* refer to the web of social relationships that surrounds an individual. Social networks are defined as the objective, structural components of support, whereas *social integration* is the degree of involvement in the network, and *social support* is considered the qualitative, or perceived, functional component. A social network is made up of persons an individual or family knows and with whom they interact. These interactions may occur frequently or infrequently and may include a large number of individuals.

Social integration is the extent to which an individual is linked to or participates in his or her social environment at difference levels (Cohen, 2004). The converse of social integration is social isolation or the lack of contact with family, friends, and others in the social network.

Social support refers to the social interactions within the network that are sensed as being available and supportive (perceived) or that actually provide support (received). The social support system for any given individual or family is usually much smaller than the social network or number of contacts. Social networks are linkages between people.

Characteristics of social networks have been described. The network characteristics have been organized into a typology along three dimensions: network, location, and resources, as shown in Table 9–1 (Moren-Cross & Lin, 2006). Network characteristics include density, size, homogeneity, and demographics. Location characteristics include degree, strength of tie, frequency, duration, intimacy, multiplicity, reciprocity, and reachability. Resource characteristics include social capital, which refers to resources embedded in the network. This typology is helpful, as it describes the characteristics that are assessed when defining an individual's social network. The most commonly studied network characteristics are network size, frequency of interactions with network members, and composition of network.

Social network is considered a static concept, as it refers to relationships across the life span. *Social convoy* is considered a more dynamic concept to describe an individual's social network (Antonucci, Ajrouch, & Janevic, 2003). The nature of an individual's relations can be depicted using a hierarchical mapping technique that has three progressively enlarging concentric circles around an inner circle. The inner circle consists of closest, inti-

TABLE 9–1   Typology of Social Network Properties

Type	Definition
Network Features	
Density	Extent individuals are connected (measured by the actual number of direct ties in the ego's network relative to the number of possible ties)
Size	Number of individuals directly and/or indirectly connected within a specified network
Homogeneity	Extent that ties are alike or different on a specified characteristic, such as race/ethnicity or socioeconomic status
Demographics	Descriptive, aggregate indicators of demographic characteristics of the network, such as the proportion of a particular race/ethnicity, or the mean income
Location Features	
Degree	Extent to which one member of the network is tied to others
Strength of tie	Whether connection between two ties is strong or weak
Frequency	How often two ties interact
Duration	How long two ties have known one another
Intimacy	Perceived emotional attachment of one tie to another
Multiplexity	Number of relationships between two particular ties, such as whether they are friends, as well as neighbors
Reciprocity	Extent to which resources are both received and given
Reachability	Average number of ties necessary to link any two members of the network
Resource Features	
Social capital	Resources embedded in a network that are accessed and/or mobilized in purposive actions. These can be material or emotional

Source: Reprinted from *Handbook of aging and the social sciences,* 6th ed, R. Binstock and L.K. George (Eds.), Jennifer L. Moren-Cross and Nan Lin, "Social Networks and Health," pp. 111–128. Copyright 2006, with permission from Elsevier.

mate relationships, such as family and longtime friends. Individuals in the middle circle may be close relatives, friends, and neighbors. The outer circle reflects contacts that are somewhat close, such as coworkers. Throughout the life span, the middle and outer circles are more likely to change, whereas the inner circle tends to be more stable. Inner circle members are difficult to replace and when they are no longer available, there is a sense of grief and loss.

Social networks are important to individuals and families to the extent that they fulfill members' needs. In addition, knowledge of the interactions of network characteristics shed light on how they influence the quantity and quality of social support. The size of the network is thought to be a major component in social support. However, the types of persons in the network who provide the support, not the network size, have been associated with satisfaction. For example, voluntary social network ties, such as friends and church membership, may be more important for well-being than obligatory social network ties, such as the family, because one usually chooses network ties that are rewarding.

SOCIAL INTEGRATION

Social integration, the extent of close family and friends and community ties, has two components: a behavioral component, or actively engaging in multiple social activities and relationships, and a cognitive component, a sense of community and identification with one's social roles. Social integration has been linked with psychological and physical well-being. Research by Cohen and Lemay (2007) indicates that social integration is related to health practices: Adults who participated more in activities drank less alcohol and smoked few cigarettes than those with lower participation. In the study, social integration was the social network index that assessed participation in 12 types of relationships they spoke to at least every two weeks, including spouse, parents, parents-in-law, children, other close family members, neighbors, friends, coworkers, fellow volunteers, and members of groups with and without religious affiliation. Reviews indicate that social integration has been associated with longer life, less severe dementia, less risk for cancer reoccurrence, survival from heart attack, fewer respiratory infections, and less depression and anxiety (see Cohen, 2004 for a review). The process by which it is associated with health is not well understood, but it is thought to promote positive psychological states (e.g., purpose, self-worth, positive effect) that induce health-promoting behavior.

SOCIAL SUPPORT

The functions provided by social relationships are considered social support. *Social support* can be defined as a network of interpersonal relationships that provide psychological and material resources intended to benefit an individual's ability to cope. Social support is perceived (emotional support) and tangible (supportive acts). Four broad categories of social support have been described: emotional, instrumental, informational, and appraisal support (Berkman, Glass, Brissette, & Seeman, 2000). Emotional support refers to the demonstration of caring, empathy, love, and trust. Instrumental support includes tangible support or actions, including goods or services. In informational support, advice is provided as well as personal information or suggestions. Last, appraisal support refers to the provision of affirmation support or constructive feedback that is useful for self-evaluation. The type of support that is beneficial at any given time may differ, depending on the nature and stage of the confronting situation. For example, emotional support may help in a crisis circumstance, whereas informational support may be more useful in assisting individuals to understand how to relate effectively with their peers. Instrumental or tangible assistance or aid provides help with specific tasks, such as the preparation of nutritious meals or transport of children to recreational activities. Appraisal or affirmation support consists of constructive feedback to help individuals realize their own strengths.

Social support must be viewed within the cultural context of social relationships (Kim, Sherman, & Taylor, 2008). This requires knowledge of cultural characteristics that shape receiving and giving support. Cultural boundaries define the various subgroups of American society, such as African-Americans, Asian-Americans, Hispanics–Latinos, and Native Americans. Within these cultural boundaries, social support operates uniquely within each social context. For example, based on the history of slavery in the African-American community and group effort needed for survival, the family and church have been the major providers of social support (Dilworth-Anderson & Marshall, 1996). Hispanic–Latino Americans and Asian-Americans are similar in that the core of their social support systems is *familism* or the family, which includes close and distant kin. Asian-Americans have rules regulating gender hierarchies (patrilineage) and respect for older adults, and use shame and harmony in giving and receiving support. In the Native American culture, social support is less well understood, as the term is not defined in many tribal languages. However, Native Americans live in relational networks that foster mutual assistance and support, and the extended family is a core feature of their network. Research with the First Nation and Inuit communities in Canada indicates that social support is a strong indicator of both positive and negative behaviors (Richmond & Ross, 2008). Their social structure reinforces an individual's sense of belonging; however, the high-density networks can also exert conformity pressures and social obligations that may promote and even normalize health-damaging behaviors.

Although many similarities in social support exist among the various American cultures, the influence of the sociohistorical context differs greatly across the different populations. Culturally sensitive theoretical views are needed to understand the role of social support as well as gender and life span differences in these populations.

Several social support systems relevant to health have been identified and described in the literature: natural support systems (families), peer support systems, organized religious support systems, organized professional support systems, and organized self-help support groups not directed by health professionals. In most instances, the family remains the primary support group.

Professional helpers who have a specific set of skills and services to offer clients offer a different type of support system. Questions have been raised about the effectiveness of their role in social support. Although professionals have access to information and resources that might not otherwise be available, they are seldom the first source of help for an individual. Family and close friends or peers are sought for advice and support initially. Health professionals are rarely included as members of an individual's social network in an assessment; they become the support system only when other sources of help are unavailable, interrupted, or exhausted. Professionals are usually unable to provide support over long periods of time. In addition, these relationships are not characterized by reciprocity; they usually involve a power differential and offer limited empathic understanding due to lack of intimacy. In spite of these limitations, professional helpers have a role to play in offering short-term support as well as providing informational support.

All support systems of a given individual or family are synergistic. In combination, they represent the social resources available to facilitate stability and actualization. Various systems will be dominant at different points in the life cycle, depending on stage of development and the stressors or challenges at hand. For example, in preadolescence and early adolescence, parents are the greatest source of support. The network shifts to a greater reliance on peers for lifestyle choices during middle adolescence with a decreased perception of parental support. Friends remain dominant in young adults. The family network and friends are important sources of support for the elderly.

Functions of Social Support Groups

The primary functions of social support groups are to augment personal strengths of members and promote achievement of life goals. The functions of social support groups in promoting health can be conceptualized in four ways, as depicted in Figure 9–1.

Social groups can contribute to health by (1) creating a growth-promoting environment that supports health-promoting behaviors, self-esteem, and high-level wellness; (2) decreasing the likelihood of threatening or stressful life events; (3) providing feedback or confirmation that actions are leading to anticipated and socially desirable consequences; and (4) buffering or mediating the negative effects of stressful events through influencing interpretation of events and emotional responses to them, thus decreasing their illness-producing potential. Support groups function to share common social concerns, provide intimacy, prevent isolation, respect mutual competencies, offer dependable assistance in crises, serve as a referral agent, and provide mutual challenge.

Social support groups conducted for persons with cancer offer insight about the unique role of social support in reducing stress (Ussher, Kirsten, Butow, & Sandoval, 2006). They provide a strong sense of community, nonjudgmental acceptance, and invaluable information, which results in empowerment and control over life. The type of group leader (professional or peer) did not matter, but whether the group provided a supportive environment and a sense of belonging, and whether it met perceived needs.

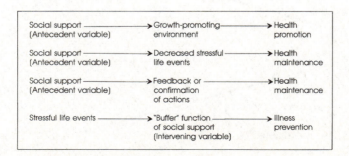

FIGURE 9–1 Possible Impact of Social Support on Health Status

Family as the Primary Support Group

The family is the primary context for learning to give and receive social support. Family cohesion, expressiveness, and lack of conflict are reflected in the supportive behaviors that family members provide to one another. Low family support and poor child–parent interactions influence the life course trajectories of young people. Family stressors, such as unemployment, welfare dependence, change in family structure (as a divorce), and crime and substance use may decrease family cohesion and increase conflict and adolescent behavioral and mental problems (Kraft & Luecken, 2009).

Family social support exerts complex effects on the physical and mental health of its members. The well-known Alameda County, California, study provided initial information about the association of social networks, social integration, social support and mortality (Berkman & Syme, 1979). Men who are single or widowed have consistently shown higher mortality rates than married men. Depressive symptoms have been associated with an adverse family environment that offers low levels of social support. Men who remain socially isolated after losing their partners are at higher risk of developing symptoms of chronic depression, whereas having supportive relationships has been associated with decreased risks for depression. Having a marital partner or, if unmarried, having socially supportive relationships reduces psychological distress, such as depression, in community living elders (Krause, 2006). Close friends, group membership, and finding life worthwhile was associated with lower mortality in the elderly, but with the passage of time, these associations decreased (Sato et al., 2008).

Instrumental support has positive effects throughout the life span. Using the convoy model (Antonucci et al., 2003), two aspects of social support networks—a greater proportion of kin and the presence of family members in the inner circle—significantly reduce distress. The interplay between family stressors and family support is depicted in Figure 9–2.

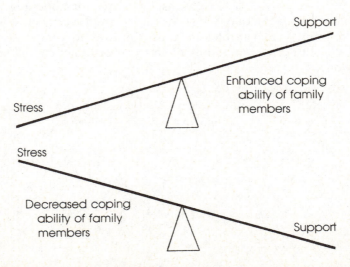

FIGURE 9–2 Family as a Source of Support or Stress

Within families, both positive and negative interactions occur. Negative interactions can be viewed as stressors, whereas positive, helpful interactions constitute support. Positive emotional bonds of the family with its social network buttress the family's competence and effective functioning. For example, in the Strong African-American Families Program, parents successfully used affectively positive parent–child relationships, consistent disciplines, and racial socialization to decrease underage drinking and prevent the development of conduct problems (Brody, Kogan, Chen, & Murry, 2008).

Social support is unequally distributed and varies by socioeconomic status. Individuals with lower socioeconomic status report less support from family and friends, and have a scarcity of emotional and tangible resources (Mickelson & Demmings, 2009). Impoverished women are especially vulnerable and less able to nurture children due to multiple issues. Many rely on minor children for support, which may result in worse well-being for the children and worse outcomes for the mother. Burdening the children decreases their well-being, which becomes an additional stress for the mother (Mickelson & Demmings, 2009). These findings point to the need to assist persons with low socioeconomic status, including impoverished women, in finding alternate network substitutions to provide social support. Family income has also been shown to mediate the effects of cortisol, a marker of stress system activity, in young adults in divorced families. Participants in higher-income divorced families had lower salivary cortisol, even after controlling for family conflict. A poverty-alleviation program in Mexico that provided instrumental support was shown to decrease salivary cortisol in children in the program compared with those who did not participate in the program (Fernald & Gunnar, 2009). This study and others point to the need to pay special attention to social support resources for persons with lower socioeconomic status (Huurre, Eerola, Rahkonen, & Hillevi, 2007).

Community Organizations as Support Groups

Characteristics of a community and its organizations have a direct bearing on the level of well-being of individuals and families who reside in it. The quality of social interaction and the life experiences of residents can contribute positively to health or negatively, resulting in social disorganization and illness. Stability within a community tends to promote close-knit ties among residents that mitigate the effects of crises on community members. Stable communities are characterized by value similarity, mutual assistance, shared trust, and concern for members.

Organized religious support systems such as churches, temples, mosques, or other religious meeting places constitute a support system for individuals as the congregations share a similar value system, a common set of beliefs about the purpose of life, and a set of guidelines for living. Even highly mobile individuals may find a support system in the local church or synagogue. The church takes primary responsibility for support to enhance the spiritual dimension of health, which includes the ability to discover and articulate one's basic purpose in life; learn how to experience love, joy, peace, and fulfillment; and discover how to help oneself and others achieve full personal potential.

Religious institutions are viewed as a source of support in the community for health and healing. This is especially true for African-Americans, as the church has been the most important institution in the community, for reasons mentioned previously. Churches represent miniature, dynamic communities that may provide childcare, meals, transportation, counseling, and other support resources. In addition, volunteer helpers are readily available. Nurses now function in the role of parish or congregational nurses in churches to support health promotion within a community setting. Parish nurses integrate concern for the spirituality of the person with holistic care within a faith-based community.

Peers as a Source of Support

Peer support systems consist of people who function informally to meet the needs of others. Many of these individuals have encountered an experience that has had a major influence in their own lives and achieved successful adjustment and growth. Because of personal insight, their advice is sought primarily in relation to resolving a problem of immediate concern with which they are familiar. Examples include the avid runner, the health-food enthusiast, or the individual who has lost a large amount of weight.

Informal support from one's peers has consistently been shown to have powerful stress-buffering and health-promoting effects, which are often greater than formal support services. Support from peers is important when there is a breakdown in an individual's usual support network. The peer shares salient similarities and possesses specific concrete knowledge that is pragmatic and derived from personal experiences. Peer support can be provided through one-on-one sessions, self-help groups, or online computer groups in diverse settings. Peer support primarily occurs without the provision of instrumental support. Peers are a valuable source of support with which the individual can identify and share common experiences. The more similar the peer relationships, the more likely the support will lead to understanding, empathy, and mutual help. Evidence suggests that peer support positively affects physical and mental health outcomes (Ali & Dwyer, 2009). In a peer-group social support clinical trial, the peer group support intervention decreased symptoms of depression, anxiety, and anger in AIDS orphans, aged 10–15 years (Kumakech, Cantor-Graee, Maling, & Bajunirwe, 2009).

Peers must be skilled in communication, active listening, and problem solving. In addition, peers need empathy with the person's difficulties and must be willing to take a supportive role. The common forms of peer support include befriending, mediation/conflict resolution, mentoring, and counseling. Peer support systems have been developed in schools and colleges to decrease aggressive acts and social isolation as well as to teach skills and promote health. Males are greatly underrepresented as peer supporters.

SELF-HELP GROUPS.   Organized support systems not directed by health professionals include voluntary service groups and self-help groups. These groups do not have an expert leader, which distinguishes them from support groups, which are led by a trained facilitator. Self-help groups are an attempt to change the behavior of members or promote adaptation to a life change such as chronic illness. They are defined by the members' expectations.

The number of self-help groups continues to increase in the United States. Self-help groups have been called "mutual help groups" to reflect the fact that group members give and receive advice, encouragement, and support (King & Moreggi, 2006). One of the main therapeutic factors is the group's ability to normalize a stigmatizing condition and to take away the embarrassment of having an undesirable behavior. This is a necessary step to making cognitive, emotional, and behavioral changes to improve life quality.

Examples of self-help groups include Narcotics Anonymous, Alcoholics Anonymous, Mended Hearts, Compassionate Friends, and physical fitness clubs. Characteristics of self-help groups include a critical mass sufficient to form a group, a form of publicity or recruitment to attract members, and a central goal or activity that gives the group purpose and sustains the investment of its members.

The question has been raised as to why individuals use self-help groups rather than other resources, such as professional services. Two possible reasons are offered: (1) Self-help groups fulfill a need for services not being offered; or (2) self-help groups arise because of disappointment with traditional medical models and lack of meaningful resources within the community.

Self-help groups are an important resource, as they enable group members to expand their social networks as well as receive informational, instrumental, emotional, and appraisal support from others. Self-help groups empower individuals by increasing self-worth, support, and affirmation. Some consider the term *self-help* misleading, because members are not involved in these groups just to help themselves. Instead, they help each other, so the term *mutual-aid group* has been suggested, which implies that each person is both a helper and receiver of help (King & Moreggi, 2006). However, self-help group members prefer the term *self-help.*

The successes of self-help groups in assisting individuals cope with different life experiences attest to their continuing viability as an integral part of community health resources. Self-care may be particularly effective for individuals who do not receive support from other relationships.

Virtual Communities as a Source of Support

Virtual communities are social units in which members interact using communication technologies that bridge geographical distance (Demiris, 2006). Virtual communities that do not include professionals function as self-help groups. Virtual communities may include educational information and discussion forums. Technologies for virtual communities include online message boards, asynchronous or synchronous communication, and videoconferencing. These communities include virtual health care delivery teams, virtual research teams, virtual disease management, and peer groups (Demiris, 2006).

Computer-mediated environments such as the Internet offer opportunities for people to expand their social networks. Evidence indicates that the Internet is a potential avenue for obtaining informational, instrumental support as well as social companionship and self-esteem support. The use of email has been shown to increase communication with family and friends as well as extend social networks to new contacts.

Research findings investigating the role of computer-mediated communication have, for the most part, been positive (Eastin & LaRose, 2005). Young people who participated in a Web-based intervention to reduce stigma and promote help seeking used it as a source of information and support for mental health issues and help seeking (Burns, Durkin, & Nicholas, 2009). However, an Internet-based resource for weight control found that social support sections were used least and received the lowest satisfaction ratings (McConnon, Kirk, & Ransley, 2009). This finding was explained by the participants' limited ability to use the Internet. Internet interventions may be complex, so they need to be tailored to the individual or group. In addition, participants must have the skills and be able to access the Internet to participate effectively.

Internet technology has been shown to be acceptable across ethnically diverse groups. However, socioeconomic status continues to be a limiting factor. Although older people are the least likely group to use new communication technologies, virtual communities may play a powerful role in meeting the informational and support needs of this group. Online support groups among the elderly have the potential to overcome many barriers, including mobility limitations, lack of transportation, and finances. Facebook, one of the best-known Web-based social networking sites, has great appeal to young adults. However, other sites have developed for older adults, such as SagaZone for adults aged 50 years and older (Godfrey & Johnson, 2009). The site features community forums to discuss topics such as health, difficult life transitions, and caregiver issues as well as other topics. Older adults are active participants.

Advanced technologies are beginning to play an important role in the provision of social support across the life span. The rapid growth of the Internet has occurred without concurrent attention to policy, ethical, and legal issues. Nurses and other health care providers must be prepared to adopt these technologies and evaluate their usefulness in health and health promotion.

ASSESSING SOCIAL SUPPORT SYSTEMS

It is important for both clients and health care providers to be aware of available sources of social support for individuals and families. Two approaches for assessing social support networks of clients are described in Chapter 4, the support system review and the emotional support diagram. These approaches can be useful in providing insight into existing support resources for both the client and nurse. When assessing the adequacy of a client's support systems, it is important to be cognizant of factors that may cause the assessments to vary. Such things as culture, stage of life-span development, social context (e.g., school, home, work), and role context (e.g., parent, student, professional) must be considered for their influence on perceived and received support.

SOCIAL SUPPORT AND HEALTH

The importance of social support to mental and physical health is now well established. Lower levels of support are consistently linked to higher rates of morbidity and mortality. However, the actual mechanisms linking social support to health are still not well understood. Several different processes have been proposed. First, the main effects hypothesis suggests that social support may be directly linked to health by promoting healthy or unhealthy behaviors, supplying information, or making available tangible resources (child care, opportunities for work). In this hypothesis, social support may foster a sense of meaning in life or be associated with more positive affective states, such as enhanced sense of self-worth and increased sense of control (Cohen, 2004). Individuals may appraise events as less threatening, resulting in less physiologic arousal.

The second way in which social support may contribute to health is by buffering the effects of stress on an individual. The stress-buffering hypothesis model of support has been most widely researched (Uchino, 2004). Social support is thought to be beneficial because it reduces the negative effects of stressful experiences on one's mental and physical health. Stress promotes negative coping patterns and activates physiological systems that place a person at risk for developing mental and physical illnesses. Social support is thought to buffer the negative effects of the stress response by promoting less threatening interpretations of adverse events and effective coping strategies (Cohen, 2004). In other words, having individuals who provide support can reduce the intensity of stress.

Research has begun to identify the physiologic mechanisms underlying the role of social support in health. Biologically, social support may intensify positive neuroendocrine and immunologic responses despite the presence of stressors. More than 20 years of research supports the relationship between social relationships and immune function (Graham, Christian, & Kiecolt-Glaser, 2007). Loneliness, divorce, small social networks, and relational conflict have been associated with adverse changes in immune function and health, whereas positive social support is associated with more adaptive immune function. Relocation (moving away from home) and a small social network have also been shown to be negatively related to immune function (Segerstrom, 2008). Research has also shown that interacting with a socially supportive individual decreases cortisol reactivity to a social stressor, providing evidence for the benefit of social support on neural and physiologic activity (Eisenberger, Taylor, Gable, Hilmert, & Lieberman, 2007). Social integration has been shown to be associated with lower levels of C-reactive protein, an inflammatory marker considered a risk factor for cardiovascular disease (Ford, Loucks, & Berkman, 2006). All of these studies provide beginning evidence for the protective biologic mechanisms of social support in promoting health.

Social support interventions have been categorized as (1) the nature of the relationship between the support provider and the participant (professional or peer), (2) unit of support (individual or group intervention), and (3) the type of intervention (building social skills or increasing network size) (Uchino, 2004). When developing social support interventions, it is important to consider the type of social support that will be the target of the intervention. Will it be emotional or informational support, or an increase in social contacts? Perceived support is a function of an individual's personality characteristic, the social environment, and an interaction between the perceiver and supporter. The kind of support, who provides the support, and contextual issues all play a role. Interventions to increase perceived support should focus on helping persons recruit supportive others into their social network by teaching them relationship-building skills.

Reviews of interventions that have been tested to improve social support indicate varying long-term results. Although many studies have been conducted, many suffer from weaknesses that limit the ability to generalize the findings. In addition, studies that were well designed showed no effects of the intervention or improvement in support. So although the intervention may have improved health or well-being, the client's naturally occurring social support did not change; therefore, the desired outcomes did not last when the intervention was completed. Social support is complex and includes characteristics of the person who needs or desires support (perceiver), characteristics of the person who gives the support (supporter), characteristics of the situation, and the interaction of these factors. All of these factors must be taken into consideration when designing interventions to improve social support.

Social Support and Health Behavior

Social support systems also influence health behavior. It is well known that significant others function as an important lay referral system for individuals in making decisions to seek professional care for health promotion, illness prevention, or care. Concurrence by the lay referral system often determines the extent to which advice from health professionals is actually followed.

Social support from spouses or partners is related to health behaviors. This relationship may be due to encouragement and support of the health behavior, including giving approval and disapproval; having control over aspects of the proposed change such as food shopping and preparation; and participating in the behavior change, such as joining an exercise program with the spouse or partner. High levels of warmth, encouragement, and assistance occur in spousal and partner support. A nonsupportive network can interfere with successful alteration of health habits by limiting the client's time and energy available for health behavior or introducing stress, which compromises healthy behaviors.

Social support has been correlated with adoption of other health behaviors or cessation of negative behaviors. Adult smokers who had attended at least one meeting of a smoking cessation program reported that both family and peer support were positively associated with behavior change (Wagner, Burg, & Sirois, 2004). Having the trust, acceptance, and support of a family member or friend increased the individual's use of the transtheoretical model process of change for smoking cessation. In a support intervention to promote smoker use of a social support help line, which included telephone counseling by an adult nonsmoking support person, smokers reported the help line acceptable and helpful (Patten et al., 2008). A support intervention using telephone coaching and an exercise support group was effective in increasing levels of physical activity and reducing body weight in African-Americans (Rimmer, Wang, Heckerling, & Gerber, 2009). A review of the literature provides evidence for the value of the family as a source of support and motivation in achieving weight goals and physical activity for children as well as adults (Gruber & Haldeman, 2009). Parental modeling and support for physical activity and fruit and vegetable consumption are important strategies in their children's behavior change. A Walking School Bus was pilot tested in an urban underserved school district for kindergarten to fifth graders to promote social interaction and physical activity to combat obesity (Kong, Sussman, Patterson, Middleman, & Hough, 2009). Initial findings indicate the program provided a supportive and safe environment and was enthusiastically received by parents and students. These types of social support programs, which target children, are needed to establish health promoting behaviors early.

Adoption and maintenance of health-behavior change over time is difficult unless the behavior is encouraged through support from family members and friends. This points to the importance of naturally occurring support and connectedness or long-term formal or informal support systems if natural ones are not available. Many retrospective studies have described the effect of social support on health behavior. However, more prospective studies are needed to identify networks of social support that promote health promotion and illness prevention behaviors.

ENHANCING SOCIAL SUPPORT SYSTEMS

Support-enhancing strategies have three goals: assisting individuals and families to strengthen existing supportive relationships, helping individuals and families establish satisfying interpersonal ties, and preventing disruption of ties from evolving into mental or physical illness.

Facilitating Social Interactions

Social skills training represents one approach to changing the characteristics of clients to enable them to develop supportive interpersonal relationships with others. Training can be conducted with individuals or groups who have similar skill deficits. Social skills training is based on the belief that socially competent responses can be learned just like other behaviors. Initially, training is directed toward assessing and modifying perceptions of appropriate behavior in social situations. In addition, persons are taught to reevaluate their thoughts about themselves in a more positive manner. Attempts are made to improve social interaction patterns through modeling, role playing, performance feedback, coaching, and homework assignments. Skills to be taught might include initiating conversations, giving and receiving compliments, handling periods of silence, recognizing nonverbal methods of communication, and handling criticism and conflict. Within the school setting, training in social skills and problem solving can be provided in the classroom to prevent the acquisition of health-compromising behaviors. To complement such work, the broader aspects of the school environment should be assessed to determine the extent to which school engagement and peer groups facilitate or inhibit healthy behaviors (Carter, Taylor, & Williams, 2007).

Enhancing Coping

A lack of social ties and support may result in serious psychological and physical problems during developmental or situational transition periods. Support groups for widows, children of separated or divorced parents, and parents who have lost a child, for example, can assist such persons to learn to cope effectively with life stress. Benefits from such programs include help in understanding emotional reactions, reducing feelings of alienation, and assisting people to move ahead into the future. Learning to cope with the stressful event using problem-focused coping strategies enables clients to manage the stress, even if it cannot be resolved.

Preventing Loss of Support and Loneliness

Preventing loneliness or social isolation is a more desirable approach than treatment of loneliness and isolation after they have occurred. Two approaches to prevention include the identification of high-risk groups and implementing interventions that focus on developing social support ties. Young, unmarried, unemployed, and low-income persons are particularly vulnerable to lack of support and loneliness. Programs can be planned to decrease aloneness and isolation, including transportation vehicles staffed by volunteers for those in need, respite programs for caretaker relief, community support groups for families, and Internet support groups that can be accessed at home.

Educational approaches to prevent loss of social support and subsequent loneliness include classroom experiences for schoolchildren to help them gain experience in making friends, working cooperatively with others, and resolving differences or conflict. A growing body of evidence over the past 30 years has substantiated that poor social functioning of children often leads to serious personal adjustment problems in later life. Most experts would agree that children require the security of positive reciprocal relationships with their peers, parents, and teachers for maximum growth and development (Carter, Taylor, & Williams, 2007).

Social disconnectedness and perceived isolation in older adults have been associated with lower levels of self-rated health (Cornwall & Waite, 2009). Older adults must build new social relationships among people they have not previously known and create new social support systems. Many older persons must learn the interpersonal skills to promote successful relationships, as well as skills needed to resolve interpersonal conflicts with people they already know (Krause, 2006). Media campaigns, such as television public service announcements about resources for formal support and the health benefits of staying connected with relatives and friends may provide cues to initiate new relationships. In addition, community programs and neighborhood activities can be designed to help persons build relationships or to reach out to others who may need emotional or instrumental support. In the Neighbors Helping Neighbors Program, community-residing older adults reported improved quality of life after receiving social and environmental services (instrumental support) (Trickey, Kelley-Gillespie, & Farley, 2008). Both computer and telephone support have become viable options, which provide support for the elderly.

Other general suggestions for enhancing social support include the following:

- Setting mutual goals with significant others to achieve common needs for support
- Constructively resolving conflict between support network members
- Offering assistance to individuals within a social network to show concern and promote trust
- Seeking counseling, if needed, to enhance marital and/or family adjustment
- Using nurses and other health professionals as community support resources
- Increasing ties to organized social groups to expand growth opportunities

Clients should be encouraged to identify specific goals to enhance personal support networks. By focusing on one or two realistic changes relevant to the goals of highest priority, clients can alter the breadth and depth of social support available to them.

OPPORTUNITIES FOR RESEARCH IN SOCIAL SUPPORT

Evidence supports the relationship between social networks and social support and health. However, inconsistencies in this body of research leave many questions to be answered, including the following:

1. Theory development is needed to identify and test antecedents and consequences of social support.
2. The specific mechanisms by which social support enhances health are not known and warrant further investigation.
3. Interventions that enhance social support need to be tested for long-term outcomes.

4. The amount or "dosage" and type of social support necessary to promote health should be explored.
5. Culturally sensitive interventions, as well as interventions across the life span, to enhance support should be developed and tested in subgroups of the population.
6. Culturally sensitive, reliable, and valid measures of social support need further development and testing.
7. Additional research is also needed on neural pathways and immune function and their relationship to social support.
8. Further investigations are needed to understand the relationship between Internet support participation and health outcomes.

Nurse scientists play a major role in social support research and should lead interdisciplinary teams to investigate these issues.

CONSIDERATIONS FOR PRACTICE IN SOCIAL SUPPORT

Although evidence is available that provides important information about social support and health, many of these findings have not been incorporated into practice. Knowledge of current evidence is necessary to be able to intervene to enhance social networks and social support. Assessment of social network and support systems should be incorporated into initial nursing assessment. In these assessments, nurses should know how to obtain culturally sensitive information from diverse populations. If the social network needs to be enhanced, the nurse should develop programs to teach clients the skills needed to develop or access supportive relationships. Finally, nurses should tap support resources such as families, friends, neighbors, self-help, Internet and telephone support groups, and community organizations to increase the potential for success in health promotion and lifestyle change.

Summary

Social support plays an important role in the health and well-being of clients. The nurse must consider the client as well as the social environment to facilitate comprehensive health promotion. Social support groups assist clients to cope with everyday hassles and major stressful life experiences. The extent to which stressful events threaten health and health-promoting behaviors may well depend on the support available from core (family) or extended (peer, community, and professional) social networks. The design and evaluation of nursing interventions to increase social support is critical. These interventions will enhance the quality of human social transactions across the life span.

Learning Activities

1. Perform a social network review with a young adult and an elderly client using the six components described in the chapter.
2. Design a plan to establish a self-help group for adolescents who are overweight. Incorporate both face-to-face and Internet group meetings into your plan.
3. Detail three strategies to increase your client's social support, based on the assessment you performed in #1, taking current sources as well as potential sources of support into consideration.

Selected Web Sites

http://MySpace.com and *http://Facebook.com*
The most popular social networking Web sites in the United States.

http://www.dailystrength.org
The largest, most comprehensive health network with access to over 500 online support groups that are anonymous and free to help people overcome personal challenges or support a loved one through a challenge.

http://www.obesitydiscussion.com
An example of a forum that targets a specific health promotion challenge. The forum provides

a place to talk about weight loss and obesity related topics and an place to get support for the diet journey.

http://www.sermo.com
An example of a professional led social networking site when physicians answer questions and collaborate or refute information submitted by colleagues.

http://caringbridge.org
An example of a Web site that connects family and friends during a serious health event and recovery. It is personal and private.

References

Ali, M. M., & Dwyer, D. S. (2009). Estimating peer effects in adolescent smoking behavior: A longitudinal analysis. *Journal of Adolescent Health, 45*(4), 402–408.

Antonucci, T. C., Ajrouch, K. J., & Janevic, M. R. (2003). The effect of social relations with children on the education-health link in men and women aged 40 and over. *Social Science & Medicine, 56*, 949–960.

Berkman, L., & Syme, S. L. (1979). Social networks, host resistance, and mortality: A nine-year follow-up study of Alameda County residents. *American Journal of Epidemiology, 115*, 684–694.

Berkman, L. F., Glass, T., Brissette, I., & Seeman, T. E. (2000). From social integration to health: Durkheim in the new millennium. *Social Science & Medicine, 51*, 843–857.

Brody, G. H., Kogan, S. M., Chen, Y., & Murry, V. M. (2008). Long-term effects of the Strong African American Families Program on youths' conduct problems. *Journal of Adolescent Health, 43*, 474–481.

Burns, J. M., Durkin, L. A., & Nicholas, J. (2009). Mental health of young people in the United States: What role can the Internet play in reducing stigma and promoting help seeking? *Journal of Adolescent Health, 45*, 95–97.

Carter, M., Taylor, B., & Williams, S. (2007). Health outcomes in adolescence: Association with family, friends, and school engagement. *Journal of Adolescence, 30*, 51–62.

Cohen, S. (2004). Social relationships and health. *American Psychologist, 59*(8), 676–684.

Cohen, S., & Lemay, E. P. (2007). Why would social networks be linked to affect and health practices? *Health Psychology, 26*, 410–417.

Cornwall, E. Y., & Waite, L. J. (2009). Social disconnectedness, perceived isolation, and health among older adults. *Journal of Health and Social Behavior, 50*, 31–48.

Demiris, G. (2006). The diffusion of virtual communities in health care: Concepts and challenges. *Patient Education and Counseling, 62*, 178–188.

Dilworth-Anderson, P., & Marshall, S. (1996). Social support in its cultural context. In G. R. Pierce, B. R. Sarason, & I. G. Sarason (Eds.), *Handbook of social support and the family* (pp. 67–79). New York: Plenum Press.

Eastin, M. S., & LaRose, R. (2005). Alt. Support: Modeling social support online. *Computers in Human Behavior, 21*, 977–992.

Eisenberger, N. I., Taylor, S. E., Gable, S. L., Hilmert, C. J., & Lieberman, M. D. (2007). Neural pathways link social support to attenuated neuroendocrine stress responses. *Neuroimage, 35*, 1601–1612.

Fernald, L., & Gunnar, M. R. (2009). Poverty-alleviation program participation and salivary cortisol in very low-income children. *Social Science & Medicine, 68*, 2180–2189.

Ford, E. S., Loucks, E. B., & Berkman, L. F. (2006). Social integration and concentrations of C-reactive protein among U.S. adults. *Annals of Epidemiology, 16*, 78–84.

Godfrey, M., & Johnson, O. (2009). Digital circles of support: Meeting the information needs of older adults. *Computers in Human Behavior, 25,* 633–642.

Graham, J. E., Christian, L. M., & Kiecolt-Glaser, J. K. (2007). Close relationships and immunity. *Psychoneuroimmunology, II,* 781–798.

Gruber, K. J., & Haldeman, L. A. (2009). Using the family to combat childhood and adult obesity. *Preventing Chronic Disease, 6*(3). Retrieved June 2009 from http://www.cdc.gov/pcd /issues/2009/jul/08_0191.htm

Huurre, T., Eerola, M., Rahkonen, O., & Hillevi, A. (2007). Does social support affect the relationship between socioeconomic status and depression? A longitudinal study from adolescence to adulthood. *Journal of Affective Disorders, 100,* 55–64.

Kim, H. S., Sherman, D. K., & Taylor, S. E. (2008). Culture and social support. *American Psychologist, 63,* 518–516.

King, S. A., & Moreggi, D. (2006). Internet therapy and self help groups: the pros and cons. In J. Gackenbach (Ed.), *Psychology and the Internet: Intrapersonal, interpersonal and transpersonal implications* (2nd ed., pp. 221–244). San Diego, CA: Academic Press.

Kong, A. S., Sussman, A. L., Patterson, N. S., Middleman, R., & Hough, R. (2009). Implementation of a walking school bus: Lessons learned. *Journal of School Health, 79,* 319–325.

Kraft, A. J., & Luecken, L. J. (2009). Childhood parental divorce and cortisol in young adulthood: Evidence for mediation by family income. *Psychoneuroendocrinology 34*(9), 1363–1369.

Krause, N. (2006). Social relationships in later life. In R. H. Binstock & L. K. George (Eds,) *Handbook of Aging and the Social Sciences* (6th ed., pp. 181–200). Boston, MA: Academic Press.

Kumakech, E., Cantor-Graee, E., Maling, S., & Bajunirwe, F. (2009). Peer-group support intervention improves the psychosocial well-being of AIDS orphans: Cluster randomized trial. *Social Science & Medicine, 68,* 1038–1043.

McConnon, A., Kirk, S. F., & Ransley, J. K. (2009). Process evaluation of an Internet-based resource for weight control: Use and views of an obese sample. *Journal of Nutrition Education and Behavior, 41,* 261–267.

Mickelson, K. D., & Demmings, J. L. (2009). The impact of support network substitution on low-income women's health: Are minor children beneficial substitutes? *Social Science & Medicine, 68,* 80–88.

Moren-Cross, J. L., & Lin, N. (2006). Social networks and health. In R. H. Binstock & L. K. George (Eds.), *Handbook of Aging and the Social Sciences* (6th ed., pp. 111–125). Boston, MA: Academic Press.

Patten, C. A., Smith, C. M., Brockman, T. A., Decker, P. A., Anderson, K. J., Hughes, C. A., et al. (2008). Support person intervention to promote smoker utilization of the QUIT-PLAN helpline. *American Journal of Preventive Medicine, 35*(6S), S479–S485.

Richmond, C., & Ross, N. A. (2008). Social support, material circumstance and health behavior: Influences on health in First Nation and Inuit communities of Canada. *Social Science & Medicine, 67,* 1423–1433.

Rimmer, J. H., Wang, A., Heckerling, P. S., & Gerber, B. S. (2009). A randomized control trial to increase physical activity and reduce obesity in a predominately African American group of women with mobility disabilities and severe obesity. *Preventive Medicine, 48,* 473–479.

Sato, T., Kishi, R., Suzukawa, A., Horikawa, N., Saijo, Y., & Yoshioka, E. (2008). Effects of social relationships on mortality of the elderly: How do the influences change with the passage of time? *Archives of Gerontology and Geriatrics, 47,* 327–339.

Segerstrom, S. C. (2008). Social networks and immunosuppression during stress: Relationship conflict or energy conservation? *Brain, Behavior, and Immunity, 27,* 279–284.

Trickey, R., Kelley-Gillespie, N., & Farley, O. W. (2008). A look at a community coming together to meet the needs of older adults: An evaluation of the Neighbors Helping Neighbors program. *Gerontology and Social Work, 50,* 81–98.

Uchino, B. N. (2004). *Social support & physical health.* New Haven, CT: Yale University Press.

Ussher, J., Kirsten, L., Butow, P., & Sandoval, M. (2006). What do cancer support groups provide which other supportive relationships do not? The experience of peer support groups for people with cancer. *Social Science & Medicine, 62,* 2565–2576.

Wagner, J., Burg, M., & Sirois, B. (2004). Social support and the transtheoretical model: Relationship of social support to smoking cessation stage, decisional balance, process use, and temptation. *Addictive Behaviors, 29*(5), 1–5.

PART 4

Evaluating the Effectiveness of Health Promotion

CHAPTER 10

Evaluating Individual and Community Interventions

OBJECTIVES

1. Describe the purpose of evaluation for health promotion.
2. Compare three approaches to evaluation and provide examples of each.
3. Discuss the types of outcomes to consider when evaluating effectiveness of health promotion interventions.
4. Describe evidence for continuing to implement programs for individuals.
5. Describe the evidence for continuing to promote community-level interventions.
6. Discuss strategies that facilitate effective health promotion interventions.

Outline

- **Purpose of Evaluation**
- **Approaches to Evaluation for Health Promotion Interventions**
  - A. Efficacy or Effectiveness Evaluation
  - B. Process or Outcome Evaluation
  - C. Mixed Methods Evaluation
- **Deciding Which Health Outcomes to Measure**
  - A. Nursing-Sensitive Outcomes
  - B. Individual, Family, and Community Outcomes
  - C. Short-Term, Intermediate, and Long-Term Outcomes
  - D. Economic Outcomes
- **Evaluating Evidence for Practice**
- **Evaluation of Interventions with Individuals and Communities**
  - A. Individuals
  - B. Community
- **Strategies for Effective Health Promotion Interventions**
  - A. Designing the Intervention
  - B. Selecting Outcomes

A scientific knowledge base to guide health promotion interventions is established by evaluating the accumulating results of health promotion programs and interventions. Evaluation information can be used to improve and implement health promotion programs that provide the most favorable outcomes for clients and communities. Our knowledge of the effectiveness of health promotion is based on research and program evaluations that have been conducted and published. Nurses and other health care professionals are continually being asked about the effectiveness of their health promotion and risk reduction efforts. This question can be answered by carefully examining research and evaluation evidence that has accumulated about a specific type of health promotion intervention or program.

PURPOSE OF EVALUATION

Evaluation, the process of collecting and analyzing information, is undertaken to learn the value of a health promotion program or intervention. Evaluations are considered decision oriented, whereas research involves generating theoretically valid knowledge (Eriksson, 2000). Evaluations serve many purposes: to assess if program objectives were achieved, to improve program implementation, to contribute to the scientific knowledge of health promotion, to provide accountability to funding agencies, and to inform policy makers (McKenzie, Neiger & Thackery, 2009). Evaluations also provide information to enable nurses and other health care professionals to make decisions about resource allocation, as ineffective programs can be eliminated and replaced with cost-effective ones that have been shown to promote change. Health promotion evaluations enable the nurse to improve the program, to make choices between health promotion activities, and to test whether a new intervention with documented effectiveness will translate to practice.

The evaluation plan must be considered during the program development process, as this enables appropriate, accurate information to be collected. Planning for evaluations is important for initial or baseline information to be obtained before the program or intervention is implemented and to be able to train those who will collect the evaluation information. Questions that may be answered by a comprehensive evaluation include the following (Ovretveit, 1998):

- Is the health promotion intervention effective in an ideal situation (efficacy)?
- Is the health promotion intervention effective in clinical practice (efficiency)?

- How does the health promotion intervention work?
- What are the intended and unintended effects (outcomes)?
- How long do the effects last?
- What resources are needed to implement the intervention or program?
- Is it cost-effective?
- Are clients satisfied?
- Who will benefit from the intervention?
- How can the program or intervention be improved?

Cost, time, and resources pose limitations on evaluations. All stakeholders must be engaged in the evaluation process, including those affected by the intervention as well as intended users. Credible evidence is critical to make accurate conclusions. In addition, performing an evaluation requires knowledge, skills, and administrative support. If these things are not present, the evaluation is unlikely to be performed successfully and produce useful results.

APPROACHES TO EVALUATION FOR HEALTH PROMOTION INTERVENTIONS

Evaluation approaches provide the road map for the systematic collection, analysis, and reporting of information. Knowledge of differences in efficacy and effectiveness studies, process and outcome evaluations, and qualitative and quantitative evaluation approaches is needed to design an appropriate plan to evaluate evidence for one's practice. Other approaches, such as systems analysis, goal-based evaluations, and decision-making evaluations, are not covered in this chapter.

Efficacy or Effectiveness Evaluation

Efficacy refers to changes in health outcomes of interventions that are achieved under ideal circumstances. The health promotion intervention is studied and evaluated under controlled or optimal conditions to demonstrate that the outcomes are due to the intervention and not to chance or other factors unrelated to the intervention. Efficacy is best demonstrated by a phase III randomized controlled trial.

The *effectiveness* of an intervention is the result it achieves in the real world, with limited resources, in entire populations or specified subgroups of a population. Effectiveness addresses the clinical usefulness of the intervention, as it is implemented and evaluated in a typical community setting, where it will eventually be applied. Effectiveness studies have also been called phase IV clinical trials.

Efficacy studies are considered less applicable to the general population because they are tested under ideal circumstances with a targeted group of clients. However, both types of evidence must be evaluated. Efficacy studies test the usefulness of interventions, followed by effectiveness studies in which the intervention is applied to real-life settings for feasibility, costs, effectiveness in actual practice, and acceptance by differing groups of clients. If the efficacy of a health promotion intervention has been scientifically tested, clinicians can then implement and evaluate its effectiveness in their client population or clinical setting.

Process or Outcome Evaluation

Process evaluations of health promotion interventions refer to verifying the content of the program and whether it was delivered as intended, whereas *outcome* evaluations focus on the results of the intervention. Process or implementation evaluations provide information to help refine the intervention or delivery of the program and define the needs and preferences of the targeted group. Variations in delivery among sites and clients are identified as well as breakdowns between what was intended and what was actually delivered.

Process evaluations provide insights into what factors might hinder or facilitate achievement of program goals. The evaluation also assesses whether the intended "dosage" of the program was delivered. *Dosage* refers to amount of exposure to the program or intervention (Thorogood & Coombes, 2000). Was the exposure strong enough to produce the desired outcomes?

Process evaluations are important tools for health promotion. *Pool Cool*, a skin cancer prevention program designed to increase skin cancer protection among children, underwent process evaluation to examine how well the program was implemented (Escoffery, Glanz, & Elliott, 2009). Results indicted the program was implemented successfully and identified factors responsible for successful program diffusion.

Outcomes evaluations focus on the results or changes brought about by the program, intended or unintended. The choice of outcomes to measure is determined by the program goals. If the goal is to achieve weight loss, weight should be measured prior to the program initiation and at the end of the program. If the program goal is primary prevention of cancer, clients should be followed for years to learn if and when cancer occurs.

In outcomes evaluations, the size of the effect of the intervention is an important question to ask. The effect size depends on multiple factors, including the size of the population that received the intervention, sensitivity of measures, time points measured, and the scope of the intervention. Small effects may be important when large numbers of people are involved. Effect size is discussed in statistical textbooks.

Mixed Methods Evaluation

The randomized controlled trial (RCT) is considered the gold standard to evaluate the efficacy of an intervention. *Precision*, *objectivity*, and *control* are commonly used terms to describe this type of research. An intervention is evaluated with measures that obtain numerical (quantitative) data, such as a test score or body weight. Results of an RCT answer the question "Did the intervention produce the intended effect?" Statistical tests are applied to the information (data) collected to see if significant differences are found between the group who received the intervention and the group who served as the control group.

Challenges in evaluating complex programs with multiple components have resulted in the use of multiple evaluation tools. Mixed methods evaluations, which incorporate both quantitative (numerical or numbers) and qualitative (words) data offer one solution (Clark, Cresswell, Gutmann, & Hanson, 2008). *Mixed method* refers to an umbrella term that encompasses multiple evaluation methods. The premise of mixed methods evaluations is that no one method is adequate to evaluate a program or intervention.

Mixed method approaches have been implemented to study the influence of social support on the health of vulnerable populations (Stewart, Makwarimba, Barnfather, Letourneau, & Neufeld, 2008). In this study, qualitative methods facilitated an understanding of vulnerable populations' support needs, support resources, intervention preferences, and satisfaction with interventions. Quantitative approaches documented the effectiveness and outcomes of the interventions and reliability and validity of the measures. The researchers concluded that participatory strategies are needed to make studies contextually appropriate and empowering to reduce health disparities. In another mixed methods design to evaluate televised health promotion advertisements, a population-based telephone survey and focus groups were used to obtain data about a Web site's credibility and participant's intention to perform healthy behaviors (Berry et al., 2009). Focus groups provided valuable information on reasons for no differences in interventions. These studies attest to the value of multiple sources of information when evaluating complex intervention.

DECIDING WHICH HEALTH OUTCOMES TO MEASURE

Measurement of the effectiveness of health promotion efforts is necessary to determine the most appropriate and cost-effective interventions. Choice of which health promotion outcomes to measure is dependent on the goals to be attained, the purpose and type of intervention, and the ability to access the information needed to measure the results of care. The challenge is to select health outcomes that are comprehensive, comparable, meaningful, and accurate in reflecting the effects of the health promotion.

Nursing-Sensitive Outcomes

Although quality of care has always been a concern for nursing, quality improvement programs have focused on structure and process. The shift to effectiveness (outcomes) poses an issue for nursing, as nurses practice in interdisciplinary teams, in which health outcomes are influenced by more than one discipline. For example, in many health promotion programs nurses, along with nutritionists, psychologists, and exercise physiologists, may all be involved in implementing the program. The challenge is to identify and measure outcomes that are influenced by nursing actions.

Nursing-sensitive outcomes reflective of health promotion and community outcomes have been identified and published (Head et al., 2004, Head, Maas, & Johnson, 2003; Ingersoll, McIntosh, & Williams, 2000). Categories of these outcomes are summarized in Table 10–1. Biologic outcomes are the most commonly used and include such things as weight, skin-fold thickness, blood pressure, and cholesterol values. Psychosocial outcomes measure patterns of behavior, communication, and relationships. Psychosocial measures may include attitude, mood, emotions, coping, and social functioning. Functional measures include activities, mobility, and self-care measures. Behavioral outcomes involve the client's activities and actions, such as participation in regular physical activity. Knowledge, the cognitive level of understanding, is a common nursing-sensitive outcome, because teaching is a major component of nursing practice.

Home functioning outcomes focus on the performance of the client and family in the home environment. Measures of this outcome may include family support and role function. Safety is a nursing-sensitive outcome, as nurses implement interventions to

TABLE 10–1	Categories of Nursing Sensitive Outcomes
Category	**Examples**
Biologic	Blood pressure
	Weight
	Laboratory values
Psychosocial	Attitudes
	Emotions
	Moods
	Social functioning
Functional	Activities of daily living
	Mobility
	Self-care
Behavioral	Actions
	Activities
Cognitive	Knowledge
Home functioning	Family support
	Family roles
Safety	Noise-free environment
Symptom control	Smoking withdrawal
Goal attainment	Behavior change
Satisfaction	Program/service contentment
Costs	Cost effectiveness

promote safe home, community, and work environments. For example, the nurse may work with clients in the community to promote safe neighborhood environment with lighted walking paths.

Symptom control outcomes involve the management of symptoms. For example, health promotion interventions for smoking cessation may need to manage symptoms associated with smoking withdrawal. Or symptoms may describe results of unsuccessful health behavior change that may need attention, such as depressive symptoms.

Goal attainment outcomes refer to assisting clients to accomplish their health promotion goals. Client satisfaction, as an outcome, is a global measure of contentment with the services provided to the client. For example, measures of satisfaction or dissatisfaction with health promotion programs provide valuable information for nurses to make changes.

Cost outcomes are also considered sensitive to nursing practice. However, the nursing profession has just begun to seriously focus on the cost-effectiveness of nursing interventions. Health promotion and risk reduction interventions offer an exciting opportunity to assess the cost-effectiveness of nurse counseling, coaching, and teaching activities.

The Nursing Outcomes Classification (NOC) is a standardized classification of patient–client outcomes developed to evaluate the effects of nursing interventions (Moorhead, Johnson, Maas, & Swanson, 2008). Seven categories have been identified: physiological health, functional health, psychosocial health, family health, health knowledge and behavior, perceived health, and community health. NOC is one of the standardized languages recognized by the American Nurses Association (ANA).

Information about the NOC system is available on its Web site (listed at the end of the chapter).

Health outcomes that reflect nursing's contribution to health promotion and risk reduction must be identified and measured. Some of these include lifestyle behaviors (dietary and physical activity behaviors), knowledge, attitudes, coping behaviors, biological changes (e.g., weight, blood cholesterol values, blood pressure), self-esteem, self-efficacy, and empowerment. Nursing's focus on positive lifestyle change and wellness places an emphasis on positive health-promoting behaviors.

Individual, Family, and Community Outcomes

Three categories or levels of outcomes can be measured: (1) individual or client focused, (2) family focused, and (3) community focused. These are described in Table 10–2.

Individual-focused outcomes measure the effects of health care interventions on individual behaviors. These outcomes can be classified as biological and holistic. Biological outcomes are physiologic changes in the client that reflect the effects of health promotion or risk reduction interventions, For example, health promotion outcomes as a result of a nutritional intervention may result in a change in weight or body mass index.

Holistic outcome measures are broad measures of behavior and health. Holistic outcomes include knowledge, lifestyle change, functional status, psychosocial functioning, perceptions, self-care, and health-related quality of life. It is important to have concrete definitions and measures that accurately reflect the definitions. Monitoring holistic outcomes is important in health promotion efforts, as these outcomes may detect change before biologic effects are observed.

TABLE 10–2   General Classification of Outcomes

Category	Types of Outcomes
Client Focused	
Biologic	Physiologic measures
	Weight
	Body mass index
Holistic	Lifestyle change
	Functional status
	Perceptions
	Self-care
	Quality of life
Family Focused	
	Support
	Resources
Community Focused	
	Empowerment
	Participation
	Health of Community

Family-focused interventions have received less attention due to the challenges in measuring the contributions of individual family members. However, family support is important to assess, as well as family cohesion and role functioning. The significant role the family plays in the development of both health-promoting and health-damaging behaviors, beginning at a very early age, is well documented. Family measures must be developed and tested, as family interventions are expected to increase.

Community outcomes are global measures in health promotion, as they focus on results of community- or organizational-level interventions. Community outcomes include community participation, empowerment, and changes in the community to support health promotion, such as biking paths and wellness centers. Community outcomes may be measured at the neighborhood or group level, rather than individual evaluations. This type of measurement poses multiple challenges but has great potential, as the health of the community following health promotion efforts needs to be known.

Short-Term, Intermediate, and Long-Term Outcomes

One reason for the lack of effectiveness of health promotion interventions may be due to measuring the outcomes at the wrong time. If information is collected immediately following the intervention, it may be too soon to capture the change in lifestyle behaviors. If the effects are measured many months following the intervention, other factors may have intervened to influence the expected results. Therefore, the timing should be planned carefully to capture the anticipated effects. Measurement at multiple time points is usually necessary. Short-term outcomes are measured immediately following the intervention. Appropriate short-term outcomes are knowledge, coping behaviors, and readiness to change. Intermediate outcomes are targeted at a period of time following the intervention when a change is expected to have occurred. Intermediate outcomes are measured soon enough following the intervention so that its effects can be accurately isolated from other possible reasons. Intermediate outcomes may be useful in reflecting attitude changes or attempts to change, although lifestyle change has not yet occurred. Long-term outcomes are the ultimate outcomes, as they are the final or end results of the health promotion intervention. Long-term outcomes include lifestyle change and improved quality of life. These long-term outcome measures may also be used to measure intermediate outcomes. When measuring long-term change, it is important to consider the intervening factors mentioned previously when interpreting the results.

Economic Outcomes

The role of economic outcomes in health promotion is important to evaluate the costs and benefits of program for consumers, health care payers, and policy makers. The inclusion of both costs and intervention effects is called a cost-inclusive evaluation and includes costs, benefits, cost-effectiveness, cost utility, and cost benefit (Yates, 2009). These are described in Table 10–3.

A cost-inclusive evaluation has three components (Herman, Avery, Schemp, & Walsh, 2009). First, costs are compared to effects (benefits). Benefits may be determined by a cost-benefit analysis, a cost-effectiveness analysis, or a cost-utility analysis. Second, the program or intervention of interest is compared with an alternative. The comparison may be an

TABLE 10–3	Cost-Inclusive Evaluation Terms	

Terms common in cost-inclusive evaluations

Term	Definition	Example
Costs	Value (typically monetary) of the amounts of different types of resources consumed to implement the program	• $1,243 per client per day of program implementation
Benefits	Value of resources produced or saved as a result of program implementation, measured in the same units as costs (typically money)	• $2,506 saved per student per semester • $11,508 in additional income per year
Effectiveness	Results of program implementation that are measured in nonmonetary units	• 10.5 fewer accidents per intersection per year • .75 quality-adjusted life years added
Cost-beneficial	Favored according to results of cost-benefit analyses	• The new program costs 74% as much as our old program, and produces similar cost-savings in criminal justice actions avoided
Cost-effective	Favored according to results of cost-effectiveness analyses	• The new program costs 74% as much as our old program, and produces significantly better increments in Quality-Adjusted Life Years for clients
Cost analysis	*Should* just measure costs *of* program implementation, but often is meant to include monetary outcomes (i.e., benefits) resulting from program as well	• $114 per client per day of outpatient services • Average of $253 was spent per treatment participant
Cost-benefit analysis (CBA)	Relationship between value of resources used by a program and value of resources produced by program. Value is measured in same, usually monetary, units for both costs and benefits	• 2.1 ratio of benefits to costs after 1 year of program operation • Net $126 per client per year • 44 min saved for every 10 min invested in prevention
Cost-effectiveness analysis (CEA)	Relationship between value of resource used in program implementation and nonmonetary outcomes produced by program	• $51 per opiate-free day • $72 per pound lost and kept off for 6 months or more

Source: Reprinted from *Evaluation and Program Planning*, Volume 32, B. T. Yates, "Cost-inclusive evaluation: A banquet of approaches for including costs, benefits, and cost-effectiveness and cost-benefit analysis in your next evaluation," pages 52–54, Copyright 2008, with permission from Elsevier.

existing program or the costs of not offering the program. Third, the stakeholders must be identified. Is the analysis for the participant, the community, or institutional stakeholders?

A simple way to describe the different types of analyses is by the questions they answer. An analysis of costs answers the question "What are the monetary costs of the resources needed to implement the program?" Cost-effectiveness analysis (CEA) answers the question "What is the most inexpensive way to achieve a given outcome?" In cost-utility analysis, the question answered is "What is the cost per quality-adjusted life years?" In cost-benefit analysis, the question answered is "What is the net benefit of a given alternative?" Economic analysis begins with merely reporting the cost of the treatment or intervention implemented. This is followed by cost-benefit analysis, which places a monetary value on a health outcome. Cost-benefit analysis compares the monetary value of resources used in the program with the value of resources produced by the program.

Cost-effectiveness analysis reflects the amount of benefit a treatment or intervention provides relative to alternative programs or no program (Yates, 2009). The purpose of CEA is to evaluate the comparative potential of expenditures on different health care interventions. CEA does not determine whether an intervention is worth its cost in some absolute sense. It provides a relative measure of which services afford the highest health benefit per dollar. The cost-effectiveness ratio (C/E), the central measure used in CEA, is the incremental price of obtaining a unit of health effect from a given health intervention when compared with an alternative intervention. Implicit in the C/E ratio is a comparison between alternatives: the intervention under study with either another intervention or no intervention. The two intervention outcomes must have a common unit of measurement to be compared. CEA is meant to be informative and identify interventions that produce the greatest health using the resources available. It is meant to provide additional information for a decision; however, it is not considered the sole determinant of the decision to use to eliminate an intervention. A sensitivity analysis may be conducted after the cost-effectiveness analysis to evaluate how the extraneous or error sources might affect the cost or effectiveness of the intervention. In cost-effectiveness study of an intervention to asses the relative efficiency of multivitamin and multimineral supplementation compared with no supplementation in adults aged 65 years and older, results indicated that the placebo intervention was less costly and as effective as the supplement intervention (Kilonzo et al., 2007). A sensitivity analysis was performed, including all outpatient and inpatient costs, including costs of emergency visits and hospital admissions. The results were not sensitive to any of the charges. The authors concluded that taking supplements is unlikely to be cost-effective in older people.

Examples of CEA studies are available in the literature. For example, a CEA for an exercise and diet intervention for overweight and obese adults with knee osteoarthritis was conducted (Sevick, Miller, Loeser, Williamson, & Messier, 2009). The diet and exercise intervention was compared with a healthy lifestyle control group, and the analysis was done from a payer perspective. Results indicated that the intervention was most cost-effective for reducing weight ($35 for each percentage point reduction in baseline body weight), and increasing physical activity ($10 for each percentage point improvement in a six minute walk test).

Cost-utility analysis is a special case of cost-effectiveness analysis that uses the expressed preference (utility) of a health state as the unit of outcome. The units reflect preferences of the population. Quality-Adjusted Life Years (QALYs), the unit of analysis in cost-utility analysis, are the incremental costs per quality adjusted life year. QALYs are estimated by multiplying length of life in a given state with the value placed on that state, on a scale ranging from complete health to the worst possible health (Buckingham & Devlin, 2009). The values are obtained with the Time Trade-Off method, in which an individual is asked to consider living for a period of time in poor health compared with some shorter period of time in complete health.

In a cost-utility analysis of the National Truth Campaign to prevent smoking in youth, finding indicated that the cost per QALYS saved was $4,302 (Holtgrave, Wunderink, Vallone, & Healton, 2009). This was cost-effective and below the cost of other prevention programs, suggesting that the national social marketing campaign improved the public's health and was cost-effective.

Several issues must be taken into consideration when deciding to perform cost-effectiveness analysis (Sullivan, et al., 2001). First, intervention studies usually include groups that are not representative of the general population. Second, intervention studies and cost-effectiveness analyses are designed for different purposes, and the distinction creates several issues. The outcomes needed for the two are usually different, sample size needs may be different, and the time frame needed may also differ. Last, adding cost-effectiveness analysis to an intervention study can be quite time-consuming, in terms of sample size, data collection, observation periods, and staff and expertise needed.

Cost-effective analysis and other economic evaluations are increasingly assuming an important role in health care policy decisions. The approach has been standardized with principles and procedures for reporting the results. Regulatory bodies now consider cost-effectiveness part of the approval process for new medications and technologies. However, the analytic techniques are not simple and have many methodological pitfalls, so only those with the expertise should conduct the analysis. Although consensus-based recommendations and a standard set of methods to improve the comparability and quality of studies have been developed, the techniques are still evolving.

EVALUATING EVIDENCE FOR PRACTICE

Current best evidence for one's practice can be obtained from many sources: a synthesis of relevant literature; international, national, and local standards of practice; cost-effectiveness analysis; clinical expertise; and patient preferences. A literature search should be conducted to see if adequate information is available to evaluate the intervention. The literature (evidence) is critically evaluated and synthesized and then integrated into one's practice to guide health promotion decisions for clients. This process is called *evidence-based practice* or *evidenced-based health promotion*. The aim of evidence-based practice is to reduce wide variations in practice, eliminate worst practices, and enhance best practices to improve quality and decrease costs. Evaluation questions to ask include the following:

- Can I trust this information (validity)?
- Will the information make an important difference in my practice (significance)?
- Can I use the information in my practice (applicability)?

Evidence-based practice involves an assessment of research-based evidence for changing practice, identifying the type of evidence needed, conducting a literature search for

---

TABLE 10–4   Steps in Evidence-Based Practice

1. Select health prevention–health promotion area of interest.
2. Identify most effective intervention for defined area.
3. Tailor intervention to client.
4. Identify potential factors that may influence outcomes.
     Client characteristics
     Demographic factors
     Family characteristics
5. Select outcomes to measure effects of intervention.
     Short term
     Intermediate
     Long term

---

evidence, critically evaluating the evidence, identifying clinically meaningful results, and translating the evidence into one's practice (Rosswurm & Larrabee, 1999; Scudder, 2006). Table 10–4 reviews the steps to help establish evidence for a practice intervention. After an evidence-based practice change is implemented, both the implementation process and expected outcomes are evaluated.

The evidenced-based process does not replace clinical expertise, as the nurse must evaluate new knowledge in light of its applicability to the target population. For example, the clinical problem might be the inability to promote physical activity in a rural setting and the potential of telehealth interventions in this setting. The literature about telehealth interventions to promote physical activity is evaluated to assess its applicability for clients in rural settings. Other considerations include the sociocultural environment of the targeted population, prior experiences with health promotion in rural settings, and available resources. If the nurse finds that the evidence is applicable and relevant, plans are made to implement and evaluate the telehealth intervention.

Adaptation is often necessary when translating evidenced-based research into practice (Cohen et al., 2008). The intervention may need to be modified to accommodate the target setting or client circumstances, and the local setting may need to be supported throughout implementation. Flexibility, without compromising fidelity to the intervention, is necessary to match the evidence with the type of approach needed.

Current best evidence can be obtained from the Cochrane Collaboration, an organization committed to improving global health through systematic reviews of the effectiveness of health interventions. The Cochrane Collaboration's Web site and other useful ones are listed at the end of the chapter.

EVALUATION OF INTERVENTIONS WITH INDIVIDUALS AND COMMUNITIES

Changes in the conceptualization of health have resulted in different approaches to promoting and evaluating wellness. One difference focuses on whether health promotion strategies concentrate on individual lifestyle changes or community-wide changes. Individual approaches identify a finite number of lifestyle areas that can be targeted for intervention. McKinlay (1975) coined the term *downstream* to describe interventions

TABLE 10–5	Levels and Types of Interventions	
Level	**Target**	**Types of Interventions**
Downstream	Individuals Curative	Education Counseling Support
Midstream	Communities Prevention	Work site programs School programs Community-based programs
Upstream	Public policy Environment	Tax incentives or deterrents Policy changes Local ordinances Laws Media campaigns

Source: Based on McKinlay's Model for Public-Health Interventions (McKinlay, J. & Marceau, L., (2000). U.S. Public Health and the 21st Century: Diabetes Mellitus.) Reprinted with permission of Elsevier, *The Lancet*, 2000, Vol. 356, pp. 757–761.

that are aimed at individuals. *Midstream* interventions describe community-based interventions and are aimed at schools, work sites, health plans, and other organizational channels, as well as entire communities or specific populations. *Upstream* health behavior interventions are those that address policy and environmental changes. Upstream strategies may include protection from environmental hazards such as asbestos in old buildings or nuclear wastes, changes in advertising of unhealthy behaviors such as antismoking campaigns, food labeling, and economic incentives such as excise taxes on liquor and cigarettes. Table 10–5 describes the three levels of interventions and suggested activities and outcomes for the three levels.

Wellness behaviors are a result of individual attitudes, beliefs, and values as well as conditions in the community. Because the three types of interventions are interrelated, success is more likely to be achieved if all are taken into consideration when planning and evaluating health promotion programs.

Individuals

Programs that target individuals provide clients with strategies for wellness and/or lifestyle change. Individuals must then maintain the new behaviors in the larger social environment, which often rewards at-risk behaviors or provides barriers to the maintenance of healthy behaviors. Low-income and disadvantaged individuals are at greatest risk for not sustaining change due to lack of resources in their social and physical environments. A challenge for nurses and health care professionals is to develop, test, evaluate, and implement models of health promotion that incorporate community, environmental, and sociocultural factors with individual behaviors to promote wellness.

Individual theoretical models of health behavior focus on attitudes, beliefs, or other characteristics within the individual that are amenable to change (see Chapter 2). Interventions promote attitudes, knowledge, and skills to change individual behaviors. Bandura's social learning theory, Prochaska and DiClemente's stages of change model, and the health belief model have been used extensively in the design and delivery of individual health promotion interventions. In a meta-analysis of 54 self-efficacy and smoking studies, self-efficacy was found to be consistently associated with future smoking abstinence, but the association was less robust than expected (Gwaltney, Metrik, Kahler, & Shiffman, 2009). Although prior reviews have found a relationship between self-efficacy and smoking, this was the first to assess the magnitude of the association. In a systematic review of 40 studies of tailored interventions conducted to provide information about cancer risk and screening, the major theories used to guide the tailoring intervention included Prochaska's transtheoretical model (20 papers), and the health belief model (11 papers) (Albada, Ausems, Bensing, & van Dulmen, 2009). Theoretically based tailored interventions were more effective than tailoring based on family history alone.

Interventions for physical activity and dietary behaviors are abundant in the literature. A systematic review of physical activity and health-related quality of life in adults found a positive effect of physical activity on health-related quality of life (Bize, Johnson, & Plotnikoff, 2007), although methodological limitations precluded a definitive statement about the nature of the association. Only 25 studies of 5,508 identified studies met criteria in a systematic review of long-term effectiveness of physical activity interventions (Muller-Riemenschneider, Reinhold, Nocon, & Willich, 2008). Although the quality of the studies varied, there was evidence for long-term increases in physical activity and fitness compared with no-intervention groups. Almost two-thirds of the studies used booster interventions, which facilitated long-term effectiveness. A review of 14 studies using pedometers to promote physical activity in children and adolescents reported an increase in physical activity in 12 of the studies, indicating they can be used to promote physical activity (Lubans, Morgan, & Tudor-Locke, 2009). Another systematic review of 26 telephone intervention for physical activity ($n = 16$) and dietary change ($n = 10$) provides evidence for the telephone as a primary intervention method (Eakin, Lawler, Vandelanotte, & Owen, 2007). Twenty studies reported significant behavioral improvements. Factors associated with positive outcomes included length of intervention (6–12 months) and number of telephone calls (12 or more).

Individual dietary interventions have also been shown to be effective. A review of 28 intervention studies to prevent childhood obesity and overweight reported that 11 trials were effective in reducing body fat (Connelly, Duaso, & Butler, 2007). Factors promoting success included regular, vigorous physical activity that was compulsory rather than voluntary. In a systematic review of clinical trials with a minimum one-year follow-up, interventions using both a reduced calorie diet and physical activity were associated with weight loss at six months (Franz et al., 2007). In studies extending to 48 months, a 3–6% weight loss was maintained, and no one regained weight to baseline. Advice-only and physical activity–only groups had minimal weight loss at all time points.

Dietary studies have also been conducted with Latinos. In a systematic review of 22 peer nutrition education and dietary behaviors, peer interventions had positive effects on diabetes self-management, breast feeding, general nutrition knowledge, and dietary intake behaviors (Perez-Escamilla, Hromi-Fiedler, Vega-Lopez, Bermudez-Millan, & Segura-Perez, 2008). In a systematic review of acculturation and diet, less acculturated Latinos reported consuming more fruit, rice, and beans, and less sugar and sugar-sweetened beverages; however, no differences in dietary fat intake were reported (Ayala, Baquero, & Klinger, 2008). The role of culturally appropriate interventions, as well as acculturation status, must be taken into account when designing interventions.

Individual strategies for health promotion warrant continued use based on the previously mentioned reviews and six systematic reviews of 112 intervention studies and 297 observational studies (Brug, van Lenthe, & Kremers, 2006). The reviews included children, adolescents, and adults for physical activity and nutrition behaviors. Factors found to be successful, on the basis of the systematic reviews, include the following:

- Social support
- Tailored information
- Boosters
- Parent role models
- Opportunities for physical activity
- Available and accessible healthy food
- Cultural sensitivity

Computer-delivered interventions for health promotion are increasing. In a review of 75 randomized control trials, participants who received the computer-delivery intervention improved their health behaviors as well as knowledge, attitudes, and interventions, compared with the control groups (Portney, Scott-Sheldon, Johnson, & Carey, 2008). The interventions were less effective for older adults, and as expected, greater intervention dose strengthened its effectiveness. The role of tailoring as well as long-term behavior change was not evaluated. A review of 49 eHealth (Internet) interventions for physical activity and dietary change reported that Internet interventions were more effective than the comparison groups in 21 (51%) of the studies (Norman et al., 2007). Mixed results are likely due to the early stage of use of these types of interventions and the need for further development and refinement.

The extensive research reviews document the need to include community and environmental factors, as well as individual factors, if nurses are going to be successful in promoting healthy lifestyles. Increased use of communication technology is also warranted. Interventions in childhood and adolescence need increased emphasis due to the early development of unhealthy behaviors, which are more difficult to change in adulthood.

Community

Community-based interventions are designed to promote wellness and behavior change in the community or target populations within the community. These types of interventions consider broader factors that influence health other than individual beliefs and attitudes. Instead, the physical and social environment in which the individual lives and works is targeted. This approach necessitates the collaboration of individuals and organizations within the community and often demands considerable resources, including time and money.

Community settings that have commonly been the site of health promotion programs include the workplace, religious institutions, and schools. The work site is appealing because of the ability to implement comprehensive programs that may result in cost savings. Process evaluations indicate that work site interventions reported in the literature vary in comprehensiveness, intensity, and duration in providing health education to employees. Work site programs for smoking cessation consistently show positive benefits (Albertsen, Borg, & Olderburg, 2006). Evidence also indicates that the work environment influences aspects of smoking behavior. Environmental changes in work site health promotion programs—such as work site walking tracks, fitness facilities, and availability of healthy food products in company restaurants and vending machines—influence both physical activity and dietary intake (Engbers, van Poppel, Chin A Paw, & van Mechelen, 2005).

Evaluations of interventions that have been implemented in barbershops and hairstylist salons for African-Americans have been conducted. These cultural institutions are ideal work sites for health promotion programs, as barbers and hair stylists are seen as trusted advisors and have long-term clients who spend time discussing various topics with peers during their visits. Evaluation of the Healthy Hair Campaign, designed to educate African-Americans about disease risks and motivate prevention behaviors, indicated that 60% of clients reported an increase in healthy behaviors (Madigan, Smith-Wheelock, & Krein, 2007). The centerpiece of the intervention was a health chat offered by stylists to educate and motivate clients to take steps to a healthy life style.

African-American barbers have been effective implementing programs to screen and refer male clients for blood pressure follow-up as well as prostate cancer screening. In an evaluation of the role of African-American barbers in measuring blood pressure and referring clients, barbers were found to take blood pressure in 85% of clients, and treatment increased from 49% to 62% (Hess et al., 2007). Barbers were trained to measure blood pressure and plot their client's blood pressure on a wallet-sized card. They offered free haircuts for returning the blood pressure cards signed by their physicians and hung posters and displays in their shops that emphasized healthy behaviors. Both studies emphasize the role of specialty work sites in community health promotion and prevention behaviors.

Churches and other places of worship have been used as sites for health promotion. Churches are a source of support for its members and provide a setting in which health promotion programs can be offered in a culturally accepted manner. In these settings, there is a higher level of volunteer involvement to assist with program implementation, so less professional involvement is needed. Religious organizations have access to large numbers of people, effective communication channels, and adequate meeting facilities, all factors that have been shown to facilitate successful delivery of health education. These settings are ideal for community participatory interventions. Findings from a community-based participatory research intervention to promote physical activity over a two-year period in 20 churches showed an increased awareness of physical activity, but no change in physical activity behaviors (Wilcox et al., 2007). The findings are discussed in light of the challenges faced when implementing community-based participatory programs. However, partnerships with faith-based communities offer an exciting avenue for health promotion, especially for some ethnic minority groups.

Another popular site for health promotion is the classroom or school, where the focus is on children and adolescents. Schools are appealing because of the amount of time students spend in this environment, they have existing facilities, and it is possible to involve the parents in health-promotion activities. This approach is based on the premise that the family, as well as peers, plays an important role in the adoption and maintenance of healthy behaviors. A comprehensive school-based health promotion program should include health instruction, health services, social support services, health education curricula, extracurricular activities that meet the needs and interests of the students, and involvement of the family. Additional program components have focused on specific behaviors, such as food service changes to promote a healthy diet or physical activity instruction and programs. These programs have begun to be implemented in preschool and elementary grades to promote health behaviors early in life. Long-term evaluation of these programs will be important.

Community health promotion occurs in neighborhoods or communities and relies on coalitions to address the targeted health behaviors, so community activation is a necessary component in implementing community programs. Activation of the community can be challenging because of the need to coordinate many agencies and develop actions that will not reflect the interests of a particular group or agency. Factors have been identified in process evaluations that facilitate community activation. These include the ability of the community coalition to provide its own vision, members who have the skills and time to work together, frequent and productive communication, and a sense of cohesion (Pluye, Potvin, & Denis, 2004). Barriers to communication and coalition building include staff that lack organizational skills, staff turnover, difficulty recruiting members, and reluctance of community members to conduct activities.

Despite the challenges and obstacles, interventions targeting the community have increased in recent years. Large-scale community interventions have been implemented to promote cardiovascular health promotion, walking in older adults, and weight control (Culos-Reed, Doyle-Baker, Paskevich, Devonish, & Reimer, 2007; DeCocker, de Bourdeaudhuij, Brown, & Cardon, 2007; Kaczorowski et al., 2008; Lee, Arthur, & Avis, 2007; Wendel-Vos, et al., 2009). In general, results have shown improvements in lifestyle factors, including physical activity levels.

Media campaigns have been found to be an effective adjunct to both individual- and community-based interventions. Message repetition is important, and presentations must be of high quality, which means that media campaigns can be expensive. However, some media programs are inexpensive, such as bill inserts, grocery bag flyers, television feature news stories, and community newspapers. Modern technology has resulted in media-based interventions that are delivered in personalized, interactive formats. A two-year national physical activity marketing campaign for children aged 9–13 years resulted in a positive influence on children's' attitudes about physical activity and increased physical activity behaviors (Huhman et al., 2007). A community-based physical activity project was disseminated through a Web site and assessed in terms of program adoption (Mummery, Schofield, Hinchliffe, Joyner, & Brown, 2006). Evidence supports the use of Web sites to disseminate programs beyond the borders of the original project. Evaluation of a mass media campaign increased awareness and understanding of the value of physical activity and promoted positive attitudes toward activity (Bauman, Smith, Maibach, & Roger-Nash, 2006). Short-term behavior change has been documented with mass media campaigns, but long-term follow up has been limited.

In summary, intervention approaches at the individual and community levels have resulted in behavior change, which is cause for optimism in health promotion. Effective individual-based programs have mainly used cognitive–behavioral theories to guide the interventions. The increased emphasis on the context in which individuals work and live has resulted in approaches that target both the individual and the community. Community health promotion programs have potential to improve health because of their ability to target large segments of the population through broad-based interventions. Community health promotion also offers many challenges in program implementation and evaluation.

STRATEGIES FOR EFFECTIVE HEALTH PROMOTION INTERVENTIONS

Strategies have been identified that increase the likelihood of effective health promotion programs. Evaluation must be considered in designing the intervention, selecting outcome measures, deciding the time frame for both implementing the intervention and measuring anticipated outcomes of the intervention. Knowledge about long-term maintenance of change, the last step in the change process of health promotion, is limited. However, strategies to increase sustainability of health promotion programs have been identified.

Designing the Intervention

Health promotion interventions are complex and usually involve multiple components. When designing programs, the nurse must assess the appropriateness of the intervention for the target population (Morley & Farewell, 2000). First, the intervention must be affordable to individuals, agencies, or communities. A program that is too expensive will result in poor participation. If the intervention is too expensive or resource intensive for community-based systems, commitment by the agency will be lacking and participation will be poor. The intervention must also be manageable and compatible with existing programs in the community. Programs that are less complex and fit with existing programs have a greater chance of being successfully implemented. Evidence of the efficacy of the intervention should be available. If the efficacy of the intervention has not been tested, results of implementing the intervention in the new group or community must be evaluated carefully.

Selecting Outcomes

Realistic, high-quality outcomes must be chosen to evaluate the program results. The outcomes of some health promotion interventions may not be known for many years. In addition, community-level outcomes are complex and often very expensive, so the decision of which end points and outcomes are realistic is a critical one. The outcome evaluation component needs careful planning so that the results are realistic, affordable, and meaningful. After a decision is made about which outcomes to measure, based on program goals, accurate measures must be chosen. Self-report measures, using paper-and-pencil questionnaires, are used in many health promotion programs. Objective measures should be used whenever possible, as they are more precise and sensitive to change for health promotion interventions, such as physical activity and dietary changes. Measurement of community-level outcomes is less well developed because of their complexity. One type of community measure is change in the community environment, such as the number of new public physical activity facilities or the number of restaurants that provide healthy choices. These broader outcomes provide information about how the program has improved the overall community, independent of behavior change of individual members.

Outcomes that can be measured when long-term outcomes may not be realistic include program participation rates. Although participation does not measure effectiveness, it provides information about the acceptance of the intervention and its implementation. Process measures are also useful to assess the implementation effectiveness. Measurement of the "delivered dose," or an assessment of aspects of the program that were implemented, and "received dose," or the number of people who participated in the program, are useful aspects of process evaluation (Sidani & Braden, 1998).

Deciding Time Frame

A realistic time frame is necessary to properly conduct the program and evaluate the results. What is realistic depends on the type, comprehensiveness, and complexity of the program and the target population. In an individual-focused intervention targeting a small group, six months may be a realistic period to implement and evaluate short-term results. However, five years may be needed to implement and evaluate a complex community-based program targeting primary schools. The time frame for a community-based program is related to acceptance and action by the community and may backfire if it is rushed.

Sustaining Behavior Change

Most of the progress in health promotion research has been in promoting health-behavior change; less progress has been seen in implementing strategies to sustain these changes. The current models of health behavior focus on how people decide to adopt health behaviors. Exceptions are Bandura's cognitive theory, which states that self-efficacy beliefs are a critical determinant of both the initiation and maintenance of behavior change, and Prochaska and DiClemente's transtheoretical model, which includes a maintenance stage. However, neither of these models of behavior change offers guidance about the process of maintenance and how it differs from initiation and adoption of behaviors (Rothman, 2000). A survey was conducted to evaluate which of the major transtheoretical model constructs distinguished between action and maintenance (Fallon, Hausenblas, & Nigg, 2005). For men, continuing to overcome barriers, the consequences of their behavior on others (social norms), and coping with negative affect were important in exercise maintenance. Women needed to focus on the belief that their family and friends benefited and their confidence to overcome the daily barriers in their exercise regimens (exercise self-efficacy). Studies like this one help researchers understand the theoretical and behavioral processes that guide successful behavioral maintenance. These factors can then be addressed and evaluated.

In weight maintenance programs, factors that have been shown to be associated with sustainability of weight loss include duration of the program, continuing contact or booster follow-up sessions, moderate to high levels of physical activity, ongoing self-monitoring of body weight and food intake (food and weight records), and self-efficacy (Carels et al., 2008; Hollis et al., 2008; Wiltink et al., 2007). Theoretically based Internet approaches have also been shown to be effective in long-term weight gain prevention (Winett, Tate, Anderson, Wojcik, & Winett, 2005). These programs have documented changes in nutritional practices, physical activity, and weight loss for up to a year.

The use of structured eating with meal replacements has shown varying success in long-term weight loss maintenance. Although some research has found greater short- and long-term weight loss, others have found no differences (Annunziato et al., 2009). Meal replacements are palatable and portion controlled, eliminate the need to choose and prepare foods, and can be incorporated into many settings. This type of diet may be very successful for those who need more structure to successfully manage their weight.

Long-term follow-up of physical activity behavior indicates that self-efficacy and positive affect predict long term behavior, as well as social support and exercise frequency (McAuley, Jerome, Elavsky, Marquez, & Ramsey, 2005; McAuley et al., 2007). Confidence (self-efficacy) consistently is shown to predict maintenance of physical activity as well as for resisting temptation to eat unhealthy foods (Riebe et al., 2005). To date, long-term results provide support for use of the theoretical constructs and models discussed in Chapter 2 for behavior change.

Sustaining health promotion programs is also a challenge, as multiple issues influence the sustainability of a program's effectiveness over time. Sustainability includes maintaining the health benefits achieved through the initial program, continuing the program long term, or building the capacity of the community that received the program (Casey, Payne, Eime, & Brown, 2009). The program must be transferred from outside agencies to the community to have a sustained effect. Sustainability is influenced by the design of the intervention and implementation factors, facilitators and barriers within the targeted community setting, and factors in the broader community environment. Sustainability is more likely to be successful when capacity building has occurred in the community and program goals have included long-term maintenance (Schierer, Hartling, & Hagerman, 2008).

Program sustainability must be conceptualized as an ongoing process that is ever changing as new knowledge is gained. An infrastructure that integrates resources should be established to support the program. These resources might include state health department units, universities, professional societies, and federal organizations. Attention to sustainability is important for the program to continue to promote health behaviors.

OPPORTUNITIES FOR RESEARCH IN EVALUATING HEALTH PROMOTION

Evaluation of health promotion programs offer many avenues for research. First, it is evident that current theories of health promotion should be expanded and tested, as most theories have not paid much attention to long-term behavior change. Continuing research is needed to identify the determinants of behavior maintenance. Socio-ecological models of health promotion, which integrate individual constructs of behavior change with social and physical environmental determinants, need further testing and evaluation.

Second, accurate and sensitive measures of behavior change are needed to evaluate community outcomes. Self-report measures of behavior change should be developed that are reliable and valid and sensitive to both short-term and long-term change. Objective measures of behavior change also need to be refined to more precisely measure dietary and physical activity behaviors, family change, and community change concepts such as empowerment. Outcome measures also must be standardized across studies of health behaviors, such as physical activity, to enable researchers and practitioners to compare findings.

Research to promote long-term maintenance has been limited. Exploratory studies are needed to answer such questions as these: "What factors promote successful maintenance of healthy behaviors?" "What factors prevent relapse?" "What are the greatest challenges encountered in maintenance?" Descriptive studies are necessary to describe factors associated with maintenance of behaviors over long periods of time as well as differences in factors that predict success in various age and ethnic groups. What role do parents play in the maintenance of their children's physical activity? Experimental studies that evaluate interventions to promote long-term maintenance are also needed. These studies should be implemented for individuals as well as in schools and work sites in the community.

CONSIDERATIONS FOR PRACTICE IN EVALUATING HEALTH PROMOTION

Health care professionals are mandated to base their practice on current research findings as well as other factors, so it is important to understand the criteria used to evaluate the evidence. Courses that teach these skills can be offered in the clinical setting or through collaboration with local chapters of professional organizations or universities. Knowledge of the evidence-based process will enable the nurse to accurately evaluate the literature and make informed decisions about the evidence.

Knowledge of effective health promotion interventions and programs provide the nurse with information to refer clients to successful programs or deliver individual- or community-based interventions that have been successful. An interdisciplinary approach has been shown to be more effective in the delivery of complex or community-based interventions.

Nurses in clinical settings must implement and evaluate new models of delivery of health promotion interventions. For example, telephone counseling and follow-up is a relatively low-cost intervention that can be effectively used to provide ongoing contact, social support, and expertise to answer questions. Telephone and Web-based interventions should become a standard component of self-help interventions and follow-up for all ages, including youths, the elderly, and rural populations.

Maintenance continues to be a major problem in health-behavior change, so nurses should follow clients carefully to identify issues and provide these individuals with ongoing support. Nurses can identify strategies through counseling and discussions with clients and their families. New strategies should be implemented and evaluated with realistic long-term follow-up.

Summary

Evaluation of health promotion programs shed light on what is most effective to promote wellness and behavior change as well as what does not work. Evaluating health promotion interventions facilitates the development of a knowledge base on which to make decisions about programs that are most effective for behavior change. The evaluation process is complex, time-consuming, and requires advanced knowledge not previously applied in practice. However, learning to evaluate the literature provides valuable information about the usefulness of individual- and community-based interventions.

Learning Activities

1. Select a health promotion intervention of interest, such as physical activity in the elderly, and using the steps in Table 10–5, evaluate the literature and establish the evidence on which to base your planned intervention.

2. Develop an evaluation plan for a health education program to teach adolescents proper nutrition.

   a. What would you consider in designing the program?

   b. Develop a process evaluation plan, describing how you will evaluate the dosage of the intervention received by the participants.

   c. Describe your outcome evaluation plan. Which outcomes will be appropriate to measure, and how will you measure them? Consider both short-term and intermediate outcomes.

   d. Describe the time frame you will use to implement and evaluate the results of the program and the rationale for choosing the particular time points.

   e. What factors do you need to consider in promoting sustainability of the change, and how will you monitor sustainability?

Selected Web Sites

Agency for Health Care Research and Quality
http://www.ahrq.gov/clinical/epcix.htm
The Web site presents summaries of published evidence for or against the use of methods to manage or prevent disease.

The Centers for Disease Control
http://cdc.gov/eval/framework.htm
The Centers for Disease Control has an evaluation framework for public and community health.

The Centre for Health Evidence
http://www.cche.net/usersguide/main.asp
The Centre for Health Evidence provides a user's guide for evidence-based practice.

The Cochrane Collaboration
http://www.cochrane.org
The Cochrane Collaboration is a global network of volunteers who conduct systematized reviews of health care interventions that are available in the Cochrane Library. It is the best single source of health care evidence.

The Health Links
http://healthlinks.washington.edu/ebp
The Health Links site contains resources for evidence-based practice.

The Joanna Briggs Institute
http://www.joannabriggs.edu.as
The Joanna Briggs Institute is a professional organization that provides resources and reviews of evidence-based nursing.

The New York State Teachers Center for Program Evaluation
http://programevaluation.org
The New York State Teachers Center for Program Evaluation provides tools for planning and conducting evaluation projects.

Penn State University
http://www.libraries.psu.edu/instruction/ebpt-07/index.hlm
The Penn State site offers evidence-based practice tutorials for nurses and other health care professionals.

References

Albada, A., Ausems, M., Bensing, J. M., & van Dulmen, S. (2009). Tailored information about cancer risk and screening: A systematic review. *Patient Education and Counselling*, 77(2), 155–171.

Albertsen, K., Borg, V., & Oldenberg, B. (2006). A systematic review of the impact of work environment on smoking cessation, relapse, and amount smoker. *Preventive Medicine, 43,* 291–305.

Annunziato, R. A., Timko, C. A., Crerand, C. E., Didie, E. R., Bellace, D. L., Phelan, S., et al. (2009). A randomised trial examining differential meal replacement adherence in a weight loss maintenance program after one-year follow-up. *Eating Behaviours, 10*(3), 176–183.

Ayala, G. X., Baquero, B., & Klinger, S. (2008). A systematic review of the relationship between acculturation and diet among Latinos in the United States: Implications for future research. *Journal of the American Dietetic Association, 108*, 1330–1344.

Bauman, A., Smith, B. J., Maibach, E. W., & Reger-Nash, B. (2006). Evaluation of mass media campaigns for physical activity. *Evaluation and Program Planning, 29*, 312–322.

Berry, T. R., Spence, J. C., Plotnikoff, R. C., Bauman, A., McCarger, L., Witcher, C., et al. (2009). A mixed methods evaluation of television health promotion advertisements targeted at older adults. *Evaluation and Program Planning, 32*, 278–288.

Bize, R., Johnson, J. A., & Plotnikoff, R. C. (2007). Physical activity level and health-related quality of life in the general adult population: A systematic review. *Preventive Medicine, 45*, 410–415.

Brug, J., van Lenthe, F. J., & Kremers, S. P. (2006). Revisiting Kurt Lewin: How to gain insight into environmental correlates of obesogenic behaviours. *American Journal of Preventive Medicine, 31*, 525–529.

Buckingham, K. J., & Devin, N. J. (2009). A note on the nature of utility in time and health and implication for cost utility analysis. *Social Science & Medicine, 68*, 362–367.

Carels, R. A., Konrad, K., Young, K. M., Darby, L. A., Coit, C., Clayton, A. M., et al. (2008). Taking control of your personal eating and exercise environment. *Eating Behaviours, 9*, 228–237.

Casey, M., Payne, W. R., Eime, R. M., & Brown, S. J. (2009). Sustaining health promotion programs within sport and recreation organisations. *Journal of Science and Medicine, 12*, 113–118.

Clark, M. P., Cresswell, J. W., Gutmann, M. L., & Hanson, W. E. (2008). Advanced mixed methods research designs. In M. P. Clark & J. W. Cresswell (Eds.), *The mixed methods reader* (pp. 161–196). Los Angeles, CA: Sage Publications.

Cohen, D. J., Crabtree, B. F., Etz, R. S., Balasubramanian, B. A., Donahue, K. E., Leviton, L. C., et al. (2008). Fidelity versus flexibility: Translating evidence-based research into practice. *American Journal of Preventive Medicine, 35*(5S), S381–S389.

Connelly, J. B., Duaso, M. J., & Butler, G. (2007). A systematic review of controlled trials of interventions to prevent childhood obesity and overweight: A realistic synthesize of the evidence. *Public Health, 121*, 510–517.

Culos-Reed, S. N., Doyle-Baker, P. K., Paskevich, D., Devonish, J. A., & Reimer R. A. (2007). Evaluation of a community-based weight control program. *Physiology and Behaviour, 92*, 855–860.

DeCocker, K. A., de Bourdeaudhuji, I. M., Brown, W. J., & Cardon, G. M. (2007). Effect of "10,000 Steps Ghent": A whole community intervention. *American Journal of Preventive Medicine, 33*, 455–463.

Eakin, E. G., Lawler, S. P., Vandelanotte, C., & Owen, N. (2007). Telephone intervention for physical activity and dietary behaviour change. *American Journal of Preventive Medicine, 32*, 419–434.

Engbers, L. H., Poppel, M., Chin A Paw, M. J. M., & van Mechelen, W. (2005). Worksite health promotion programs with environmental changes: A systemic review. *American Journal of Preventive Medicine, 29*, 61–70.

Eriksson, C. (2000). Learning and knowledge-production for public health: A review of approaches to evidence-based public health. *Scandinavian Journal of Public Health, 28*, 298–308.

Escoffery, C., Glanz, K., & Elliot, T. (2009). Process evaluation of the *Pool Cool* diffusion trial for skin cancer prevention across two years. *Health Education Research, 23*, 732–743.

Fallon, E. A., Hausenblas, H. A., & Nigg, C. R. (2005). The transtheoretical model and exercise adherence: Examining constructs associations in later stages of change. *Psychology of Sport and Exercise, 6*, 629–641.

Franz, M. J., van Wormer, J. J., Crain, A. L., Boucher, J. L., Histon, T., Caplan, W., et al. (2007). Weight-loss outcomes: A systematic review and meta-analysis of weight-loss clinical trials with a minimum 1-year follow-up. *Journal of the American Dietetic Association, 107,* 1755–1767.

Gwaltney, C. J., Metrik, J., Kahler, C. W., & Shiffman, S. (2009). Self-efficacy and smoking cessation: A meta-analysis. *Psychology of Addictive Behaviors, 23,* 56–66.

Head, B. J., Aquilino, A. L., Johnson, M., Reed, D., Mass, M., & Moorhead, S. (2004). Content validity and nursing sensitivity of community-level outcomes from the Nursing Outcome Classification (NOC). *Journal of Nursing Scholarship, 36*(3), 251–259.

Head, B. J., Maas, M., & Johnson, M. (2003). Validity and community health nursing-sensitivity of six outcomes for community health nursing with older clients. *Public Health Nursing, 20*(5), 385–398.

Herman, P. M., Avery, D. J., Schemp, C. S., & Walsh, M. E. (2009). Are cost-inclusive evaluations worth the effort? *Evaluation and Program Planning, 32,* 55–61.

Hess, P., Reingold, J., Jones, J., Leonard, D., Haley, R., Freeman, A., et al. (2007). Barbershop as hypertension detection referral and follow-up centers for young men with hypertension. *Hypertension, 49,* 1040–1046.

Hollis, J. F., Gullion, C. M., Stevens, V. J., Brantley, P. J., Appel, L. J., Ard, J. D., et al. (2008). Weight loss during the intensive intervention phase of the weight-loss maintenance trial. *American Journal of Preventive Medicine, 35,* 118–126.

Holtgrave, D. R., Wunderink, K. A., Vallone, D. M., & Healton, C. G. (2009). Cost-utility analysis of the national truth campaign to prevent youth smoking. *American Journal of Preventive Medicine, 36,* 385–388.

Huhman, M. E., Potter, L. D., Duke, J. C., Judkins, D. R., Heitzler, C. D., & Wong, F. I. (2007). Evaluation of a national physical activity intervention for children. *American Journal of Preventive Medicine, 32,* 38–43.

Ingersoll, G. L., McIntosh, E., & Williams, M. (2000). Nurse-sensitive outcomes of advanced practice. *Journal of Advanced Nursing, 32*(5), 1272–1281.

Kaczorowski, J., Chambers, L. W., Karwalajtys, T., Dolovich, L., Farrell, B., McDonough, B., et al. (2008). Cardiovascular Health Awareness Program (CHAP): A community cluster-randomized trial among elderly Canadians. *Preventive Medicine, 46,* 537–544.

Kilonzo, M. M., Vale, L. D., Cook, J. A., Milne, A. C., Stephen, A. I., Avenell, A., et al. (2007). A cost-utility analysis of multivitamin and multimineral supplements in men and women aged 65 years and over. *Clinical Nutrition, 26,* 364–370.

Lee, L., Arthur, A., & Avis, M. (2007). Evaluating a community-based walking intervention for hypertensive older people in Taiwan: A randomized controlled trial. *Preventive Medicine, 44,* 160–166.

Lubans, D. R., Morgan, P. J., & Tudor-Locke, C. (2009). A systematic review of studies using pedometers to promote physical activity. *Preventive Medicine, 48,* 307–317.

Madigan, M. E., Smith-Wheelock, L., & Krein, S. L. (2007). Healthy hair starts with healthy body: Hair stylist as lay health advisors to prevent chronic kidney disease. *Preventing Chronic Diseases* (serial online) retrieved from http://www.cdc.gov/ped/issues2007/jul/06_0078.htm

McAuley, E., Jerome, G. L., Elavsky, S., Marquez, D. X., & Ramsey, S. N. (2005). Predicting long-term maintenance of physical activity in older adults. *Preventive Medicine, 37,* 110–118.

McAuley, E., Morris, K. S., Motl, R. W., Hu, L., Konopack, J. F., & Elavsky, S. (2007). Long-term follow-up of physical activity behavior in older adults, *Health Psychology, 26,* 375–380.

McKenzie, J. F., Neiger, B. L., & Thackery, R. (2009). *Planning, implementing and evaluating health promotion programs. A primer* (5th ed.). Boston: Pearson Benjamin Cummings.

McKinlay, J. B. (1975). A case for re-focusing upstream: The political economy of illness. In A. J. Enelowm & J. B. Henderson (Eds.), *Applying behavioral science to cardiovascular risk* (pp. 7–18). Seattle, WA: American Heart Association.

Moorhead, S., Johnson, M., Maas, M., & Swanson, E. (2008). *Nursing Outcomes Classification (NOC)* (4th ed.). St. Louis, MO: Mosby.

Morley, R., & Farewell, V. (2000). Methodological issues in randomised controlled trials. *Seminars in Neonatology, 5,* 141–148.

Muller-Riemenschneider, F., Reinhold, T., Nocon, M., & Willich, S. N. (2008). Long-term effectiveness of interventions promoting physical activity: A systematic review. *Preventive Medicine, 47,* 354–368.

Mummery, W. K., Schofield, G., Hinchliffe, A., Joyner, K., & Brown, W. (2006). Dissemination of a community-based physial activity project: The case of 10,000 steps. *Journal of Science and Medicine, 9,* 424–430.

Norman, G. J., Zabinski, M. F., Adams, M. A., Rosenberg, D. E., Yaroch, A. L., & Atienza, A. A. (2007). A review of eHealth interventions for physical activity and dietary behavior change. *American Journal of Preventive Medicine, 33,* 336–345.

Ovretveit, J. (1998). Evaluation purpose, theory and perspectives *Evaluating health interventions* (pp. 24–47). Bristol, PA: Open University Press.

Perez-Escamilla, R., Hromi-Fiedler, A., Vega-Lopez, S., Bermudez-Millan, A., & Segura-Perez, S. (2008). Impact of peer nutrition education on dietary behaviors and health outcomes among Latinos: A systematice literature review. *Journal of Nutrition and Education Behavior, 40,* 208–225.

Pluye, P., Potvin, L., & Denis, J. L. (2004). Making public health programs last: Conceptualising sustainability. *Evaluation and Program Planning, 27,* 121–133.

Portney, D. B., Scott-Sheldon, L., Johnson, B. T., & Carey, M. P. (2008). Computer-delievered interventions for health promotion and behavioral risk reduction: A meta-analysis of 75 randomized controlled trials 1988–2007. *Preventive Medicine, 47,* 3–16.

Riebe, D., Blissmer, B., Greene, G., Caldwell, M., Ruggiero, L., Stillwell, K. M., et al. (2005). Long-term maintenance of exercise and health eating behaviors in overweight adults. *Preventive Medicine, 40,* 769–788.

Rosswurm, M. A., & Larrabee, J. H. (1999). A model for change to evidence-based practice. *Image: Journal of Nursing Scholarship, 31*(4), 317–322.

Rothman, A. J. (2000). Toward a theory-based analysis of behavioral maintenance. *Health Psychology, 19*(1) (Suppl.), 64–69.

Schierer, M. A., Hartling, G., & Hagerman, D. (2008). Defining sustainability outcomes of health programs: Illustrations from an online survey. *Evaluation and Program Planning, 31,* 335–346.

Scudder, L. (2006). Using evidence-based information. *The Journal of Nurse Practitioners, 2*(3), 180–185.

Sevick, M. A., Miller, G. D., Loeser, R. F., Williamson, J. D., & Messier, S. P. (2009). Cost-effectiveness of exercise and diet in overweight and obese adults with knee osteoarthritis. *Medicine & Science in Sports & Exercise, 41*(6), 1167–1170.

Sidani, S., & Braden C. (1998). Intervention variables. *Evaluating nursing interventions: A theory-driven approach* (pp. 105–137). Thousand Oaks, CA: Sage Publications.

Stewart, M., Makwarimba, E., Barnfather, A., Letourneau, N., & Neufeld, A. (2008). Researching reducing health disparities: Mixed methods approaches. *Social Science & Medicine, 66,* 1406–1417.

Sullivan, S. D., Liljas, B., Buxton, M., Lamm, C., O'Byrne, P., Tan, W., & Weiss, K. (2001). Design and analytic considerations in determining the cost-effectiveness of early interventions in asthma from a multinational clinical trial. *Controlled Clinical Trials, 22,* 420–437.

Thorogood, M., & Coombes, Y. (2000). Use of process evaluation during project implementation: Experience from the CHAPS project for gay men. In *Evaluating health promotion: Practice and methods* (pp. 84–98). Oxford: Oxford University Press.

Wendel-Vos, W., Dutman, A. E., Verschuren, M., Ronckers, E. T., Ament, A., Assema, P., et al. (2009). Lifestyle factors of a five-year community intervention program: The Hartslag Limburg intervention. *American Journal of Preventive Medicine, 37,* 50–56.

Wilcox, S., Laken, M., Bopp, M., Gethers, O., Huang, P., McClorin, L., et al. (2007). Increasing physical activity among church members: Community-based participatory research. *American Journal of Preventive Medicine, 32,* 131–138.

Wiltink, J., Dippel, A., Szczpanski, M., Thiede, R., Alt, C., & Beutel, M. L. (2007). Long-term weight loss maintenance after inpatient psychotherapy of severely obese patients based on a randomized study: Predictors and maintaining factors of health behavior. *Journal of Psychosomatic Medicine, 62,* 691–698.

Winett, R. A., Tate, D. F., Anderson, E. S., Wojcik, J. R., & Winett, S. G. (2005). Long-term weight gain prevention: A theoretically based Internet approach. *Preventive Medicine, 41,* 629–641.

Yates, B. T. (2009). Cost-inclusiveness evaluation: A banquet of approaches for including costs, benefits, and cost-effectiveness and cost-benefit analyses in your next evaluation. *Evaluation and Program Planning, 32,* 52–54.

PART 5

Health Promotion in Diverse Populations

CHAPTER 11

Self-Care for Health Promotion Across the Life Span

OBJECTIVES

1. Differentiate between self-care and self-management.
2. Contrast the focus of self-care in children and adolescents with young, middle aged, and older adults.
3. Discuss the steps in the self-care empowerment process to promote health.
4. Describe the role of the Internet in self-care to promote health.

Outline

- Self-Care or Self-Management
- Self-Care and Health Literacy
- Orem's Theory of Self-Care
- Self-Care to Promote Health Throughout the Life Span
  - A. Self-Care for Children and Adolescents
  - B. Self-Care for Young and Middle-Aged Adults
  - C. Self-Care for Older Adults
- Goals of Health Education for Self-Care
- The Process of Empowering for Self-Care
  - A. Mutually Assess Self-Care Competencies and Needs
  - B. Determine Learning Priorities
  - C. Identify Short- and Long-Term Objectives
  - D. Facilitate Self-Paced Learning
  - E. Use Positive Reinforcement to Increase Perceptions of Competence and Motivation for Learning
  - F. Create a Supportive Environment for Learning
  - G. Decrease Barriers to Learning
  - H. Evaluate Progress Toward Health Goals
  - I. Other Considerations in Self-Care Empowerment

- The Role of the Internet in Self-Care Education
- Opportunities for Research in Self-Care
- Considerations for Practice in Self-Care
- Summary
- Learning Activities
- Selected Web Sites
- References

Professional nurses play a major role in enhancing clients' capacity for self-care throughout their life span. Nurses have long recognized the right of individuals and families to be informed and active participants in their care. Broad-based efforts to activate the general public for self-care must be spearheaded by nurses in collaboration with other health professionals and community members. Activation of consumers to "take charge" of their health is based on the assumptions that consumers must:

1. Be actively involved in solving their health problems
2. Make rational and informed decisions about their health and health care
3. Develop competencies and skills that foster creativity and adaptation amid changing life circumstances
4. Strive for greater mastery over environmental conditions that influence health and well-being
5. Promote public policy to build healthy communities
6. Advocate for financing plans that pay for self-care education for all people.

Individuals, families, and communities should be empowered for health promotion. Advances will be achieved when all groups work in concert to make health promotion a coherent social movement that influences the quality and cost of health care.

SELF-CARE OR SELF-MANAGEMENT

Self-care is a universal requirement for sustaining and enhancing life and health. Self-care directed toward health promotion can be defined as deliberate activities initiated or performed by an individual, family, or community to achieve, maintain, or promote maximum health and well-being (Orem, 2001). Care of self and others to maximize health includes actions to minimize threats to personal health, self-nurturance, self-improvement, and continued personal growth. Self-care approaches embody the notion of empowerment and autonomy. Self-care changes the balance of power in health promotion by challenging the "top-down" approach to promote health (Boote, Telford, & Cooper, 2002). Active involvement in self-care is widely acknowledged as an important strategy for achieving national health goals. The government initiative Healthy People 2020 emphasizes the importance of prevention and health promotion (see http://www.healthypeople2020.gov). Self-care is the basis for implementing health promotion and prevention strategies.

Self-care is considered the predominant and basic form of primary care. Engaging in self-care means taking responsibility for one's health and well-being. Self-care includes eating a healthy diet, exercising, getting adequate rest, and avoiding harmful substances and environments, as well as other behaviors to enhance well-being. Characteristics of self-care include the following:

- It is situation and culture specific.
- It involves the capacity to make choices and act.
- It is influenced by knowledge, skills, values, motivation, and self-efficacy.
- It focuses on aspects of health under individual control (Ganz, 1990).

Self-care and *self-management* are used interchangeably. However, they are not the same. *Self-management* is an individual's ability to detect and manage symptoms, treatments, physical and psychosocial consequences, and lifestyle changes associated with living with a chronic illness (Barlow, Wright, Sheasby, Turner, & Hainsworth, 2002). In self-management, an individual participates in activities to manage the illness, such as adjusting medication, eating special foods, or taking direct action, such as making a doctor's appointment. In self-management, clients and families assume responsibilities that were previously carried out by health professionals (Redman, 2007).

The components of care have been described as a continuum (Chambers, 2006). At one end of the continuum is self-care, or individual responsibility to promote one's health and well-being. Next is self-management to manage the illness, and then *shared care*, when health care professionals and clients work together to manage the health condition. Last on the continuum is *dependent care*, which occurs in an acute illness episode resulting in little opportunity for self-care. Self-care to promote health across the life span will continue to gain significance as consumers challenge the superiority of the traditional paternalistic medical model in health care and health policy.

Client activation, a concept similar to self-management, refers to capability and willingness to manage one's health and health care (Hibbard et al., 2008; Hibbard, Mahoney, Stock, & Tusler, 2007). Activation has been measured with the Patient Activation Measure, a scale that assesses self-reported knowledge, skills, and confidence for self-management (Hibbard, Mahoney, Stockard, & Tusler, 2005). The authors of the scale suggest there are four stages in the process of activation (Hibbard et al., 2005). These overlap with Prochaska's stages of change:

Stage 1:   Clients do not play an active role in their own health (Precontemplation).

Stage 2:   Clients do not have the knowledge to understand their health or health recommendations (Preparation).

Stage 3:   Clients take action but lack confidence and skills to support new behaviors (Action).

Stage 4:   Clients have adapted new behaviors but may be unable to maintain newly adopted behaviors due to life stressors (Maintenance).

Social environments may be precursors to activation, as individuals in supportive, less stressful environments report higher levels of activation and are engaged in more health-promoting behaviors (Hibbard et al., 2008). Further research is needed with the activation concept to more fully understand its complementary role with self-care and self-management.

SELF-CARE AND HEALTH LITERACY

Self-care for health promotion requires that clients have the knowledge and competencies needed to maintain and enhance health independently of the medical system (Wilkinson & Whitehead, 2009). An individual's ability to obtain, process, and understand information is essential to being an informed consumer who can make appropriate decisions for self-care, health, and well-being. Limited literacy skills have been associated with less knowledge and skills, negative health behaviors, and less access to screening and preventive health services (Yin, Forbis, & Dreyer, 2007). Four domains of an individual's set of capabilities have been cited in the definition of health literacy: cultural and conceptual knowledge, speaking and listening skills, reading and writing skills, and numeracy skills, or the ability to understand and use numerical and mathematical information. *Functional health literacy* refers to reading and writing skills that enable clients to function effectively on a daily basis, and *interactive literacy* refers to the cognitive and social skills needed to enable individuals to find meaning and apply new information to changing circumstances (Nutbeam, 2000). In addition, *critical literacy* involves advanced cognitive skills to be able to critically evaluate and use information to gain greater control over the situation. Clients must be able to schedule appointments; read, understand, and complete written forms and questionnaires; provide explanations; and follow instructions to learn new skills.

The client's reading and comprehension levels should be assessed prior to conducting health education to promote self-care. Health literacy screening questions can be asked using available measures, such as the Health Activities Literacy Scale. Health information should be written at a level the client and all family members can understand. Interventions to promote understanding include the following:

- Oral communication strategies
- Plain language materials
- Pictorial illustrations
- Audiovisual aids
- Group educational sessions
- Tailored sessions (Yin et al., 2007)

Health literacy is an empowerment strategy to enable individuals and families to take responsibility for their health. Health literacy empowers individuals to gain control over the personal, social, and environmental determinants of their health. Health literacy skills enable clients and families to participate fully in health promotion activities and practice self-care behaviors to promote wellness (Nutbeam, 2008).

OREM'S THEORY OF SELF-CARE

In Orem's Self-Care Nursing Model, three types of self-care requisites are described: (1) universal, (2) developmental, and (3) health deviation requirements (Orem, 1995, 2001). Universal self-care requirements include sufficient air, water, food, elimination, a balance between activity and rest, a balance between solitude and social interaction, protection from hazards, and protection of human functioning and development. Developmental self-care requirements fall into two categories:

1. Maintenance of living conditions that support life processes and promote development or progress toward higher levels of organization of human structure and maturation.
2. Provision of care either to prevent the occurrence of deleterious effects of conditions that can effect human development or to mitigate or overcome these effects from various conditions.

Three concepts are central to the model: self-care, self-care agency, and basic conditioning factors (Orem, 2001). Orem's definition of self-care is provided in a previous section of the chapter. *Self-care agency* refers to the complex capabilities needed to perform self-care, such as knowledge and skills. Self-care agency includes foundational capabilities such as memory, self-concept, and self-awareness; and power capabilities specific to self-care actions, such as motivation and decision making. *Basic conditioning factors* influence an individual's self-care and self-care agency and include age, developmental state, life experiences, sociocultural background, resources, and health state. Self-care activities are learned in everyday life. The nurse is concerned with universal and developmental requirements, although health deviation requirements, such as knowledge and skill needs for self-management in illness, must be attended to if they arise.

In Orem's model, individuals perform self-care to meet needs and demands consistent with their age, maturation, experience, resources, and sociocultural background. In her model, three systems are described within professional practice: a compensatory system, a partially compensatory system, and an educative-developmental system. In the *compensatory system*, the nurse provides total care for the client. This can be considered dependent care and is most common in acute-care settings, such as hospitals during acute illness episodes. The *partially compensatory system* of care is implemented when the nurse and the client share the responsibility for care (shared care). Care during rehabilitation from illness is partially compensatory. In contrast, the *educative-developmental system* gives the client primary responsibility for personal health, with the nurse functioning as a consultant. The educative-developmental system is compatible with self-care in health promotion. Orem's (2001) model of self-care has been criticized because it is based on the assumption that individuals are able to exert control over their environments in the pursuit of health. However, many individuals and families do not have control over their physical and social environments, two components that influence health promotion behaviors. Therefore, it is important to evaluate this assumption when applying the model to environments in which the ability to change factors may be limited.

The educative-developmental system of nursing practice is a reimbursable service by health payers. Major areas of educative-developmental nursing for self-care include enhancing clients' capacities for exercise and physical fitness, nutrition and weight control, stress management, risk reduction, maintenance of social support systems, avoidance of injurious and violent behaviors and substance abuse, and environmental modifications in homes, schools, work sites, and communities to reduce barriers to health and strengthen health-enhancing features. Education, counseling, and environmental interventions directed to these ends are a shared responsibility that includes the federal government, state and local governments, policy makers, health care providers, community leaders, and individuals.

SELF-CARE TO PROMOTE HEALTH THROUGHOUT THE LIFE SPAN

Self-Care for Children and Adolescents

Children represent the potential for a healthy society. This population faces multiple challenges, as the assumption that school-aged children are healthy is no longer valid. The prevalence of obesity in industrialized societies continues to increase, and childhood obesity is now a global epidemic with far-reaching consequences for the health of our nation (Williamson et al., 2008). Childhood is a critical period for the adoption of healthy behaviors and a health-promoting lifestyle. Behaviors are developed and learned based on developmental level, social and physical environment, and personal experiences. Thus, health promotion efforts need to begin before unhealthy behavior patterns solidify.

Childhood is a developmental period during which social and cognitive skills for autonomous decision making and health behaviors are developed. As with adults, health behaviors can be linked to family support; socialization through family, schools, and media; and socioeconomic variables. The family environment plays a significant role in self-care for health promotion through positive, stable childhood experiences. A supportive family shapes the child's behavior through the use of rewards and punishment in behavior choices. Family role modeling of self-care behaviors has also been shown to facilitate the development of healthy behaviors such as physical activity. Socioeconomic status plays a significant role in health behaviors, as increased socioeconomic status enables the family to provide resources, such as a more affluent school system, nutritional food choices, and access to multiple physical activities.

Parents exert influence over their child's health-promoting behaviors by serving as a role model, providing encouragement, and providing transportation and financial resources to participate in physical activity programs. Children in the 3rd grade were followed until the 12th grade to predict adolescent smoking based on the number of parents who smoked (Peterson et al., 2006). Having one parent who smoked substantially increases the risk that children will become daily smokers. This risk is almost doubled when two parents smoke. Home-based interventions that target parents as well as the children can increase physical activity in sedentary children (Trost & Loprinzi, 2008). Parent involvement in school-based programs has also been shown to be effective for physical activity and nutrition. Although it is often difficult to involve the parents due to work and other commitments, the success of these programs warrants the effort.

The family also influences eating patterns. In the United States National Longitudinal Study of Adolescent Health, parental obesity was associated with children in school grades 7 through 12 being overweight or obese as a young adult (Crossman, Sullivan, & Benin, 2006). Dietary patterns, such as regular breakfast eating, that are established in childhood and adolescence continue into adulthood. Eating breakfast regularly has been shown to have multiple positive effects. However, breakfast is the most frequently skipped meal in young people. Parental breakfast eating and living in a two-parent family have been shown to be associated with adolescent breakfast consumption (Pearson, Biddle, & Gorely, 2009). Research has also shown that adolescents in nontraditional families (single parent, step-parent, no parent) are more likely to display unhealthy eating behaviors such as skipping breakfast and lunch, eating fewer vegetables, and eating more fast foods than adolescents in traditional (two-parent) households (Stewart & Menning, 2009). Nonresident father involvement increased healthy eating behaviors. Parents must be encouraged to be positive role models for their children for successful health-promoting dietary self-care behaviors.

Schools have traditionally concentrated on the role of peer pressure in the adoption of self-care behaviors, rather than focusing on health in the curriculum, beginning in the early school years. However, efforts have been expanded, based on research showing that targeted education can make a difference in adoption of healthy behaviors. Schools can reach most children and adolescents, have trained personnel who are interested in health promotion, have an organizational structure and facilities, and are capable of interacting with the community (Trost & Loprinzi, 2008). The results of three large school-based programs led the U.S. Task Force on Community Preventive Services to recommend implementing programs that increase the length of activity levels in school-based physical educational classes. The successful programs taught self-care skills for physical activity and included the family in the intervention.

Teacher-led and self-led programs to promote physical activity for bone health in teenage girls have been compared (Murphy, Dhuinn, Browne, & O'Rathaille, 2006). Although both types of programs resulted in improvements in physical activity, only the self-led groups sustained the exercise after the intervention. Self-care health promotion in schools can be effective to increase longer-term behavior change, although teacher-led programs can also be effective in changing behavior.

Children and adolescents should participate in more vigorous activities and reduce time in sedentary activities. For example, computer and television use time can be limited daily, and participation in community and family outdoor physical activities planned and fostered. At both the family and community levels, new physical activity programs must be developed and fostered that involve participation by peers as well as family members. In this group, walking instead of riding should be rewarded. The "Walking School Bus" mentioned in Chapter 8 is an example of promoting physical activity.

Adolescence is a critical period of physical, cognitive, emotional, and social development in a dynamic and uncertain period between childhood and adulthood. Developmentally, it is a time characterized by change and transitions. The primary biological transition is puberty. Cognitively, adolescents begin to think more abstractly. However, as children, they lack the ability to apply their cognitive skills to solving problems in stressful situations. The mismatch between biological and social maturity has implications for behavioral choices under stress, such as being pressured by peers to drink alcohol or experiment with illegal drugs. Socially, the family remains an important source of support. Parents can play a positive role in providing emotional support and encouragement and promoting healthy peer interactions, as peers also serve as important role models. The Strong African-American Families Program is an example of an intervention to deter negative adolescent behaviors (Brody, Kogan, Chen, & Murry, 2008). Children who received the intervention, which focused on positive parent–child relationships and communication along with consistent discipline, had fewer conduct problems and were less likely to begin drinking alcohol.

Adolescents are considered a high-risk group for engaging in risky and health-damaging behaviors, such as cigarette smoking, alcohol use, illicit drug use, early sexual activity, and physical aggression. Critical parental factors include communication, values, monitoring and control, and support. The social environment of adolescents has an important influence on development of health-damaging or health-promoting behaviors. Connectedness to family and school is protective against developing health-compromising behaviors (Carter, McGee, Taylor, & Williams, 2007). Students who reported high levels of family connectedness and school engagement reported fewer health risk behaviors. A school climate in which the adolescents were emotionally engaged and that students perceive as fair had a positive association with fewer negative behaviors. Connectedness to friends (peers) was associated with greater health compromising behaviors. Stronger connection in family and community contexts during adolescence predicts greater civic engagement as young adults, including a greater likelihood of voting, participation in community volunteer services, and involvement in social groups (Duke, Skay, Pettingell, & Borowsky, 2009). The importance of parental factors has resulted in the development of adolescent health-promotion programs with a parent component. Although these programs vary in the amount of parental involvement, results indicate that programs that strengthen parent–adolescent relationships result in self-care that promotes healthy adolescent behaviors.

Children and youth who have dropped out of school or are homeless need special attention in developing self-care behaviors for health promotion. Homeless youth do not benefit from family ties and depend on peers for support. Education sessions may have to take place in parks, food kitchens, or homeless shelters. Children of one-parent families as well as "latchkey youth" of two working parents may also require special attention. Special sensitivity to the lack of resources for daily living, lack of parental influence and supervision, and low levels of motivation because of life conditions is critical for promoting a healthy lifestyle.

The rapid developmental changes that occur for children and adolescents and the emerging behavioral patterns that will carry into adulthood make the preschool and school-age years a critical time to enhance skills for health-promoting behaviors. Many groups and persons influence the lifestyle behaviors of children and adolescents, including family members, peers, religious groups, popular entertainers, athletes, teachers, and other adults in their lives. Peer groups play a critical role in molding lifestyles for school-aged children, particularly adolescents. When peers reinforce the active health consumer role, peer pressure becomes a positive force. Parents serve as powerful role models of health and health-related behaviors. Approaches to enhance the health-promoting behaviors of children and adolescents should focus on both families and peer groups. This dual approach is critical, because values, attitudes, beliefs, and behaviors of both families and peers influence children's and adolescent's lifestyles.

Self-Care for Young and Middle-Aged Adults

Two contextual factors shape the health of young adults, aged 18–24 years: (1) a prolonged transition to adult roles and responsibilities and (2) the weakening of the family support safety net (Park, Mulye, Adams, Brindis, & Irwin, 2006). Young adults pursue multiple pathways, such as college, military service, employment, parenthood, and marriage. Each of these paths has its unique set of role expectations and potential barriers to health. Many health problems peak during this period, including homicide, motor vehicle injuries, substance abuse, and sexually transmitted infections. Almost all (98%) of first-year university students in law, teaching, and medicine reported from one to four risk behaviors related to diet, physical activity, alcohol consumption, and smoking (Keller, Maddock, Hannover, Thyrian, & Basler, 2008). Although there is diminishing parental involvement during the transition to adulthood, evidence describing the health status of this group indicates that parent, community, and institutional support is needed to address this period.

Young and middle-aged adulthood is the time in the life cycle when many persons are intensely involved in careers and child rearing. The momentum of everyday life and demands of dependent others may leave little time for focusing on health in the absence of an illness crisis. Strengthening support within the family for self-care is particularly important at this time. Adults must accept responsibility for modeling and teaching children competent self-care, increasing family self-care knowledge and skills, and learning how and when to access health care resources for the family. Adult learners bring many assets to self-care education, including life experiences, self-direction in learning, problem- or interest-centered (as opposed to subject-centered) learning needs, and interest in immediate rather than delayed application. Self-care education for adults consists of the following components (Whitehead & Russell, 2004):

1. Provide time to express feelings.
2. Express a supportive attitude.
3. Reinforce client self-esteem.
4. Provide access to health information.
5. Teach self-care skills that can be applied immediately.
6. Present alternative views on health issues.
7. Offer all views related to complementary self-care therapies.
8. Provide timely feedback and reinforcement.
9. Offer flexible learning pathways.

Adults who are aware of their own needs for self-care may be more effective in reducing the stress inherent in multiple societal roles, including family and work responsibilities. Systematically planning health promotion activities into daily routines at work or with family members can both enhance health in a busy lifestyle and model healthy lifestyles to family members. For example, physical activities can be planned prior to dinner rather than watching television. Or, if feasible, children can walk to school, rather than be driven. Adequate attention to self-care during the young and middle-aged years promotes optimal productivity and life satisfaction and lays the groundwork for a healthy and productive retirement and old age.

Activities of everyday life shape and influence the health of family members. Family practices either promote or hinder the development of good health habits and well-being in children. Life transitions (e.g., having children, beginning paid work) are associated with physical inactivity in women, as well as the social roles of women that carry expectations of caring for their families (Cockerman, Hinote, & Abbott, 2006). Nurses should accommodate the social context and implement interventions within the family that take into consideration family demands, employment status, educational levels, and available resources to promote self-care for healthy behaviors for parents and their children.

Self-Care for Older Adults

Older adults are the fastest growing population group in the United States. Research indicates that chronic health problems associated with old age can be prevented or postponed and controlled with health behaviors such as regular exercise and good nutrition (Schuit, 2006). Physically active older adults maintain health functioning longer than sedentary adults and report higher levels of subjective well-being (Garatachea et al., 2009). Exercise can enhance the self-esteem of older adults and in some cases decrease depression and anxiety. Sedentary activity, such as television viewing, can be replaced with physical activity. This approach is as useful as it has been in children and young adults. Psychological barriers such as loneliness and depression are common in the elderly. Health barriers may include limited mobility or vision and hearing difficulties. Regular participation in physical activity has the potential to reduce the burden of chronic diseases and disability and improve quality of life in this group.

Self-care for older adults focuses on maximizing independence, vigor, and life satisfaction. The ability for self-care is high for many older adults, and most function well. Personal autonomy, the ability to make self-directed choices, is important in older adults (Matsui & Capezuti, 2008). The older person is a partner in the self-care educational process, rather than a passive recipient. Nurses should provide information that promotes informed decision making and independence. Self-care education must also take into account the physical, sensory, mobility, sexual, and psychosocial changes that accompany aging as well as feelings of isolation, dissatisfaction, and helplessness. Personality and coping styles do not seem to change significantly with age. Thus, persons who develop positive coping skills early in life are able to meet social demands in later years, find meaning in life, and direct energy to appropriate self-care activities. Older individuals who have been characterized as information seekers have more effective health-promoting behaviors. Other patterns linked with health-promoting behaviors and well-being include positive perceptions of one's health and aging, education, social integration, involvement in groups and organizations, and contact with family members (Lyyra, Leskinen, Jylhä, & Heikkinen, 2009; Meléndez, Tomás, Oliver, & Navarro, 2009).

Retirement is a significant life event that presents a major challenge for the older population financially, socially, and emotionally. The challenges are likely to be magnified, as the length of time an individual will live following retirement continues to increase. Employment is a fundamental role central to an individual's identity, so retirees may feel they have lost an important role if it is not replaced with new activities (Pinquart & Schindler, 2007). The process begins in preretirement and continues into postretirement. Appropriate self-care in the form of anticipatory planning in the preretirement phase is associated with successful adaptation. Gioiella's (1983) self-care actions that facilitate healthy retirement are still timely:

1. Plan ahead to ensure adequate income.
2. Develop friends not associated with work.
3. Decrease time at work in the last years before retirement by taking longer vacations, working shorter days, or working part-time.
4. Develop routines, including adequate physical activity, to replace the structure of the workday.
5. Rely on other people and groups in addition to spouse to fill leisure time.

6. Develop leisure-time activities before retirement that are realistic in energy and monetary cost.
7. Anticipate that exhilaration will be followed by ambivalence before satisfaction with one's retirement lifestyle develops.
8. Assess living arrangements, and if relocation is necessary, expend time to develop new social networks.
9. Expect job role loss to have a short-term effect on self-esteem and one's marital relationship.

Retired adults often have more time available to pursue personal wellness than younger adults. They should be challenged to use the time productively and counseled about resources available within the community to facilitate healthy behaviors.

The fastest growing segment of the population in the United States is the group aged 85 and older. Less than one-fourth of persons in this age group live in nursing homes, so these individuals need safe, health-promoting communities as well as support services to assist them in continuing activities that focus on quality versus quantity of life. With adequate support from families, friends, and health professionals and access to resources, older adults are able to remain in their own home throughout their old age.

Older adults are at risk for consuming inadequate diets and decreasing functional capacity due to decreased mobility. Barriers to healthy diets and physical activity must be identified and addressed by health professionals as well as policy makers. Homebound community-dwelling elderly should be encouraged to go outdoors on a regular basis to maintain functional capacity (Shimada et al., 2009). Community-based interventions in senior centers are ideal places to promote physical activity and healthy eating behaviors. In an intervention based on the health belief model for older adults in senior centers in Georgia, chair exercises and promotion of walking improved physical function (Fitzpatrick et al., 2008). An intervention to increase fruit and vegetable intake in the Georgia senior centers also resulted in an increased consumption of fruits and vegetables and fewer perceived barriers (Hendrix et al., 2008).

Health and well-being in old age depends on freedom from disease, adequate functional status, and sufficient social and environmental supports. Promotion of self-care activities to maintain and improve functional status includes strategies for safe mobility and prevention of falls, and activities to promote social functioning and social integration. All evidence to date indicates that the elderly can become physically fit. However, it is much easier to remain physically active if self-care behavior is developed earlier in life.

Self-care for health promotion in older women needs attention because of different experiences of aging and old age in women. Women live longer than men and are more likely to live their later years alone with substantially lower incomes, more vulnerability to poverty, and more chronic health conditions than men in the same age group (U.S. Department of Health and Human Services, 2009). Women are also more likely to have no or inadequate insurance coverage, resulting in barriers to health care (Ogburn, Voss, & Espey, 2008). Institutional environments and living alone are negative influences on the performance of health behaviors. Many challenges and opportunities are presented for women as they age. Nurses and the health care system must respond to the issues that prevent elderly women from being able to participate in healthy behaviors, such as fear of leaving the security of their home, lack of transportation, and inadequate financial resources. Neighborhood deprivation, the socioeconomic conditions of the older person's residence, also effects the person's participation in leisure-time physical activity. Low cost interventions such as walking groups can be implemented in communities. Frameworks that take into account the social context in which women live their lives, as well as their perceptions of their health and well-being must be incorporated into all health promotion activities.

GOALS OF HEALTH EDUCATION FOR SELF-CARE

Education of the public for self-care has begun to be a viable and visible focus for federal health expenditures. Only a small percentage of the federal budget is actually spent on health-education activities. Within the federal government, the Office of Disease Prevention and Health Promotion, the Office on Smoking and Health, the Office of Women's Health, the Center for Minority Health, and the Centers for Disease Control and Prevention are examples of major agencies focused on meeting the health-education needs of the public. National goals for health education regarding self-care are not well articulated in a single document but exist in numerous documents that address various self-care issues, such as those related to cardiovascular health, mental health, child development, nutrition, and elimination of health disparities.

Health policy makers and health professionals must be sensitive to the extent to which problems of literacy and poverty present barriers to health education and self-care. Approaches to self-care education that use community workers and communication media (e.g., radio) are important in educating low-literacy populations about self-care needs and strategies. Competent self-care must also be economically plausible to individuals and families living in poverty. This requires coordination of public, private, and volunteer services to provide coherent self-care education and options to facilitate responsible yet low-cost health promotion programs and services, such as walking and jogging trails and peer support groups for adolescents and adults who are trying to change unhealthy behaviors.

THE PROCESS OF EMPOWERING FOR SELF-CARE

Personal empowerment is a strategic issue in health policy (Lemire, Sicotte, & Pare 2008). Empowerment is a process through which individuals gain mastery over their lives (Aujoulat, d'Hoore, & Deccache, 2007). The aim of empowerment is to enable clients to take proactive actions to promote the positive aspects of their lives. Health empowerment has an intrapersonal dimension, or self-reliance through individual choice, as well as an interpersonal dimension. The interpersonal dimension may incorporate professionals or the collective (community). In the nurse–client relationship, empowerment is a process of communication and education in which knowledge, values, and power are shared. In the intrapersonal dimension, empowerment is a process of personal transformation (Aujoulat et al., 2007). When individuals are empowered, they have the self-efficacy, knowledge, and competence to take proactive actions to reach their health promotion goals. Empowerment is a health-enhancing process, as it emphasizes rights and abilities rather than deficits and needs of individuals and communities. Characteristics of the empowering relationship include the following:

- Continuity
- Patient centered
- Relatedness
- Autonomy
- Shared decision making

In empowered relationships, health professionals are not in control; they are facilitators, as client choice, shared decision making, nonjudgmental responses, and experiential learning are part of empowerment-based interventions. Self-care results when clients determine their own goals and the strategies to reach these goals.

The process of empowering health education for self-care is multidimensional and complex. The client brings a unique personality and learning style, established social interaction patterns, numerous group affiliations, cultural norms and values, proximal and distal environmental influences, and a level of readiness to adopt self-care behaviors. The nurse also brings innate personality characteristics, values, attitudes, and social circumstances that affect the nature of the interaction. The self-care education process as a collaborative endeavor between client and nurse is depicted in Figure 11–1. The interaction for self-care education brings the professional expertise of nurses and other health care professionals together with the knowledge and goals of the client. Mutual assessment of health care competencies, strengths, and needs by the client and nurse will enable the client to prioritize the learning activities, set the pace of learning, establish long- and short-term goals, and identify any interpersonal and environmental support needed for learning. Barriers to learning and implementing self-care behaviors are identified and directly addressed with clients. Failure to identify and decrease barriers can result in frustration and a lack of progress toward the self-care goals. For example, barriers to obesity management

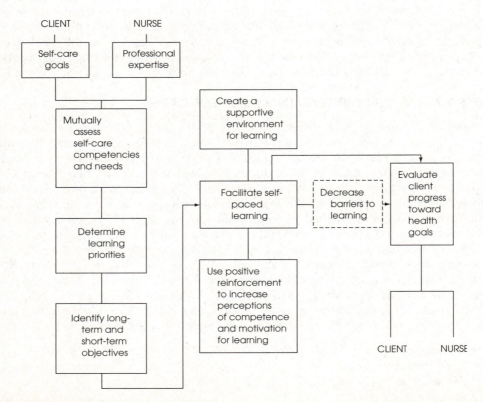

FIGURE 11–1 The Self-Care Education Process

that have been identified include low socioeconomic status, time constraints, intimate saboteurs, and attitudes and beliefs (Mauro, Taylor, Wharton, & Sharma, 2008). Lack of attention to these barriers results in a sense of failure, low self-efficacy, and low self-esteem.

Mutually Assess Self-Care Competencies and Needs

The client often comes to the encounter with certain self-care goals in mind. Competencies related to these goals can be assessed through informal discussion, health-knowledge checklists (Figure 11–2), or structured tests of knowledge in specific content areas. Informal discussions are recommended for low-literacy clients or individuals who are uncomfortable with paper-and-pencil tasks. Observation of actual behavior can also provide useful insights, if this is possible.

The activated client is motivated to seek health information that will assist in self-care. Apathy, lack of interest, and inattention should alert the nurse to a lack of motivation. Reasons for lack of interest should be explored so that interventions can be designed to increase motivation.

In the list below, please check those behaviors that you are comfortable in performing for yourself without assistance from others.

_____ Counting my pulse at the wrist for 1 minute

_____ Counting my pulse at the neck for 1 minute

_____ Selecting comfortable and appropriate shoes for brisk walking or jogging

_____ Selecting appropriate clothing for walking or jogging activities

_____ Planning a progressive schedule of exercise to meet my personal needs

_____ Indicating the ideal weight range for my height

_____ Calculating my maximal heart rate during exercise

_____ Planning time for exercise that is convenient and possible

_____ Selecting warm-up exercises that I could do before brisk walking or running

_____ Selecting procedures for cooling down after vigorous exercise

_____ Exercising at least five times a week for 30 minutes

_____ Integrating physical-fitness activities with my recreational interests

_____ Maintaining a record of my progress in physical activity over a period of several months

_____ Eating appropriately before or after vigorous exercise

_____ Avoiding injuries during exercise

FIGURE 11–2   Health-Knowledge Checklist for Exercise and Physical Fitness

Determine Learning Priorities

Deciding where to begin is often a dilemma when the client needs information about many health topics and behaviors. The empowerment process enables the client to make decisions about what they wish to know and what is important to them. Sometimes their priority may not be the area of greatest threat to personal health. As an example, a client may smoke but be more interested in starting to exercise than in quitting smoking. Although the nurse may believe that smoking constitutes a more serious threat to the health of the client than a sedentary lifestyle, it is important that client choice be honored. If an exercise program is implemented, the client may develop a heightened awareness of the negative impact of smoking on lung capacity and physical endurance. At a later point, the client may exhibit readiness to discuss approaches to smoking cessation based on concrete experiences with the health- and activity-compromising effects of smoking.

Identify Short- and Long-Term Objectives

Mutual identification of both short- and long-term objectives is important in self-care education. Long-term objectives guide large segments of learning. Short-term objectives identify the specific content or activities that must be progressively mastered to meet long-term objectives. The objectives should be realistic, not too easy to result in boredom, and not too difficult to cause discouragement. An example of a Goal and Objectives Identification Form is presented in Figure 11–3. The form enables the client to check each objective as it is attained and maintain awareness of the desired behavioral and health outcomes. Both the nurse and the client should retain a copy for continuing reference and update.

Facilitate Self-Paced Learning

The pace at which clients learn depends on personal motivation, assertiveness, perseverance, skills, and learning styles. The pace of learning may also vary with age, health status, and educational level. Self-pacing is important to enable the client to be self-directed and maintain control over the learning process. The pace at which the client meets each short-term objective will vary, and expectations of both the client and the health professional should be adjusted accordingly. The important factor is not how rapidly knowledge or skill is attained but the extent of mastery.

Health Goal: Increased Physical Fitness	
Long-Term Objective: To take a brisk walk for 30 minutes five times a week	
Related Short-Term Learning Objectives	**Objectives Attained**
1. Demonstrate how to check my pulse at the neck by counting beats for 10 seconds and multiplying by six. 2. State heart rate that I should achieve during exercise. 3. Demonstrate two warm-up exercises to use before walking. 4. Demonstrate two cool-down exercises to use after brisk walking. 5. Construct a weekly schedule for brisk walking. 6. Map out three different and interesting routes to take when walking.	

FIGURE 11–3   Goal and Objectives Identification Form

The nurse must be realistic about teaching and learning and accept both good and bad days in clients of all ages. Sometimes the nurse and client will be elated with the results, sometimes discouraged. When efforts are less rewarding than anticipated, the pace of learning should be reviewed carefully and renegotiated. Focusing on resources of the client, rather than deficits, is also important to maintain motivation. It is possible that expanding the time frame for learning will facilitate success. This is especially true for young children and adolescents, who have less experience in the learning process than adults.

Use Positive Reinforcement to Increase Perceptions of Competence and Motivation for Learning

In education for self-care, the client, nurse, and family play important roles in reinforcement. The nurse should be attuned to small steps in client progress and use positive reinforcement such as praise and compliments frequently to enhance the client's feelings of success in developing competence in self-care. Immediate feedback needs to be provided to correct errors in performance. When error feedback is intermingled with positive reinforcement, it is helpful and nonthreatening, and enhances intrinsic motivation. Immediate and consistent reinforcement facilitates rapid learning and results in client satisfaction from learning. After learning has occurred, intermittent reinforcement of the desired response strengthens the behavior, making it more resistant to extinction.

Family support is critical to successful behavior change. Family members must learn to serve as sources of support for one another in developing health behaviors. For example, achievement of a specific goal may be rewarded by a family outing or the family spending time at home together in a favorite activity. It is important for the family to maintain a balance between support and pressure, which will be negatively perceived. By providing mutual support, a sense of healthy interdependence rather than crippling dependence is created within the family.

Actual performance of new behaviors that lead to success is a powerful strategy to strengthen self-efficacy (perceived confidence) (de Bourdeaudhuij & Sallis, 2002). Other sources of self-efficacy (e.g., modeling, observational learning, verbal persuasion) can be learned from the nurse during the educational sessions.

Clients should learn to practice self-reward or self-reinforcement in the health education process. Self-reward of one's own efforts and achievements is important, because much of the time reinforcement for self-care cannot be given by others. Rewards can be tailored to personal preferences. Use of foods or negative behaviors for reinforcement should be discouraged. Client should also learn to use internal self-reinforcement such as self-praise and self-compliment. Learning to use internal self-reward in an appropriate manner permits the client to be less dependent on the availability of tangible objects to facilitate the learning process.

Create a Supportive Environment for Learning

The health-education environment for self-care is vitally important to the success of educational efforts (Hubley, 2006). If a clinic is used for health education, the classrooms should be warm, comfortable, and informal. Tables, chairs, and sofas should be placed in a conversational setting. Pictures and textured materials should be used to create a supportive and nonthreatening climate. Visual aids such as flip charts or bulletin boards should be at a comfortable height to use while seated in a chair. If very young children are present during the sessions, an area with toys and books may need to be provided for their use. This will minimize distraction of the parents. If children are old enough to be included in the sessions, they should be actively involved. Often, use of bright colors and interesting figures or designs on flip charts will amuse children and maintain their interest. Children can play an important role in reinforcing learning or in reminding parents and other family members to engage in the recommended behaviors.

To the extent possible, materials available in the home should be used in teaching. If a client is expected to use a booklet on low-cholesterol foods to prepare meals at home, the booklet to be used should be the basis for instruction. If the client is learning relaxation techniques, audiotapes and videos for practice must be usable in the client's home. They should be demonstrated in the classroom or clinic and questions answered regarding their use. Well-illustrated materials should be supplied liberally to the client to take home to provide reinforcement of knowledge and skills gained during health-education sessions. Pictures are especially important for clients with low health literacy.

The minimum time span needed for most health instruction is 15 to 30 minutes, and either individual or small-group teaching methods may to be used. Groups should be kept small (four to six individuals) to facilitate interaction and attention to the specific needs of group members. A combination of group and individual instruction is often helpful. A combined approach allows for efficient use of professional time yet meets the unique educative-developmental needs of clients.

Decrease Barriers to Learning

Barriers to learning can result from various sources: personal values, beliefs, and attitudes; lack of motivation; poor self-concept; and inadequate cognitive or psychomotor skills, to name a few. If the client is not making progress, the environment should be explored for barriers. In addition, individual and family barriers should be assessed and reduced or eliminated.

Strategies to manage obstacles to healthy behavior should be an integral part of the health-education plan. In this way, problems are addressed systematically, and progress in decreasing barriers can be periodically assessed. The client may be unaware of what is inhibiting progress or reluctant to share information with the nurse. A climate of trust facilitates effective communication and enables the client to discuss perceived and real obstacles to learning and performance.

Evaluate Client Progress Toward Health Goals

Evaluation is a collaborative process by which the nurse and client judge the extent to which short- and long-term objectives and goals have been attained. Evaluation involves direct or indirect assessment of behavior change. When the target behaviors are observed during limited clinic or home visits, it must be kept in mind that this may not reflect actual behaviors. Self-report behavior change is also limited, as clients may not be completely honest, or they may ascribe a "halo effect" to themselves, seeing their performance as more frequent or more intensive than it actually is.

A combination of methods should be used to evaluate progress. These may include: checklists of objectives (see Figure 11–3), client daily records, laboratory measurements, paper-and-pencil tests, verbal questioning, and direct observation. The primary purpose of evaluation is to provide an accurate picture of the progress that clients have made in attaining their health goals. The desired outcome from self-care education is knowledge and skills to enhance self-care behaviors and promote a healthy lifestyle.

Other Considerations in Self-Care Empowerment

Each client's desire for change must be assessed. Some individuals do not want to be responsible for their own self-care but instead wish to function in a highly dependent role. Their desire for self-care competence may have been frustrated by their experiences in the health care system, which may have made them feel dependent and helpless. Before initiating a health education program, it is critical to assess the extent to which clients desire to assume responsibility for their own health when they are given the opportunity to gain the knowledge and skills to do so.

Clients' conceptualization of health will also decide the content to share in self-care health promotion education. When health is defined as maintaining stability or avoiding overt illness, prevention behaviors such as immunization, self-examination for signs of cancer, and periodic multiphasic screening may be most important. When health is defined as self-actualization or well-being, emphasis may be placed on physical activity, relaxation techniques, enhancing self-awareness, or developing aspects of self that represent untapped potential.

THE ROLE OF THE INTERNET IN SELF-CARE EDUCATION

The growth and improvement in Internet technology has made it an essential part of everyday life. Millions of people are now seeking health information and finding self-help groups of people who want to learn from each other (King & Moreggi, 2007). Internet virtual communities fulfill the need for affiliation, information, and support. The potential of the Internet as a platform for self-empowerment through development of feelings of competence and control is beginning to be realized (Lemire et al., 2008). Extensive information is accessible on almost any topic that was not traditionally available. The information can be accessed at any time in almost any geographic location. This has important implications for persons living in rural or inaccessible areas, who are homebound, and who work. The quality of health information available is highly variable, indicating that clients need to learn to evaluate the information.

The Internet is still inaccessible to many who do not have adequate financial resources or lack computer or health literacy skills. The "digital divide" refers to the gap in computer and Internet access between groups based on income, age, and education (Demiris, 2006). Emerging issues that will have to be addressed by this technology include the possibility of diminished involvement in face-to-face interactions with family members and friends as well as weakening attachments to one's local environment with greater access to remote people and places. Privacy and confidentiality of information remains a major challenge that has not been solved.

A layperson usually leads self-help groups that meet online. These virtual electronic networks enable persons with similar health interests to converse and pose questions, provide mutual information and support, and minimize feelings of isolation (King & Moreggi, 2007). Nurses should share knowledge of effective programs and Internet sites that will strengthen their clients' role in their self-care.

Advantages of online self-help groups have been identified (King & Moreggi, 2007). These groups are convenient to access, and there is increased access of diverse members, including people in rural or remote areas. They provide access to peers with similar interests and issues, and the embarrassment of public speaking is removed. In addition, lasting relationships may be formed. Disadvantages include misunderstanding that may result from text-based relationships; few controls to prevent erroneous information; absence of rules and guidelines; and ethical issues related to identity, deception, privacy, and confidentiality.

Mass education available through advanced technology is changing the way the public obtains health information and relates to health professionals. Young persons perceive the Internet as a primary source of information, not an adjunct to traditional informational modes. Nurses should work to ensure that the information revolution is used to empower individuals and communities and is accessible to those who do not currently benefit because of poverty or other social, environmental, and cultural conditions. In addition, health care professionals must monitor the content and quality of the sites they recommend. Last, formal evaluation of participant's health outcomes and satisfaction with information must be conducted. Formal evaluations will provide evidence of the effectiveness of this application to health promotion. Virtual communities may empower clients; however, the evidence is not yet sufficient.

OPPORTUNITIES FOR RESEARCH IN SELF-CARE

Although self-care has been practiced for centuries, it did not become the focus of research for health professionals until the 1980s. The theoretical work by Orem (2001) has been the primary driving force in nursing for empirical work on the various dimensions of self-care and related nursing care systems. Opportunities for research in self-care include the following:

1. Develop and test new models of self-care that account for sociocultural and environmental antecedents across the life span.
2. Develop interventions to test the effects of self-care practices for preschool children.
3. Conduct longitudinal studies to describe the long-term health care outcomes of self-care behaviors in preschool children, adolescents, and young adults.
4. Develop and test health literacy intervention to increase self-care behaviors in low-income groups.
5. Test culturally appropriate interventions to enhance self-care among diverse individuals and families.
6. Conduct intervention studies to increase self-care health behaviors in community-dwelling older persons.

CONSIDERATIONS FOR PRACTICE IN SELF-CARE

The nurse's role as facilitator, resource, and teacher has become more important than ever, as clients are asked to assume more responsibility for their health. Development of health-promoting behaviors at a young age and maintenance of these behaviors throughout the life span is critical. A multidisciplinary team approach is needed to implement health promotion programs in schools, at work sites, and in community locations that are easily accessible. These programs should target the individual, the family, and social and environmental factors in the community that facilitate or inhibit adoption of self-care behaviors. Strategies that strengthen family communication and support should be implemented to promote adoption of healthy behaviors in children and adolescents. The nurse should encourage school systems to include instruction for healthy nutrition and regular physical education. Opportunities should be created for after-school sports and other activities. Partnerships with community organizations are needed for children and adolescents as well as the elderly. Self-care education is complex. However, use of new technologies, such as the Internet, and active involvement of individuals and their family members in the educational process can help ensure the adoption of healthy behaviors.

Summary

Empowerment for self-care emphasizes the competencies of clients for self-direction and self-responsibility in planning and managing self-care activities. Environmental constraints that impair self-care must be addressed and resolved to optimize client success. Educative-supportive care will enable clients to achieve their health goals. The nurse, a resource person, can enhance the client's success in acquiring knowledge and skills in self-care. Further research on self-care within the context of health promotion will provide important information for facilitating optimum self-care across the age continuum.

Learning Activities

1. Plan a preschool-based intervention with parent involvement to promote a decrease in television viewing by children.
2. Develop an intervention to increase physical activity in community-dwelling older persons.
3. Describe how you would evaluate the effectiveness of the older person physical activity program with short- and long-term goals.

Selected Web Sites

Children and Adolescents
Bright Futures
http://www.brightfuturesd.org

Center for Disease Control Adolescent and School Health
http://cdc.gov/nccdphp/dash/

National Institute of Child Health and Human Development
http://nih.gov/nichd

Young and Older Adults
Health and Age
http://healthandage.com

Healthfinder
http://healthfinder.gov

HealthWeb
http://healthweb.org

MEDLINE plus
http://medlineplus.gov

National Institute on Aging
http://www.nih.gov/nia

National Women's Health Education Center
http://4women.gov

Senior Net
http://seniornet.org

References

Aujoulat, I., d'Hoore, W., & Deccache, A. (2007, April). Patient empowerment in theory and practice: Polysemy or cacophony? *Patient Education and Counseling, 66*(1), 13–20.

Barlow, J., Wright, C., Sheasby, J., Turner, A., & Hainsworth, J. (2002). Self-management approaches for people with chronic conditions: A review. *Patient Education & Counseling, 48*, 177–187.

Boote, J., Telford, R., & Cooper, C. (2002). Consumer involvement in health research: A review and research agenda. *Health Policy, 61*, 213–236.

Brody, G. H., Kogan, S. M., Chen, Y., & Murry, V. M. (2008). Long-term effects of the Strong African American Families Program on youths' conduct problems. *Journal of Adolescent Health, 43*, 474–481.

Carter, M., McGee, R., Taylor, B., & Williams, S. (2007). Health outcomes in adolescents: Associations with family, friends, and school engagement. *Journal of Adolescent Health, 30*, 51–62.

Chambers, R. (2006). The role of the health professional in supporting self care. *Quality in Primary Care, 14*, 129–131.

Cockerman, W. C., Hinote, B. P., & Abbott, P. (2006). Psychological distress, gender, and health lifestyles in Belarus, Kazakhstan, Russia, and Ukraine. *Social Science & Medicine, 63*, 2381–2394.

Crossman, A., Sullivan, D. A., & Benin, M. (2006). The family environment and American adolescents' risk of obesity as young adults. *Social Science & Medicine, 63*, 2255–2267.

de Bourdeaudhuij, I., & Sallis, J. (2002). Relative contribution of psychosocial variables to the explanation of physical activity in three population-based adult samples. *Preventive Medicine, 34*, 279–288.

Demiris, G. (2006). The diffusion of virtual communities in health care: Concepts and challenges. *Patient Education and Counseling, 62*, 178–188.

Duke, N. N., Skay, C. L., Pettingell, S. L., & Borowsky, I. W. (2009). From adolescent connections to social capital: Predictors of civic engagement in young adulthood. *Journal of Adolescent Health, 44*, 161–168.

Fitzpatrick, S. F., Reddy, S., Lommel, T. S., Fischer, J. G., Speer, E. M., Stephens, H., et al. (2008). Physical activity and physical function improved following a community-based intervention in older adults in Georgia senior centers. *Journal of Nutrition Education, 27*, 135–154.

Ganz, S. B. (1990). Self-care: Perspectives from six disciplines. *Holistic Nursing Practice, 4*, 1–12.

Garatachea, N. M., Molinero, O., Martínez-García, R., Jiménez-Jiménez, R., González-Gallego, & Márquez, S. (2009). Feelings of well being in elderly people: Relationship to physical activity and physical function. *Archives of Gerontology and Geriatrics, 48*(3), 306–312.

Gioiella, E. C. (1983). Healthy aging through knowledge and self care. *Aging Previews, 3*(1), 39–51.

Hendrix, S. J., Fischer, J. G., Reddy, R. D., Lommel, T. S., Speer, E. M., Stephens, H., et al. (2008). Fruit and vegetable intake and knowledge increased following a community-based intervention in older adults in Georgia senior centers. *Journal of Nutrition Education, 27*, 155–178.

Hibbard, J. H., Greene, J., Becker, E. R., Roblin, D., Painter, M. W., Perez, D. J., et al. (2008). Racial/ethnic disparities and consumer activation in health. *Health Affairs, 27*, 1442–1453.

Hibbard, J. H., Mahoney, E. R., Stock, R., & Tusler, M. (2007, August). Do increases in patient activation result in improved self-management behaviors? *Health Services Research, 42*(4), 1443–1463.

Hibbard, J. H., Mahoney, E. R., Stockard, J., & Tusler, M. (2005, December). Development and testing of a short form of the patient activation measure. *Health Services Research, 40*(6), 1918–1930.

Hubley, J. (2006). Patient education in the developing world: A discipline comes of age. *Patient Education and Counseling, 61*, 161–164.

Keller, S., Maddock, J. E., Hannover, W., Thyrian, J. R., & Basler, H. (2008). Multiple health risk behaviors in German first year university students. *Preventive Medicine, 46*, 180–195.

King, S. A., & Moreggi, D. (2007). Internet self-help and support groups: The pros and cons of text-based mutual aid. In J. Gackenbach (Ed.) *Psychology and the Internet: Intrapersonal and Transpersonal Implications*, 2nd ed., pp. 221–244. Boston: Academic Press.

Lemire, M., Sicotte, C., & Pare, G. (2008). Internet use and the logics of personal empowerment in health. *Health Policy, 88*, 130–140.

Lyyra, T-M., Leskinen, E., Jylhä, M., & Heikkinen, E. (2009, January–February). Self-rated health and mortality in older men and women: A time-dependent covariate analysis. *Archives of Gerontology and Geriatrics, 48*(1), 14–18.

Matsui, M., & Capezuti, E. (2008). Perceived autonomy and self-care resources among senior center users. *Geriatric Nursing, 29*, 141–147.

Mauro, M., Taylor, V., Wharton, S., & Sharma, A. M. (2008). Barriers to obesity treatment. *European Journal of Internal Medicine, 19*, 173–180.

Meléndez, J. C., Tomás, J. M., Oliver, A., & Navarro, E. (2009, May–June). Psychological and physical dimensions explaining life satisfaction among the elderly: A structural model examination. *Archives of Gerontology and Geriatrics, 48*(3), 291–295.

Murphy, P. A., Dhuinn, M. N., Browne, P. A., & O'Rathaille, M. M. (2006). Physical activity for bone health in inactive teenage girls: Is a supervised teacher-led program or self-led program best? *Journal of Adolescent Health, 39*, 508–514.

Nutbeam, D. (2000). Health literacy as a public health goal: A challenge for contemporary health education and communication strategies into the 21st century. *Health Promotion International, 15*, 259–267.

——— (2008). The evolving concept of health literacy. *Social Science & Medicine, 67*, 2072–2078.

Ogburn, T., Voss, C., & Espey, E. (2008). Barriers to women's health: Why is it so hard for women to stay healthy? *Medical Clinics of North America, 92*, 993–1009.

Orem, D. E. (1995). *Nursing: Concepts of practice* (5th ed.). St Louis: Mosby.

——— (2001). *Nursing: Concepts of practice* (6th ed.). New York: Mosby.

Park, M. J., Mulye, T. P., Adams, S. H., Brindis, C. D., & Irwin, C. E. (2006). The health status of young adults in the United States. *Journal of Adolescent Health, 39*, 305–317.

Pearson, N., Biddle, S. J. H., & Gorely, T. (2009, February). Family correlates of breakfast consumption among children and adolescents: A systematic review. *Appetite, 52*(1), 1–7.

Peterson, A. V., Leroux, B. G., Bricker, J., Kealey, K. A., Marek, P. M., Sarason, I. G., et al. (2006, May). Nine-year prediction of adolescent smoking by number of smoking parents. *Addictive Behaviors, 31*(5), 788–801.

Pinquart, M., & Schindler, I. (2007). Changes in life satisfaction in the transition to retirement: A latent-class approach. *Psychology and Aging, 22*, 442–455.

Redman, B. K. (2007). Responsibility for control: Ethics of patient preparation for self-management of chronic disease. *Bioethics, 21*, 243–250.

Schuit, A. J. (2006). Physical activity, body composition and healthy aging. *Science & Sports, 21*, 209–213.

Shimada, H., Ishizaki, T., Kato, M., Morimoto, A., Tamate, A., Uchiyama, Y., et al. (2009, April 9). How often and how far do frail elderly people need to go outdoors to maintain functional capacity? *Archives of Gerontology and Geriatrics,* doi.10.1016/j.archger.2009.02.015.

Stewart, S. D., & Menning, C. L. (2009). Family structure, father involvement, and adolescent eating patterns. *Journal of Adolescent Health, 45*(2), 193–201.

Trost, S. G., & Loprinzi, P. D. (2008). Exercise: Promoting health lifestyles in children and adolescents. *Journal of Clinical Lipidology, 2*, 162–168.

U.S. Department of Health and Human Services. (2009). *Women's Health and Mortality Chartbook: 2009 Edition.* Washington, D.C.: DHHS Office on Women's Health.

Whitehead, D., & Russell, G. (2004). How effective are health education programs? Resistance, reactance, rationality and risks: Recommendations for effective practice. *Internal Journal of Nursing Studies, 41*, 163–172.

Wilkinson, A., & Whitehead, L. (2009). Evolution of the concept of self-care and implications for nurses: A literature review. *International Journal of Nursing Studies 46*(8), 1143–1147.

Williamson, D. A., Champagne, C. M., Harsha, D., Han, H., Martin, C. K., Newton, R., et al. (2008, September). Louisiana (LA) Health: Design and methods for a childhood obesity prevention program in rural schools. *Contemporary Clinical Trials, 29*(5), 783–895.

Yin, H. S., Forbis, S. G., & Dreyer, B. P. (2007). Health literacy and pediatric health. *Current Problems in Pediatric Adolescent Health Care, 37*, 258–286.

CHAPTER 12

Health Promotion in Vulnerable Populations

OBJECTIVES

1. Discuss the major factors that play a role in health disparities.
2. Describe the concept of equity in health to eliminate health disparities.
3. Discuss the social determinants of both individual and population health that are relevant to health equity.
4. Describe the continuum of interpersonal skills necessary for cultural competence.
5. Discuss the factors to consider in designing health promotion programs for vulnerable populations.
6. Describe strategies to ensure culturally competent programs.

Outline

- Health Disparities in Vulnerable Populations
- Promoting Health Equity
- Health Care Professionals and Cultural Competence
- Designing Culturally Competent Health Promotion Programs
- Strategies for Culturally Appropriate Interventions
- Opportunities for Research with Vulnerable Populations
- Considerations for Practice with Vulnerable Populations
- Summary
- Learning Activities
- Selected Web Sites
- References

The values, attitudes, culture, and life circumstances of individuals who are poor, socially marginal, or culturally different from the traditional mainstream of society, and the communities in which they reside, must be recognized when planning health promotion and prevention activities. Taking into account the factors that reflect the diversity of these populations is key to promoting successful behavior change.

In spite of the improvements in health in the United States in recent years, disparities in health between the majority (white) population and minority populations persist. Health disparities are the differences in the incidence, prevalence, mortality, and burden of diseases and other adverse health conditions that exist among certain groups of populations in the United States. Health disparities are the diseases, disorders, and conditions that disproportionately afflict individuals who are members of racial, ethnic minority, underserved, and other vulnerable groups, such as those in geographic (rural) areas who are socially and physically isolated by the low-density dispersed population and limited community resources and services. A report by the National Center for Health Statistics continues to document these disparities for certain racial and ethnic groups in its annual report on the health status of the nation (National Center for Health Statistics, 2009). Disparities in health are believed to be the result of complex interactions among genetic variations, environmental factors, and personal health behaviors (Centers for Disease Control, Office of Minority Health & Health Disparities [CDC, OMHD], 2008; Giger et al., 2007). Major reasons for the disparities include socioeconomic factors, language, discrimination, access to care, environmental hazards, and cultural barriers. Achievement of health equity and elimination of disparities to improve the health of all groups is an overarching goal of Healthy People 2020 (see http://www .healthypeople.gov/hp2020/advisory/phaseI/summary/htm). Although many of the major causes of health disparities need the input of society and government, development of health promotion programs tailored for diverse individuals and communities is a realistic goal for nursing.

HEALTH DISPARITIES IN VULNERABLE POPULATIONS

Vulnerable populations are diverse groups of individuals who are at greatest risk of poor physical, psychological, and/or social health outcomes. Vulnerable populations are more likely to develop health problems, usually experience worse health outcomes, and have fewer resources to improve their conditions. Various terms have been used to describe vulnerable populations, including underserved populations, special populations, medically disadvantaged, poverty-stricken populations, and American underclasses (Aday, 1999). Vulnerable groups include persons who experience discrimination, stigma, intolerance, and subordination and those who are politically marginalized, disenfranchised, and often denied their human rights. Vulnerable populations may include people of color, the poor, non-English-speaking persons, recent immigrants and refugees, homeless persons, mentally ill and disabled persons, gay men and lesbians, and substance abusers.

Societal and environmental factors play major roles in characterizing vulnerable populations. Specifically, low socioeconomic status has been documented to be the most consistent predictor of disease and premature deaths. Class-related inequities in mortality rates for three-fourths of all deaths are observed across the life span in almost every country in the world (Marmot, Friel, Bell, Houweling, & Taylor, 2008). Those at greatest risks for increased morbidity and mortality are ethnic and racial minorities, two highly vulnerable groups (CDC, OMHD, 2008). Although there is great diversity among minority populations, overall, minorities have substantially lower incomes than whites. Income is a powerful variable that explains health status. Higher incomes facilitate access to care, better housing in safer neighborhoods, and increased opportunities for healthy food purchases as well as health-promotion programs. In addition, low-status occupations expose individuals to physical health hazards. The poverty rate continues to be almost three times greater for blacks (24.5%) and Hispanics (21.5%) than for whites (8.2%) (DeNavas-Walt, Procter, & Smith 2008). Educational attainment is also lower in minority groups. High-risk behaviors have been inversely correlated with lower educational levels. Higher education levels also enable persons to obtain health-related information at understandable levels.

Socioeconomic status (SES) accounts for much of the observed disparities in health, as a socioeconomic gradient exists for almost every health indicator for every racial and ethnic group (Hesdorffer & Lee, 2009; Marmot, 2007; National Center for Health Statistics, 2009). The effects of low socioeconomic status are long lasting. Low socioeconomic status in childhood has been associated with poorer health in adulthood (Hersdorffer & Lee, 2009). The effects are apparent in risk factors in adults, such as smoking, obesity, elevated blood pressure, and sedentary lifestyle. The cumulative wear and tear of the adverse experiences of living in poverty, with its multiple challenges, results in allostatic load and chronic illnesses. Allostatic load and the theory of allostasis have been used to document the lifetime stress on the body, which eventually results in disease and poor health (see Chapter 8). Individuals who are part of a group that has been poor over several generations and suffer ongoing discrimination and frustration without substantial upward movement, may feel powerless and perceive their conditions differently from recently arrived immigrants who are poor but hopeful about their future. Black–white differences in infant low birth weight and infant mortality have existed for decades; and in blacks, it is twice that of whites (CDC, 2008). Differences persist even when the effects of social class, prenatal care, and living conditions are controlled, or when only middle-class populations with access to care are studied. These findings may be explained by allostatic load.

The health status of Hispanics has declined among immigrants as their stay in the United States increases and with succeeding generations. Rates of infant mortality, adolescent pregnancy, and cigarette, alcohol, and illicit drug use have all increased with acculturation. Hispanics are almost twice as likely to die from diabetes than non-Hispanic whites and have higher rates of high blood pressure and obesity than non-Hispanic whites (CDC, 2008). Acculturation may increase risk factors, as cultural beliefs and lifestyles are abandoned to assimilate the values and practices of the dominant society.

Access to care can be measured by the proportion of a population that has health insurance. Racial and ethnic minorities are much more likely to be underinsured or lack health insurance (DeNavas-Walt et al., 2008). When they do have insurance, it is likely to be public insurance, primarily Medicaid. Health insurance contributes to the amount and type of health services obtained. Lack of health insurance has important implications for health promotion and prevention efforts, such as screening and access to wellness programs. Insurance status has been correlated with reported health status. Those who rated their health as fair or poor were more likely to be uninsured than those who rated their health as good or excellent. Racial and ethnic minorities also experience greater barriers in accessing care, have more difficulty getting an appointment, and wait longer during appointments. These factors are compounded by the fact that many minority communities mistrust the government and government-controlled programs.

Thus, financial and nonfinancial barriers to access care exist for vulnerable populations. These barriers must be eliminated to improve and promote healthy lifestyles and access to quality health care.

PROMOTING HEALTH EQUITY

Achieving health equity means that everyone has the opportunity to attain their full health potential and no one is disadvantaged from achieving their potential because of social, demographic, or geographic differences (International Society for Equity in Health, 2000). Health disparities can be eliminated through the promotion of health equity, which minimizes avoidable disparities between groups of people who have different levels of underlying social advantage (Braveman, 2006; Marmot, 2007). Most of the literature on health disparities in this country focuses on racial/ethnic differences in health and "closing the gap;" less use of the phrase "achieving health equity." However, equity in health places emphasis on multiple influences on individual and population health and draws attention to the multilevel challenges that need to be addressed (Marmot et al., 2008).

Health is a product of multiple factors superimposed on genetic predisposition, so achieving equity in health is a complex process, encompassing social and physical environmental changes, policy, and education (Starfield, 2006). Influences on individual health that should be addressed are shown in the model in Figure 12–1.

Concepts in the model amenable to health care provider interventions include the community context, behaviors, chronic stress, and health services received. In addition, societal influences on population health also must be addressed. These factors, which

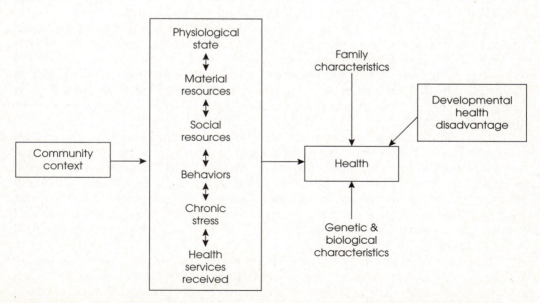

FIGURE 12–1   Social Influences on Individual Health   *Source*: "State of the Art in Research on Equity in Health," in *Journal of Health Politics, Policy and Law,* Volume 31, no. 1, p. 15. Copyright, 2006, Duke University Press. All rights reserved. Used by permission of the publisher.

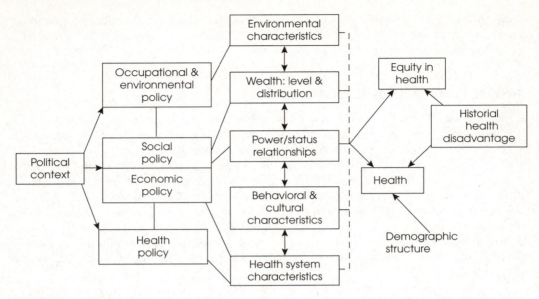

FIGURE 12–2   Societal Influences on Population Health   *Source*: "State of the Art in Research on Equity in Health," in *Journal of Health Politics, Policy and Law*, Volume 31, no. 1, p. 15. Copyright, 2006, Duke University Press. All rights reserved. Used by permission of the publisher.

are illustrated in the model in Figure 12–2, stress the role of the political context for policy changes to promote health equity. At the population level, health care professions should be actively involved in promoting policy changes locally as well as nationally. Health education plays an important role in changing behaviors at all levels.

All stakeholders must be included in the pursuit of health equity, including individuals, families, communities, health professionals, and policy policy-makers. Short- and long-term goals must be established, and process targets are necessary to monitor progress. Continuing professional education is needed to create new health knowledge and apply research findings through partnerships with community organizations, policy makers, and different levels of government (Johnson et al., 2008).

Primary care offers an avenue for achieving health equity, as interventions are directed at individuals versus diseases (Starfield, 2007). Primary care was established as a framework for health in the 1960s with the World Health Organization Declaration of Alma Alta. Primary care involves first contact, continuous, coordinated, decentralized care to address health promotion and disease prevention (Solheim, McElmurry, & Kim, 2007). Primary care is complex and requires community engagement and respect for individual and family viewpoints. It is an efficient, rational way to provide essential care to all people.

Investments in a primary care infrastructure have been shown to produce health equity at a lower cost. Primary care services in community health centers can reach socially disadvantaged, racial/ethnic minorities and isolated groups. Nurses have been pioneers in leading primary health care interdisciplinary teams and conducting community-based initiatives to promote community participation in health, provide health care and education, and advocate for communities. Primary care will continue to increase in value, and nurses will play a major role in promoting behavior change as primary care providers.

Nurses can implement multiple psychosocial, environmental, and community-level interventions (Cox, 2009). Traditional educational programs to teach health promoting behaviors, social support groups, and stress reduction strategies are all individual- and family-level practice interventions. Attention to the client's working conditions, household and neighborhood hazards, community resource groups, and availability of healthy foods and physical activity areas bring attention to environmental factors that can be changed by working with communities and work sites. Other community interventions include organization of walking groups, community lectures, and health fairs. Empowerment is central to all of these interventions (Marmot, 2007). People need control over their lives and the ability to participate in decisions that influence their lives. Empowerment also means having the material resources and a political voice to change their communities.

The Centers for Disease Control (CDC) Office of Minority Health and Health Disparities (OMHD) and the National Institutes of Health (NIH), and the Center for Minority Health and Health Disparities (NCMHD) were established to lead national efforts to reduce and ultimately eliminate health disparities. The NCMHD supports research to eliminate the disproportionate burden of ill health among minority Americans. African-Americans, Asians and Pacific Islanders, Hispanics and Latinos, and Native Americans are recognized groups who suffer from health disparities. What has not been as visible is a national discussion of social determinants of health and the involvement of all levels of government to develop and implement policy to achieve health equity. No simple solutions are easily available to achieve health equity. However, nurses, as frontline providers with a person–environment perspective, can implement culturally competent individual-, family-, and community-based programs to begin to address this complex issue.

HEALTH CARE PROFESSIONALS AND CULTURAL COMPETENCE

Expertise in cultural competence and sensitivity to differences among cultures is a needed skill, considering the diversity of vulnerable populations and the number of interacting factors operating to create health disparities. *Cultural competence* is defined as appropriate and effective communication that requires one to be willing to listen and learn from members of diverse populations and the provision of information and services in appropriate languages, at appropriate comprehension and literacy levels, and in the context of the individual's health beliefs and practices (Giger et al., 2007). In culturally competent health-promotion programs, the beliefs, interpersonal style, attitudes, and behaviors of individuals and families are respected and incorporated into program planning, implementation, and evaluation activities. Cultural competence is the conscious adaptation of one's practice to be consistent with the culture of the client (Purnell, 2002). All health care professionals should be aware of their own cultural values and beliefs and recognize how these influence their attitudes and behaviors toward another group.

Bushy describes cultural–linguistic competence as a continuum of interpersonal skills ranging from ethnocentrism on one end of the continuum to enculturation at the other end of the spectrum (Bushy, 1999). *Ethnocentrism*, one anchoring point on the continuum, refers to assumptions or beliefs that one's own way of behaving or believing is the most preferable and correct one and the standards by which all cultural groups will be judged. This view devalues the beliefs of other cultural groups or treats them with suspicion or hostility. *Cultural awareness*, the next stage on the continuum, refers to an appreciation of and sensitivity to another person's values, beliefs, and practices. Next, *cultural knowledge* refers to gaining understanding and insight of different cultures. The continuum progresses to *cultural change* and then *cultural competence*, the level at which the health care provider is aware, sensitive, and knowledgeable about another's culture, and has the skills to employ appropriate health promotion activities. *Enculturation*, the opposite anchoring point on the continuum, refers to fully internalizing the values of the other culture. Enculturation is evident when the health care provider develops culturally sensitive health-promotion programs in collaboration with individuals in the cultural group and incorporates members of the cultural group to deliver and evaluate the intervention. A similar cultural competence scale continuum ranges from cultural destructiveness to cultural proficiency, in which culturally competent care is delivered (Engebretson, Mahoney, & Carlson, 2008).

Developing cultural competence is not a linear process. Progress depends on life's experiences, exposures to other cultures, and receptivity to learning about new cultures. Acquisition of cultural competence skills is an ongoing process to ensure the delivery of health promotion interventions that are appropriate, acceptable, and meaningful for persons of diverse backgrounds. Diversity is embedded in cultural competence, but it is just one component. Accepting and understanding differences in customs and patterns of thinking are ways in which diversity is valued.

Health care providers must have culturally appropriate communication skills in their interactions with clients to build a trust relationship so that they can obtain the information needed to develop interventions or manage issues of concern to the client. The culturally competent communication (CCC) model emphasizes verbal and non-verbal skills, recognition of potential cultural differences, incorporation of and adaptation to cultural knowledge, and negotiation/collaboration (Teal & Street, 2009). Verbal skills should reflect respect and empathy, non-judgmental concern and interest, reflections, and follow-up questions. Non-verbal behaviors should reflect respect, concern, and interest in the client's well being. Skills include active listening and focusing on the client. Recognizing potential cultural differences entails monitoring potential cultural misunderstanding to prevent crossing cultural boundaries. Observing the client's reactions, asking for the client's perceptions, and exploring client preferences and understanding are useful strategies. The nurse must use previously learned cultural knowledge to adapt to the information provided by the client. This means acknowledging differences and developing information and priorities based on client input and preferences. Communication skills for negotiation and collaboration, the last step in the cultural communication model, require awareness and adaptability to come to a shared understanding and agreed-upon priorities. Shared decision making is important, as the client is a partner in this communication model. Advanced communication skills and cultural awareness enable the nurse to avoid stereotyping clients and ignore cultural issues. If the nurse is working with a translator, an additional layer of complexity is added. Translators need to be both content and contextual experts who can be sure they are using the language the client needs (McCaffree, 2008). They need to work in the native language, understand the dialect, and understand the context in which the words are being used.

In summary, health professionals need to challenge their own practices and cultural values and develop effective, contextually appropriate communication skills to avoid reinforcing stereotypes and successfully manage the client encounter.

DESIGNING CULTURALLY COMPETENT HEALTH PROMOTION PROGRAMS

Characteristics of vulnerable populations that may affect successful health promotion efforts need to be identified in order to achieve goals established by the nurse and client. Huff and Kline (1999) categorize these factors as demographic, cultural, and health care system variables. These factors are listed in Table 12–1. Culturally relevant interventions related to some of the characteristics are described in Table 12–2.

Demographic factors are self-explanatory. Language is probably the most salient demographic difference among diverse groups, so knowledge of language spoken is a key feature in the delivery of wellness programs. The inability to communicate creates barriers in accessing wellness and screening programs, as well as health care. Inability to communicate may also result in errors or inappropriate care. In English-speaking minority clients, communication may be problematic, as clients may not fully understand the information and avoid further verbal communication to get their questions answered. The National Institutes of Health Office of Minority Health's published standards for cultural and linguistic services address the need to provide language assistance services, including interpreter services, and verbal and written notices of clients' rights in their preferred language, and to assure competent language assistance to those with limited English proficiency.

Geographic location is another major factor to consider, as the physical environment plays a major role in promoting healthy behaviors (Ryan-Nicholls, 2004). Poor

---

TABLE 12–1   Characteristics to Assess in Vulnerable Populations

Demographic Factors	Cultural Factors	Health Care System Factors
Age	Age	Access to care
Gender	Gender, Class	Insurances, Financial resources
Ethnicity	Worldview	Response to illness
Primary language spoken	Primary language spoken	Orientation to prevention services
Religion	Religious beliefs, practices	Perception of need for services
Education, literacy level	Communication patterns	Distrust of Western medicine
Occupation, income	Social customs, values	Experience with system
Area of residence	Traditional health beliefs and practices	Western vs. folk health beliefs and practices
Transportation	Dietary preferences and practices	Communication concerns
Duration in United States	Generation in United States	

Source: Adapted from Huff, K. M., & Kline, M. V., 1999, *Promoting Health in Multicultural Populations: A Handbook for Practitioners.* Thousand Oaks: Sage Publications. Reprinted by permission.

TABLE 12–2 Culturally Relevant Intervention Strategies for Vulnerable Populations

Characteristic	Strategy
Communication	• Assess primary language spoken, knowledge of English, literacy level • Use same language as target culture • Understand cultural meanings of health terms • Explore cultural explanations of health • Use culturally specific medias to deliver messages • Involve community in developmental activities
Family relationships	• Understand role of family and extended family in health • Involve family in health promotion activities • Assess religion and its role in family • Acknowledge role of church and incorporate church network
Time orientation	• Explore time orientation of target culture • Understand meaning of "clock" time • Tailor message to dominant time orientation (i.e., present, past, future)
Access/acceptance of health promotion programs	• Assess barriers to accessibility of health promotion programs • Assess environmental resources of community • Use existing community sites to deliver programs, such as churches and schools • Incorporate health promotion activities into ongoing community activities • Explore cultural values about participating in health-promotion activities such as exercise

Source: Adapted from Keller, C., & Stevens, K., 1997, "Cultural Considerations in Promoting Wellness," *Journal of Cardiovascular Nursing, 11*(3), 15–25.

urban neighborhoods are likely to be associated with areas that are unattractive or unsafe. Research on "walkability" indicates that attractive, aesthetically pleasing settings are more conducive to physical activity (Floyd, Crespo, & Sallis, 2008). Fear may be a major factor in limiting outside activities due to drug sales or violence. Poor neighborhoods have fewer services available, such as clinics or community centers and public transportation. In addition, limited grocery stores result in higher prices paid for fresh fruits and vegetables that may be scarce and of lesser quality.

Cultural factors that may affect the success of health education also should be identified. Some cultures may believe that life is predetermined, and nothing can be done to change things. Social customs and norms described previously in nonverbal communication—including touching, shaking hands, eye contact, or smiling—may have different connotations. Religious practices may also serve as potential barriers, and certain practices may need to be taken into consideration when planning for health promotion. For example, prayer and chanting, dancing rituals, and purification ceremonies are important in the Native American culture to re-establish harmony in one's physical, mental, and spiritual life. The nurse must work within the cultural religious framework in the health promotion encounter.

Communication, body language, and word meanings vary across cultures. In low literacy groups, abstract concepts may not be understood, so traditional written communication is not appropriate. Health-promotion programs are more successful when they are delivered in the same language of the participants. Therefore, persons who represent the target culture and speak the same language should be involved in development and implementation of interventions. In addition, culturally specific newspapers and radio and televisions stations can be targeted to deliver health messages in the meaningful appropriate language. Many people will hide their illiteracy due to the stigma attached, so it should never be assumed that someone can read or follow written or complex verbal instructions. Functional literacy is the ability to read at a fifth-grade level. In the United States, almost half of the population are either functionally illiterate or possess marginal literacy skills.

Programs that meet the health literacy needs of vulnerable populations must be carefully designed (Kreps & Sparks, 2008). The message must appeal to the key beliefs, attitudes, and values of the group, using familiar and acceptable language and images. Messages need to be presented multiple times using narratives and visual illustrations to capture attention and reinforce content. Tailored cultural messages that use client information are more effective than standard communication. Last, communication channels that are familiar to the client and are easily accessible are more effective. For example, the radio may be more effective than the Internet, as clients may not have access to computers. An important question to ask is this: Who is the most credible person to deliver the message? The nurse? Other family members? Peers?

Family relationships and the concept of family differ across cultures. In some cultural groups, it is common for the family to include more than the immediate relatives. The needs of the family have priority over the needs of the individual in some cultures, such as Asians and Hispanics. In these groups, support from family members is more important than external support, so family members should be intimately involved to support the individual in lifestyle change or wellness interventions. Family-oriented approaches using family and extended family networks, rather than individual ones, are more likely to be successful in behavior change in African-American and Hispanic cultures. In cultures where the woman's role is subordinate, it may be important to emphasize the value of behavior change of the woman for the entire family. Family networks may also include church relationships in certain cultures because of the social support and communication networks offered. In these cultures, the church is an effective place to implement health-promotion programs. In addition, knowledge of and respect for religious customs is important to promote desired outcomes. Educational strategies should capitalize on the powerful effects of family and church networks to promote behavior change.

Time orientation refers to how the perception of time varies among cultures. Kluckhohn and Strodtbeck (1961), two anthropologists, identified three major time orientations that exist in every society: past, present, and future. A past orientation is based on the importance of tradition. In Asian and Native American cultures, deceased relatives are part of the extended family, so the perspective of a deceased family member may be incorporated into their health practices. In the present orientation, the focus is on the here and now. A present orientation is common in vulnerable populations, as the focus is on surviving today and short-term consequences, so the future may have no meaning. Persons with a present orientation have more difficulty changing behaviors, as the current activity is the priority. The future orientation emphasizes planning for time extending from the present. Middle-class Americans are considered to be future oriented, as they work and plan for retirement, often delaying present gratification. Health promotion programs may appeal to future-oriented persons who want to be healthy in their retirement. On the other hand, these people may be so busy working for the future that they do not prioritize health and wellness. Knowledge of one's dominant time orientation as well as adherence to "clock" time will eliminate misunderstanding of responses to appointments. Nurses also need to understand how the individual prioritizes time to plan for successful attendance at programs and screening services. Strategies should consider the individual's time orientation. For example, present-oriented persons need help in connecting their present lifestyle behaviors with future consequences. Asking for examples of persons in their family or community who may be suffering from the consequences of an unhealthy lifestyle may help make the connection.

Health care system factors are also important to assess prior to health promotion efforts. Vulnerable populations have problems accessing care and participating in interventions because of costs, distance, transportation, and language. Missed appointments or program sessions may not mean the individual is not interested in health promotion. Transportation or childcare may not be available, or bilingual support may not be adequate. Acceptance of interventions depends on multiple factors, including lack of trust, interactions with health care providers, and incorporation of cultural values and lifestyle of the community. Culturally sensitive approaches based on individual and family values enhance access and acceptance of health interventions. Focus group or individual interviews in the target community enable the nurse to learn culturally relevant information on which to base interventions. Factors that influence the success of these interviews include interviewer communication skills, the participant's ability and willingness to communicate, and contextual factors, such as the location, time commitment, and cultural customs (Birks, Chapman, & Francis, 2007). Community priorities, problems, and resources must be identified and resources allocated to promote successful health promotion efforts. Churches or other sites within the community should be used whenever possible to facilitate easy access as well as a comfortable environment. Mobile clinics that go door to door to screen and provide information are another option.

The Office of Minority Health Resources Center's standards for culturally and linguistically appropriate health care services are also relevant for the delivery of health promotion programs; these are summarized in Table 12–3. Health care providers have accepted the need for culturally competent programs. Programs that improve the quality of life of individuals in the community will lead to the development of competent communities, in which members can identify and begin to solve their own issues.

Giger and Davidhizar (2002) suggest that health promotion needs vary across diverse groups based on six cultural phenomena. These phenomena, which can be used to assess clients prior to any health promotion activities: include communication, space, social organization, time, environmental control, and biological variations (Giger et al., 2007). *Communication* and *time* are similar to the prior discussion of these concepts. *Space* refers to the area surrounding a person's body that determines the personal boundaries. Individuals in various cultures differ in their need for personal space. *Social organization* refers to patterns of behavior that provide explanations for actions related to life events such as birth, illness, and death. *Environmental control* refers to direct activities that influence the natural environment. Last, *biological*

**TABLE 12–3   Recommended Standards for Culturally Appropriate
Health Promotion Programs**

1. Acquire the attitudes, behaviors, knowledge and skills needed to work respectfully and effectively with individuals in a culturally diverse environment.
2. Use formal mechanisms to involve communities in the design and implementation of health promotion programs.
3. Develop strategies to recruit and retain culturally competent staff who are qualified to address the health promotion needs of the racial and ethnic communities.
4. Provide ongoing education and training in culturally and linguistically competent program delivery.
5. Provide all participants with limited English proficiency programs conducted in their primary language.
6. Translate and make available signage and commonly used written educational material.
7. Ensure that the participants' birthplace, religion, cultural dietary patterns, and self-identified race-ethnicity are documented.
8. Undertake assessments of cultural competence, integrating measures of satisfaction, quality and outcomes of health promotion programs.

Source: Reprinted from *Public Health Reports,* 115, D. Chin, "Culturally Competent Health Care," 25–33, Copyright 2000, with permission from Royal Institute of Public Health.

variations refer to genetic differences that exist within a racial group. Assessment of the six cultural phenomena enables nurses to respond to the needs of vulnerable populations with appropriate interventions.

STRATEGIES FOR CULTURALLY APPROPRIATE INTERVENTIONS

Strategies to make health promotion programs and materials more culturally appropriate have been described. These strategies are based on the experiences of health care professionals working with diverse populations. Krueter, Lukwago, Bucholtz, Clark, and Thompson (2002) have divided the strategies into six categories, including (1) peripheral, (2) evidential, (3) linguistic, (4) constituent involving, (5) sociocultural, and (6) cultural tailoring.

Peripheral strategies involve packaging programs or materials to give the appearance of cultural appropriateness (Kreps & Sparks, 2008). Colors, images, pictures, or titles are used to reflect the social and cultural world of the targeted group. Thus, the materials are seen as familiar and comfortable. Materials that are matched to one's culture also help establish credibility and create interest, increasing acceptance and receptivity of the information.

Evidential strategies are those used to present information to increase the perceived relevance of the topic for the specific cultural group. For example, provision of information on the prevalence of diabetes has been used to raise awareness of the issue and promote lifestyle change. The message becomes more meaningful when it is perceived to be applicable to those who are receiving the message.

When materials and programs are provided in the dominant language of the cultural group, *linguistic* strategies are applied. As mentioned earlier, appropriate language is essential to effective communication. Strategies, such as translating materials or delivering the program in the target culture's native language, are essential. Guidelines are available for translating information from one language to another.

Constituent-involving strategies are implemented to capitalize on the experiences of those within the target population. For example, training and using peers or lay helpers as well as professional members of the target population provides the nurse with additional knowledge about cultural beliefs and values. Lay health advisors serve as role models and advocate for community members. They have been used extensively in the Hispanic/Latino community to eliminate health disparities (Rhodes, Foley, Zometa, & Bloom, 2007).

Socio-cultural strategies involve building on the group's values and beliefs. The program is developed to be culturally sensitive for the target population. Implementing socio-cultural strategies facilitate the cultural meaningfulness of the material or programs. For example, interventions to change dietary behaviors in African-Americans with type II diabetes may be more successful when the church site or beauty site is used, as both of these places have meaning and familiarity. Programs that are culturally meaningful have been shown to be more effective to change behavior in vulnerable populations.

Cultural tailoring strategies are described as any combination of change strategies intended to reach an individual based on characteristics unique to that person (Canino, Vila, Normand, Acosta-Perez, Ramirez, Garcia, & Rand et al., 2008). Change strategies are based on an assessment of the individual. Targeted strategies differ from tailored strategies, in that the group is the focus when targeted strategies are used. Targeted and tailoring strategies should be used in combination. When individual differences are small, the group can be the major target. When differences within the culture need attention, cultural tailoring strategies that focus on the individual are also needed.

In summary, multiple strategies have been documented to facilitate the development and implementation of culturally appropriate interventions. Effective communication is a core concept. Using interpreters, bilingual staff, and lay health advisors; integrating the cultural values of the family and community; culturally tailoring health information; and attending to health literacy issues are all key strategies to promote health in vulnerable groups.

OPPORTUNITIES FOR RESEARCH WITH VULNERABLE POPULATIONS

Although evidence documents the adverse health outcomes caused by health disparities, research to eliminate disparities and promote health equity is limited due to the multilevel, complex nature of the multiple determinants. New methodologies are needed to investigate multilevel interventions that target sociocultural, behavioral, and environmental systems. Although the antecedents or determinants of health disparities have been described, aggregate level measures of many of the concepts need clarification or development. The effects of changing policies to increase social capital, socioeconomic status, and access and quality of care on health outcomes need rigorous investigation. Interventions that target subpopulations such as adolescents, women, the elderly, and rural residents also should be designed and tested, as these subgroups have received less attention.

Interdisciplinary research teams are crucial in research to address health disparities. Community interventions should be implemented to evaluate community changes that enhance health. Health policy research is also a priority as new policies are needed, and the effects of policy changes in achieving health equity need to be evaluated.

Research is also needed to study resilience factors in vulnerable populations that block the health-damaging effects of poverty.

Vulnerable groups have traditionally been underrepresented in research for many reasons, including ineffective recruitment and retention strategies, lack of attention to culturally sensitive measures, literacy levels, and lack of trust. Recruitment of entire communities is an even bigger challenge, but this is critical to the evaluateion of large-scale change.

CONSIDERATIONS FOR PRACTICE WITH VULNERABLE POPULATIONS

Nurses have multiple opportunities and challenges with vulnerable populations because of the diversity, poverty, and increased risks factors for disease. Prior to working with diverse populations, nurses must first examine their own attitudes and values and how these may either facilitate or impede culturally appropriate health-promotion client encounters. Next, they should make a commitment to become culturally competent as they work with vulnerable groups. Effective communication and knowledge to design successful programs can be learned through courses and practice. Lifestyle change in vulnerable populations is complex due to such factors as potential language difficulties, educational level, poverty, unsafe housing or neighborhoods and different cultural beliefs. Broader concepts, such as social capital, need to be considered. In addition, identification of potential barriers is important when planning programs that encourage and facilitate healthy lifestyles.

Summary

In the past century, tremendous progress was made in the health of the American people due to basic improvements, such as safe drinking water, advances in sanitation, the availability of more nutritious food, and advances in medical care. However, the health status of poor and minority populations has lagged behind the health of white Americans. In addition, at all levels of income, health and illness follow a social gradient, with lower socioeconomic state levels being associated with poorer health. Vulnerable populations have diverse threats to health that require attention from clinicians, researchers, and policy makers. Although the contributing factors are multiple and complex, many components are amenable to nursing input. Nurses, as holistic care providers, are well positioned to take a critical leadership role in designing and implementing culturally competent health promotion programs to help achieve health equity for diverse populations.

Learning Activities

1. Perform an assessment of a specific cultural group of your choice using concepts in the Social Influences on Individual Health Model (Figure 12–1).
2. Develop a plan describing how you would become culturally competent in a culture different from your own.

3. Develop a program to promote physical activity in Mexican American women using strategies discussed in the chapter.

Selected Web Sites

National Center for Minority Health and Health Disparities
http://www.ncmhd.nih.gov
The mission of the NCMHD is to promote minority health and to lead, coordinate, and assess the efforts of the National Institutes of Health's efforts to reduce and ultimately eliminate health disparities.

Office of Minority Health and Health Disparities
http://www.cdc.gov/omhd
The Centers for Disease Control Office of Minority Health and Health Disparities aims to eliminate health disparities for vulnerable populations.

National Center for Health Statistics
http://cdc.gov/nchs
The National Center for Health Statistics is the nation's primary resource for information about America's health.

Healthy People 2020
http://www.healthypeople.gov/hp2020
Healthy People 2020 describes the comprehensive set of national public health objectives for the next decade. The U.S. Department of Health and Human Services has released new objectives every decade since 1980.

Healthier US
http://www.healthierus.gov
The Healthier US initiative is a national effort to improve people's lives and reduce the costs of disease and promote community health and wellness.

EthnoMed
http://ethnomed.org
EthnoMed contains information about cultural beliefs and other related issues pertinent to the health care of recent immigrants.

Diversity Rx!
http://www.diversityrx.org
Diversity Rx promotes language and cultural competence to improve the quality of health care for minority, immigrants, and ethnically diverse communities.

The Cross Cultural Health Program
http://www.Xculture.org
The Cross Cultural Health Program is a training and consulting organization to enhance the abilities of health professionals to provide culturally competent and linguistically appropriate care.

References

Aday, L. A. (1999). Vulnerable populations: A community-oriented perspective. In J. G. Sebastian & A. Bushy (Eds.), *Special populations in the community: Advances in reducing health disparities* (pp. 313–330). Gaithersburg, MD: Aspen Publications, Inc.

Birks, M. J., Chapman, Y., & Francis, K. (2007). Breaching the wall: Interviewing people from other cultures. *Journal of Transcultural Nursing, 18*, 150–156.

Braveman, P. (2006). Health disparities and health equity: Concepts and measurement. *Annual Review of Public Health, 27*, 168–194.

Bushy, A. (1999). Resiliency and social support. In J. G. Sebastian & A. Bushy (Eds.), *Special populations in the community: Advances in reducing health disparities.* (pp. 144–192). Gaithersburg, MD: Aspen Publications, Inc.

Canino, G., Vita, D., Normand, S., Acosta-Perez, E., Ramirez, R., Garcia, P., et al. (2008). Reducing asthma health disparities in poor Puerto Rican children: The effectiveness of a culturally tailored family intervention. *Journal of Allergy and Clinical Immunology, 121*, 665–670.

Centers for Disease Control, Office of Minority Health & Health Disparities. (2008). Retrieved from http://cdc.gov/omhd

Cox, K. J. (2009). Midwifery and health disparities: Theories and intersections. *Journal of Midwifery and Women's Health, 54*, 57–64.

DeNavas-Walt, C., Proctor, B. D., & Smith, J. C., U.S. Census Bureau. (2008). *Current population reports*, P60–235, *income, poverty, and health insurance coverage in the United States: 2007*. Washington, D.C.: U.S. Government Printing Office.

Engebretson, J., Mahoney, J., & Carlson, E. D. (2008). Cultural competence in the era of evidence-based practice. *Journal of Professional Nursing, 24,* 172–178.

Floyd, M. F., Crespo, C. J., & Sallis, J. F. (2008). Active living research in diverse and disadvantaged communities: Stimulating dialogue and policy solutions. *American Journal of Preventive Medicine, 34,* 271–274.

Giger, J., & Davidhizar, R. E. (2002). The Giger and Davidhizer transcultural assessment model. *Journal of Transcultural Nursing, 13,* 185–188.

Giger, J., Davidhizar, R. E., Purnell, L., Harden, J. T., Phillips, J., & Strickland, O. (2007). American Academy of Nursing expert panel report: Developing cultural competence to eliminate health disparities in ethnic minorities and other vulnerable populations. *Journal of Transcultural Nursing, 18,* 95–102.

Hesdorffer, D. S., & Lee, P. (2009). Health, wealth, and culture as predominant factors in psychosocial morbidity. *Epilepsy & Behavior, 15,* 536–540.

Huff, R. M., & Kline, M. V. (1999). *Promoting health in multicultural populations* (pp. 3–22). Thousand Oaks, CA: Sage Publications.

International Society for Equity in Health. (2000). Retrieved from http://www.iseqh.org

Johnson, S., Abonyl, S., Jeffrey, R., Hackett, P., Hampton, M., McIntosh, T., et al. (2008). Recommendations for action on the social determinants of health: A Canadian perspective. *The Lancet, 372,* 1690–1693.

Kluckhohn, F. R., & Strodtbeck, F. L. (1961). *Variation in value orientations.* Westport, CT: Glenwood Press.

Kreps, G. L. L., & Sparks, L. (2008). Meeting the health literacy needs of immigrant populations. *Patient Education & Counseling, 71,* 328–332.

Kreuter, M. W., Lukwago, S. N., Bucholtz, D. C., Clark, E. M., & Thompson, V. S. (2002). Achieving cultural appropriateness in health promotion programs: Targeted and tailored approaches. *Health Education and Behavior, 30*(2), 133–146.

Marmot, M. (2007). Achieving health equity: From root causes to fair outcomes. *The Lancet, 370,* 1153–1163.

Marmot, M., Friel, S., Bell, R., Houweling, T., & Taylor, S. (2008). Closing the gap in a generation: Health equity through action on the social determinants of health. *The Lancet, 372,* 1661–1669.

McCaffree, J. (2008). Language: A crucial part of cultural competency. *Journal of the American Dietetics Association, 108,* 611–613.

National Center for Health Statistics. (2009). *Health, United States, 2008 with chartbook.* Hyattsville, MD: U.S. Govern-ment Printing Office.

Purnell, L. (2002). The Purnell model for cultural competence. *Journal of Transcultural Nursing, 13*(3), 183–196.

Rhodes, S. D., Foley, K. L., Zometa, C. S., & Bloom, F. R. (2007). Lay health advisor interventions among Hispanics/Latinos: A qualitative systematic review. *American Journal of Preventive Medicine, 33,* 418–427.

Ryan-Nicholls, K. (2004). Health and sustainability of rural communities. *Rural and Remote Health, 4,* 1–11.

Solheim, K., McElmurry, B. J., & Kim M. J. (2007). Multidisciplinary teamwork in U.S. primary health care. *Social Science & Medicine, 65,* 622–634.

Starfield, B. (2006). State of the art in research on equity in health. *Journal of Health Politics, Policy and Law, 31,* 11–32.

Starfield, B. (2007). Pathways of influence on equity in health. *Social Science & Medicine, 64,* 1355–1362.

Teal, C. R., & Street, R. L. (2009). Critical elements of culturally competent communication in the medical encounter: A review and model. *Social Science & Medicine, 68,* 533–543.

PART 6

Approaches for Promoting a Healthier Society

CHAPTER 13

Health Promotion in Community Settings

OBJECTIVES

1. Differentiate between promoting the health of individuals and promoting the health of the family as a unit.
2. Describe four components of a successful school health-promotion program.
3. Discuss four advantages of the workplace as a setting for health-promotion programs.
4. Justify the rationale for nursing-managed health centers to increase their emphasis on health promotion.
5. Describe factors that facilitate successful community health promotion programs.
6. Discuss the domains of expertise needed to develop community partnerships.

Outline

- Health Promotion in Families
- Health Promotion in Schools
- Health Promotion at the Work Site
- Health Promotion in Nurse-Managed Health Centers
- The Community as a Setting for Health Promotion
- Creating Health Partnerships
- The Role of Partnerships in Education and Research
- Opportunities for Research in Community Settings
- Considerations for Practice to Promote Health in Diverse Settings
- Summary
- Learning Activities
- Selected Web Sites
- References

The value of health promotion services for improving the health of populations is recognized worldwide. However, insurers continue to be reluctant to include health promotion benefits in their reimbursement plans. There is also constraint on public sector resources, leading to increased pressure to demonstrate the cost effectiveness of health promoting services and activities. Integrated services are needed in a variety of settings if people of all ages are to benefit from quality, gender, and culturally sensitive health promoting care. Services should be delivered at sites where people spend the majority of their waking hours.

This chapter provides an overview of health-promotion settings from families and schools to the community at large. Partnerships to foster promotion services in the community, as well as multi-agency collaboration and the role of research in promoting a healthier society, are also described as keys to fostering healthy lifestyles within diverse communities.

HEALTH PROMOTION IN FAMILIES

Health values and attitudes and health-related behaviors are learned in the family context. Factors that influence values, attitudes, and behaviors include the family structure, employment patterns, gender and age differences, stage of parenting, family dynamics, communication patterns, power relations, and decision-making processes (Christensen, 2004). Just as individuals must assume responsibility for their own health status, families must assume similar responsibilities for the health of the family as a unit. The essential role of the family is to build human capital by investing in the health, education, values, and skills of its members to enable them to have productive roles in society (Wakefield & Poland, 2005). The family is the major social unit responsible for socialization of children, so it is an ideal target for health-promotion and prevention planning efforts.

Traditional approaches to families have focused on either family structure or family functioning. The structural approach defines how family members operate by their relationship to each other, such as a parent. Family functioning describes what families do together to meet their needs within a context of mutual responsibility.

Another theoretical approach for understanding families is an "eco-cultural" approach, which places a strong emphasis on how families maintain their everyday routines (Christensen, 2004). Three factors are assessed in the eco-cultural approach: (1) family concerns, such as earning a living, neighborhood safety, and transportation, and how the family balances these issues with efforts to sustain daily routines; (2) the meaningfulness or moral and cultural significance of everyday routines; and (3) the congruence or balance among the needs and goals of the family. This approach enables the nurse to obtain a detailed view of the health practices of families, as it describes if family routines hinder or promote the development of a health promotion-prevention plan.

The following questions generate information about family values, beliefs, and lifestyle: (1) How does the family define *health*? (2) What health-promoting behaviors does the family engage in regularly? (3) What health-promoting behaviors are particularly enjoyable to family members? (4) Do all family members engage in these behaviors, or are patterns of participation highly variable in the family?

(5) Is there consistency between stated family health values and their health actions? (6) What are the explicit or implicit health goals of the family? (7) What factors are operating to prevent health-promoting behaviors? (8) What resources are available to facilitate health-promoting behaviors?

Variant family forms are common in today's society. Family units may be traditional two-parent families, one-parent families (often mother only), blended families (parts of two preexisting families), extended families (nuclear plus a relative, often older), augmented families (additional members, not blood relations), married adults, and unmarried adults (blood and nonblood relations). The nurse working with families must be sensitive to both the commonalities and differences across varying family forms. Understanding the milieu for the promotion of health in nontraditional families is essential to successful family health-promotion planning.

The family is a pivotal unit to decrease risky behaviors and increase healthy behaviors among its members. Families exert three types of influences: cultural/attitudinal, such as church attendance or school engagement; social/interpersonal, including social support; and intrapersonal, such as self-esteem, coping, and depression. Fewer disruptive behaviors of children are seen in families when parenting skills improve and marital problems are resolved. Families demonstrate a spectrum of abilities, insights, and strengths. The challenge for the nurse is to assist the family unit in identifying relevant health goals, planning for positive lifestyle changes, and capitalizing on their strengths to achieve desired health outcomes.

Family-centered collaborative negotiation has been shown to be effective in facilitating behavior change in addressing childhood obesity. A collaborative partnership, rather than a prescriptive one, engages parents and supports parent–child relationships while enhancing motivation to change health behavior (Tyler & Horner, 2008).

HEALTH PROMOTION IN SCHOOLS

Because the majority of the nation's children are enrolled in elementary and secondary schools, school-based health promotion programs can be effective in increasing the health-promoting behaviors among children and adolescents before certain behavior patterns solidify. Schools should be health-enhancing environments that build resilience and assist children in developing healthy behaviors, such as positive nutrition and regular exercise habits.

Teachers and school health personnel set the normative expectations for healthy behaviors and serve as role models for health-enhancing lifestyles. Positive peer influences should be nurtured to foster health-promoting rather than health-damaging behaviors. Parents who are interested and involved in creating healthy school environments and model healthy lifestyles are also crucial to the success of school-based health promotion programs.

The earliest programs to target health promotion in schools focused on the individual and provided information about potential health threats and risks of certain behaviors. In the second phase of program development, the influence of parents, peers and other environmental influences began to be addressed. Both phases were based on the assumption that individuals determine their lifestyle. Most school-based interventions focused on specific topics—such as physical activity, smoking cessation, or dietary behaviors—and were based on individual-level theories, such as social cognitive theory, to promote change. These programs usually provided health education within the confines of the school curriculum. More recently, researchers have fully recognized the influences of the social and physical environment and are incorporating them into school-based programs. More diverse theories are also being applied that consider the social context.

The "Five Cs"—competence, confidence, character, connection, and caring/compassion—are key attributes of positive youth development. Programs that focus on developing these attributes assist children and adolescents in developing into healthy, productive adults. Key features of effective programs take into account both the individual and the social context and have a vision of positive development; focus on participation in all facets of the program, including design, conduct, and evaluation; and conduct programs in accessible, safe settings. In addition, they recognize the interrelated challenges facing children and adolescents: They integrate support services, provide training to adult leaders, emphasize life skills development, incorporate program evaluation, and pay attention to group diversity (Lerner & Thompson, 2002).

The Gatehouse Project targeted three aspects of the school social context: security, communication, and participation (Patton, Bond, Butler, & Glover, 2003). Schoolwide strategies, such as mentoring programs, promotion of positive classroom climates, and introduction of a curriculum to promote social and emotional skills, were the main components. Substantial positive changes were noted in behaviors of children in the intervention schools, including a reduction in health risk behaviors. The findings document the value of including both the individual and the social context of the school, where young people spend more than a third of their waking hours.

A study to evaluate a school-based teen obesity prevention intervention included seven schools with 551 teens. The intervention was a commercially produced PowerPoint nutrition education presentation given in two 30-minute periods over a week. Significant improvements occurred in knowledge, intention to maintain body weight because of importance to friends, and intention to eat fewer sweets and fried foods. Program satisfaction scores were also high (Abood, Black, & Coster, 2008). It is unknown if the participants followed their intent to improve weight and food selections with actual behavior change.

Many schools programs to promote healthy behaviors in children and youth have been implemented with varying degrees of success. The Child and Adolescent Trial for Cardiovascular Health was one of the largest school-based health education studies conducted in the United States (McCullum-Gomez, Barroso, Hoelscher, Ward, & Kelder, 2006). The study included a curriculum component augmented by a family component, a physical activity component, a school food service component, and a program to promote smoke-free school policies. An evaluation five years after the intervention showed that environmental changes can be maintained to support healthy behaviors. However, compliance was less than desired. The researchers concluded that staff training is a significant factor in achieving institutionalization of these programs. The Gold Medal Schools Program in Utah supports school policies to increase health food choices and physical activity in third- through fifth-graders (Jordan et al., 2008). Students in Gold Medal schools reported less consumption of soft drinks and an increase in the days they walked or bicycled to school. Such programs suggest that they can positively affect health behaviors of young children.

Physical activity, a major public health concern, has been the focus of school-based interventions across all ages. These interventions are based on the rationale that physical activity during childhood may enhance health, both in the short term and throughout later life. A pilot study to increase physical activity in preschool resulted in an increased structured time for physical activity and improved motor skills in three- to five-year-olds (Williams, Carter, Kibbe, & Dennison, 2009). The active school model, called "Action School-BC," was designed to promote cardiovascular health in elementary school children. Children in the intervention group had a 20% greater fitness level and 5.7% lower blood pressure (Reed, Warburton, MacDonald, Naylor, & McKay, 2008). After-school programs have also been shown to increase physical activity and other health behaviors when physical activity is incorporated in the after-school setting (Beets, Beighle, Erwin, & Huberty, 2009). The success of a senior school physical activity intervention was mediated by exercise self-efficacy in girls (Lubans & Sylva, 2009). In other physical activity interventions for adolescent girls, self-efficacy, perceived barriers and benefits, and commitment have been identified as mediators to successful outcomes (Taymoon & Lubans, 2008). A better understanding of gender differences in school-aged males and females is needed in health promotion (Östlin, Eckermann, Shanker Mishra, Knowane, & Wallstam, 2006), as well as barriers to implementation and participation in school-based programs.

Promoting physical activity in middle-school girls was emphasized in a study involving 36 schools in six geographically diverse areas of the United States. Schools and communities were targeted to increase opportunities, support, and incentives to increase physical activity (Webber et al., 2008). In the third year of the project, the effectiveness of a staff-directed intervention versus school and community leader–led interventions was measured. Physical activity level of the girls slightly improved in the community leader–led intervention. No differences were observed in fitness or percent body fat in the two groups, indicating various types of interventions are effective (Webber et al., 2008).

Another effort to increase physical activity in schools focused on the impact of re-designed play ground environments, using multicolored playground markings and physical structures. The intervention improved moderate to vigorous and vigorous physical activity in children's school recess physical activity levels (Ridgers, Stratton, Clark, Fairclough, & Richardson, 2006a; Ridgers, Stratton, Fairclough, & Twisk, 2006b). Increasing the appeal of the physical environment to children is another strategy for developing lifelong physical activity behaviors.

The tradition of fitness testing in schools has been challenged due to the limitations in the setting, including variability of motivation, external conditions, self-efficacy in testing, and group dynamics (Naughton, Carlson, & Greene, 2006). Sports-specific settings are considered ideal settings, but participation of school-aged children in physical activities outside the school setting is limited. An alternative strategy proposed for school-based testing is to focus on physical activity instead of fitness.

Health-promoting behaviors are acquired more readily in childhood when routines and habits are being formed. Habits or behaviors developed in childhood are more likely to persist as an integral part of lifestyle than changes made in health behaviors later in the adult years. Development of healthy behaviors in very young children is critical to increasing the prevalence of healthy lifestyles in the total population.

HEALTH PROMOTION AT THE WORK SITE

The escalating costs of health insurance benefits have motivated employers to implement work site prevention and health-promotion initiatives to control costs and maintain a healthy and productive workforce. The number of workplace health promotion programs has grown substantially in the past decades, and continued growth is likely to be based on the cost effectiveness and positive outcomes of health promotion programs. The financial impact of one comprehensive multisite workplace health promotion program showed a cost savings of more than $15 for each $1 it cost to offer the program (Aldana, Merrill, Price, Hardy, & Hager, 2005).

There was a negative relationship between absenteeism and participation with program participants averaging three fewer missed workdays than those who did not participant in any programs (Aldana et al., 2005). This finding was supported in a meta-analysis of studies that examined the effects of participation in a workplace wellness program in which participation was associated with job satisfaction and deceased absenteeism (Parks & Steelman, 2008). Work sites offer access to large numbers of adults and serve as a vehicle for delivering interventions at multiple levels, including individual, interpersonal, environmental, and organizational levels.

Work site programs have the potential to (1) increase healthy behaviors, (2) increase productivity, (3) decrease absenteeism, (4) decrease use of expensive medical care, and (5) lower disability claims, ultimately resulting in a more productive and globally competitive workforce. Comprehensive programs are more likely to have successful long-term results if they address risk reduction counseling, modify workplace policies, and make changes in the physical work environment.

Work site wellness programs range from annual events, such as health fairs, to ongoing comprehensive programs. Some programs are only available to employees of a certain rank, or the work site may subsidize membership at an independently operated facility. Programs typically include on-site exercise capabilities and opportunities to improve diet, stop smoking, control substance abuse, relieve stress, and control obesity. A multifaceted on-site program is likely to attract and retain a broader spectrum of workers and is more cost-effective. Offering a variety of health-promotion programs at the work site and using differing approaches increases the appeal of the program to employees of varying cultural backgrounds and ages. Although work site programs are increasing in major corporations, they remain rare in companies that employ fewer than 50 people (Parks & Steelman, 2008).

Work site programs create a cultural milieu that supports health-promoting behaviors. For example, smoke-free workplaces have made major contributions to declines in cigarette smoking in both the United States and Australia. Policy changes also have resulted in a decrease in exposure of nonsmokers to environmental tobacco smoke at the work site.

Workplace programs have access to employees during the workday over an extended period of time and the opportunity to modify policies and promote environmental change to enhance employees' healthy behaviors. The potential is increased to modify social norms and increase interpersonal support for coworkers who are motivated to change. Last, employers have opportunities to offer incentives to reward healthy behaviors.

Change in the workplace culture is important to achieve broad-based support for health-promotion programs. Examples of changes at the work site include (1) availability of health materials, (2) healthier foods in cafeteria and vending machines, (3) healthier snacks at meetings, (4) discounted rates at fitness centers for employees and families, (5) periodic health screening, and (6) on-site health fairs.

Work site programs offer a range of approaches to promote wellness. Work site behavioral skill interventions have been shown to increase physical activity and enjoyment of exercise, if employees are encouraged to exercise and are taught behavioral skills to maintain exercise such as goal setting, time management, self-talk, social support building, relapse prevention, and environmental modification (Parks & Steelman, 2008). In addition, work site–based initiatives to increase fruit and vegetable consumption have been effective.

A 12-week group and individual nutrition and fitness program was tested for its effects on weight management, and hematological and anthropometric measures for 148 men and women. Participants set individual health behavior and nutritional goals and had individual counseling. Participants experienced weight loss and deceased cholesterol level, blood pressure reading, and waist circumference, demonstrating that wellness programs in the workplace can be effective. Effectiveness seems to increase if programs are based on a social ecological approach, address multiple risk factors for change, and integrate families and neighborhoods (Stoler, Touger-Decker, O'Sullivan-Maillet, & Debchoudhary, 2006). Nurses should identify barriers and facilitators to change within work sites, as well as key policy and program components that are most effective in promoting change.

Including families in work site health promotion programs is of interest because many employers also pay health care costs for family members. Smokers are more likely to have spouses who smoke, and individuals with physically active spouses are more likely to be active themselves. Their children are also likely to be more active. Teachers have also been invited from local schools to participate in work site programs to ensure consistency and integration of health promotion concepts across schools and work sites. This effort, if expanded, may give rise to "seamless" health promotion programming in communities, which would accelerate behavior change efforts across the life span.

The major weakness of work site programs is that they attract only a limited number of employees. The primary motivator for participation in workplace health-promotion programs is concern for one's health (Stoler et al., 2006). Many workers may hesitate to identify health problems that are not evident, as they may fear loss of their job and/or privacy. Program planners should assess workers to learn their concerns related to their health without invading privacy. Barriers to participation include time commitment, availability of on-site facilities and programs, and lack of interest (Mobley, Lawyer, Faith, & Mobley, 2007). Nurses who are employed in work settings are challenged to offer many health promotion programs and to integrate health promotion into the work culture so that as many employees as possible can benefit.

Work site health promotion programs are projected to expand in the future, as healthy lifestyles help contain health care costs. Programs that include physical, mental, and social health increase the overall effectiveness of the company as well as the health and life quality of the employee. Exciting possibilities exist for integrating these programs into a coordinated community effort. In a 12-week lifestyle modification program that was implemented in the community, workers' job satisfaction increased through the acquisition of new ways of coping with stress and increased support from others in the community (Ohta, Takigami, & Ikeda, 2007).

HEALTH PROMOTION IN NURSE-MANAGED HEALTH CENTERS

Nurse-managed community health centers represent an ideal setting for offering a spectrum of services, including health promotion and prevention counseling, behavioral interventions to promote healthy lifestyles, and screening to detect health risks.

The hallmark of nurse-managed community health centers is primary care, delivered by nurses. A focus on "the individual and family" rather than "the presenting illness" has enhanced the appeal of nurse-managed centers to deliver care to a growing segment of the population. Many families prefer health care from nurse practitioners in a setting that is user-friendly and respectful of their unique assets and needs.

Nurse-managed centers provide family-oriented, culturally sensitive care to diverse populations. They include direct care services, health education classes, small-group support sessions, and family and individual counseling. Many families need assistance with healthy parenting or meeting the health promotion needs of family members. Lifestyle health behaviors are reinforced in the family, and interventions that engage parent(s) and support parent–child relationships are more likely to be successful. A collaborative relationship between the nurse practitioner and the parent or adult caregiver facilitates health-promoting behavior in the individual and family unit (Tyler & Horner, 2008).

Computerized systems to track client outcomes are needed to collect information to evaluate the quality and cost-effectiveness of health-promotion services and programs delivered in nurse-managed centers. These data will also provide evidence needed to document services for reimbursement purposes.

An example of a successful nurse-managed center is the University of South Carolina Children and Family Healthcare Center. The center opened in 1998 with a limited mission to provide primary health care for children placed in protective custody of the state because of abuse or potential abuse. The Center expanded to offer comprehensive services to children and families in the surrounding community. Pediatric and family nurse practitioner faculty members provide immunizations, well baby checkups, and health promotion and preventive services for children and adults, as well as 24-hour primary care services. The Center also serves a large population of adolescents who are in foster care.

Located in a former strip mall in a low-income area, the Center continues to experience a growing client base. Reimbursement from Medicaid, other third-party reimbursement, private pay, various state and federal programs, and grants and contracts assist the Center to maintain fiscal stability (see the Center's Web site listed at the end of the chapter).

Nurse-managed centers are located in diverse environments so they are accessible to populations served. Some centers are located at or near schools to help meet the health needs of children and adolescents in a confidential and developmentally appropriate manner. Nurse-managed centers are also located in malls, pharmacies, and low-income housing developments to provide access to people where they congregate or spend time when not at school or work. Nurse-managed centers offer care that enhances the health and well-being of all family members, interdisciplinary care, access to social services, and integrated care that covers the life span of families and individuals.

The continued national emphasis on cost containment in health care has made nurse-managed centers appealing as an integral component of the health care system. Evaluation of nurse-managed centers indicates that clients are highly satisfied with services, have improved health outcomes, believe they receive high-quality health care, and realize cost savings (Turner & Stanhope, 2008). Opportunities to link university nursing programs and nurse-managed centers are particularly attractive, as the latest scientific developments may be implemented to improve services through evidence-based practice. In addition, the primary practice settings are ideal clinical practice sites for nursing students to observe the care provided by advanced practice nurses and doctors of nursing practice.

Nurses must address legislative impediments that constrain the establishment of nurse-managed centers and the provision of reimbursed health promotion and prevention services to individuals and families (King, 2008). Nurse-managed centers are uniquely positioned in the health care system to negotiate with managed care organizations to be primary care providers to a growing segment of the population. Both professional and lay organizations should continue concerted efforts to bring nurse-managed community health centers into the mainstream of health-promotion and prevention services.

THE COMMUNITY AS A SETTING FOR HEALTH PROMOTION

Changing the health behavior of communities rather than individuals is based on the premise that community organizing and community building are central to community health education and promotion (Minkler, 2004). Community-based health promotion and prevention programs encompass a range of activities such as (1) health education, (2) risk reduction intervention programs, (3) environmental awareness and improvement programs, and (4) initiatives to change laws or regulatory policies to be supportive of health.

Four basic values influence the success of health care professionals who work in communities (Minkler, 2004). Skills and values needed in the community are not the same as those that have been effective in the traditional health care system. Values underlying a community approach are as follows:

1. Health care professionals respect the wisdom of the community.
2. Health care professionals share health information in an understandable form.
3. Health care professionals use their capacities, skills, contacts, and resources to empower the community.
4. Health care professionals focus on capacities, not needs and deficiencies.

Community activation, a health promotion strategy, includes organized efforts to increase community awareness and consensus about health problems, coordinate health promotion partnerships to plan environmental change, allocate resources across organizations within the community, and promote citizen involvement in these processes.

Community activation matches programs to community needs identified by those who reside in the community. The community is a "living" organism with interactive webs among organizations, neighborhoods, families, and friends. The challenge of community activation is to involve community members in all aspects of planning to achieve goals they have defined.

An implementation model for community programs should be responsive to issues and problems raised during program planning. Four principles facilitate community capacity building and ownership of the project (Potvin, Cargo, McComber, Delormier, & Macaulay, 2003):

1. Community members are integrated as equal partners.
2. Intervention and evaluation components must be integrated.
3. Organizational and program flexibility is necessary to be responsive to demands in the community environment.
4. The program should be a learning project for all involved.

These principles have been confirmed in multiple community projects; having ongoing knowledge of the community and viewing the community as a true partner is essential to the success of the project. A community partnership takes time, people, and resources and must be based on honesty and respect. Community programs are dynamic processes defined through an ongoing negotiation process among all members.

Sporting clubs have been proposed as an effective communitywide strategy to increase participation in physical activity in Australia. Changing the focus of clubs from program formats directed toward increasing participation and competitiveness to sports clubs as settings to promote positive physical, mental, and social benefits requires support from club members. Researchers found that the overriding factor affecting the success of change was the presence or absence of planning (Eime, Payne, & Harvey, 2008). Community planners can learn from these findings: As the number of sport clubs and other large-scale organized physical activities grow in the United States, they are ideally situated to institutionalize health promotion programming.

Community-based health promotion programs offer an excellent approach to reach impoverished communities with limited resources. A community-based intervention was implemented in five communities to improve low-income parents' interaction with their children (Powell & Peet, 2008). Improved parenting skills contributed to the children's participation in daily family functions and strengthened the family and community.

Health promotion services must be provided where people live, work, worship, and play. Offering nutrition services in churches and mammography screening in malls brings valuable services to people in real-life settings. The synergy of bringing community strengths and resources together and the empowerment that results from early successes warrant continued attention to designing and planning innovative and culturally sensitive health promotion programs communitywide.

Integrating evidence-based clinical and community strategies is necessary to improve the health of the community. Additional research is needed to develop strategies and systems to integrate clinical and community preventive strategies in program planning and policy development (Ockene et al., 2007).

CREATING HEALTH PARTNERSHIPS

Health partnerships across settings are a major strategy to optimize the health of communities. Partnerships promote continuity of care in health promotion and prevention and synergistic use of resources to achieve optimal effectiveness and efficiency. Partnerships may consist of any combination of work sites, schools, nursing centers, other health agencies, and universities working together to improve the health of an entire community.

A *community partnership* is defined as a relationship between collaborating parties (people and organizations), committed to work together to achieve a common purpose (Jenerette et al., 2008). Community partnerships recognize the value of community members, corporate leaders, and health care providers working together to create health care systems that are user-friendly, accessible, and culturally sensitive. Partnerships optimize the combined resources of all partners so that mutually valued goals are achieved. Health partnerships use community organizations to achieve health empowerment; improve health in socially, racially, and culturally diverse communities;

and eliminate health disparities (Powell & Gilliss, 2005). Thus, community health partnerships incorporate an ecological approach.

Partnerships have been organized around a variety of community concerns, including adolescent pregnancy, violence, substance abuse, and chronic kidney disease. For example, a community-partnered approach was implemented to enhance chronic kidney disease awareness, prevention, and early intervention. Academic, community leaders, patients, caregivers, faith-based organizations, and health care professionals partnered to develop shared goals and interventions to achieve an infrastructure, shared objectives, and diverse work groups to reduce the burden of chronic kidney disease (Vargas et al., 2008).

In successful health partnerships, a relationship is established that clearly communicates respect for the community's right to identify problems and potential solutions to those problems. Initially, the community's norms for participation must be assessed with the following questions:

1. Is current community problem solving an individual or collective effort?
2. How in touch are citizens with each other?
3. What are the units of interaction (e.g., neighborhoods, townships, housing complexes)?
4. Does crime or other factors deter citizens from interacting?

Some communities have established structures for community planning to address health concerns. Current patterns of citizen involvement, existing relationships among community organizations, and organizations known for activating community involvement (churches, recreation centers, and service clubs) are analyzed to learn how partnerships for health promotion might be shaped in any given community. For some communities, flexible coalitions are the appropriate organizing framework to address community health needs, whereas for others, a leadership board or council is needed to combine the power of key community activists.

An important goal of community partnerships for health promotion is empowerment. Community empowerment is defined as social-action processes in which individuals and groups act to gain mastery over their lives through changing their social and political environment (Minkler, 2004). Members of a partnership create conditions that empower their joint efforts. Community partnerships for health promotion have the potential to bring about institutional and policy changes that affect many people. The commitment of partnerships to the broader goals of positive social, structural, and individual change is essential to improving the overall health of communities.

Building partnerships requires substantial time and effort. Putting collaborative partnerships into practice is complex and represents a challenge for all the stakeholders involved in the partnership. It is important for stakeholders to acknowledge their diverse interests in the early stages of the partnership and implement strategies to address any cultural gaps that exist. Principles that should be addressed include the following:

1. Find the right mix of ownership and control among partners.
2. Recognize the assets of all partners.
3. Develop relationships based on mutual trust and respect.
4. Acknowledge and honor different partner agendas.

5. Acknowledge the difference between community input and active community involvement.
6. Resolve ethnic, cultural, and ideological differences between and among partners (Straub et al., 2007; Vargas et al., 2008).

A shared vision among partners creates a common identity and a shared purpose. A *vision* is an image of what partners see as outcomes of their collaboration. A shared vision facilitates a shared mission that identifies the primary reasons for existence of the partnership. An example of a mission statement is as follows:

To assist individuals and families in the community in adopting healthy lifestyles and to assist the community in developing culturally sensitive, cost-effective health promotion and prevention services.

The potential for fostering healthier lives for citizens of all ages lies in the power of partnerships that are multisectoral and reach beyond the bounds of traditional medicine. Partnerships enable members to appropriately plan, implement, and evaluate community-based health promotion interventions. Health access and status of adolescents and young adults who were disconnected from traditional education and work settings were studied (Tandon Marshall, Templeman, & Sonenstein, 2008). The authors concluded that given the high levels of health risks in this population, the community must be a major player in meeting health needs of adolescents by integrating health promotion activities into youth employment and training programs in the community (Tandon et al., 2008).

A community organization approach to health promotion partnering is based on concepts of self-determination, shared decision making, bottom-up planning, community problem solving, and cultural relevance. The philosophy underlying this approach is that health promotion is likely to be more successful when the community at risk identifies its own health concerns, develops its own intervention programs, forms a board to make policy decisions, and identifies resources for program implementation. Communities that are empowered through organization and active participation in partnerships develop the skills and abilities to solve problems that compromise their health and well-being.

Community health partnerships bring greater rationality to health care expenditures by advocating funding prevention and health promotion services by national, state, and private insurers. Politically active partnerships can redirect public and private health care dollars so that funds are allocated with an emphasis on population-based health care services and clinical preventive services. Community participation and enlightened health policy are key elements for successful community health partnerships.

THE ROLE OF PARTNERSHIPS IN EDUCATION AND RESEARCH

Multidisciplinary education and collaborative practice experiences with community residents help prepare health profession students for the diversity of health care roles they will assume over their careers. As care moves from traditional institutions (except for the critically ill) to the community, knowledge and skills to function in diverse community settings are essential to meet the health needs of individuals, families, and communities. Gaining access to community educational experiences for students and faculty is a win–win situation for both nursing programs and communities (Kushto-Reese, Maguire, Silbert-Flagg, Immelt, & Shaefer, 2007). For example, students in the early stages of baccalaureate nursing education can experience various aspects of the role of community health worker by distributing health education materials in a community, participating in screening programs, helping organize health fairs, and collecting health data from communities. Advanced baccalaureate students with a greater understanding of the role of culture and socioeconomic level on health behaviors can provide education classes at schools and work sites, assist community residents to identify environmental health risks, and provide self-care education to groups of individuals who have similar health-risk profiles.

Graduate students, faculty, and community member representatives provide a strong team for training community health workers in underserved communities. To build a successful cohort of community health workers, nursing programs must (1) establish rapport with the community; (2) collaborate with the community to assess health needs; (3) hire individuals from the community to gain the trust and participation of community residents; (4) share program ownership and decision making with community health care workers, empowering them to develop program goals; (5) facilitate program flexibility so workers are able to adapt to changing needs; and (6) closely link workers with community health and social service agencies so that professional backup is available as necessary.

The need has never been greater for nursing programs to take an active role in developing enduring health promotion partnerships. The holistic view of nursing provides the orientation necessary to work collaboratively with communities to accomplish health goals. The escalating need for reform in health care and the economic pressures for cost-effective, multidisciplinary, high-quality care places nurses in a unique position to make changes in community health care systems.

Community–academic health partnerships are also valuable allies in research. Partnering with universities throughout all stages of assessing, planning, and conducting health promotion interventions creates a sense of community ownership and takes advantage of the expertise of university faculty. Research community–academic partnerships foster enthusiastic participation, attentiveness to recruitment, thoughtful interpretation of findings, and commitment to dissemination of results to the community (Currie et al., 2005).

OPPORTUNITIES FOR RESEARCH IN COMMUNITY SETTINGS

There is no single method to evaluate the success of interventions that go beyond the individual level. Nurse scientists should apply diverse evaluation strategies that are effective for families, schools, and communities as units of analysis. Attention to process as well as outcome evaluation is also needed to identify strategies that are most effective in promoting healthy behaviors. Suggested opportunities for research include the following:

1. Describe health promotion and disease prevention beliefs and practices in diverse families and communities as a basis for designing culturally sensitive interventions.
2. Test the synergistic affects of school, family, and community health-promotion efforts for adolescents on individual- and community-level health outcomes.
3. Identify facilitators and barriers to participating in work site programs.
4. Test community partnership strategies that optimize community and environmental change.

5. Design and test valid and reliable community-level health outcome measures.
6. Develop uniform methods and measures to assess cost outcomes across a range of programs and communities.

Some evidence suggests that community partnerships make a difference in health practices and the health of the community (Currie et al., 2005). However, few systematic studies have been conducted to test the effectiveness and sustainability of community partnerships, particularly in communities with underserved populations. Partnership interventions must be carefully documented to identify the effective components. Multiple measures should be used to assess the behavioral, social, and environmental outcomes of partnership activities.

CONSIDERATIONS FOR PRACTICE TO PROMOTE HEALTH IN DIVERSE SETTINGS

Multiple settings offer opportunities to provide health promotion services. Nurses with an understanding of community health issues and problems are ideally suited to provide leadership in the design, development, implementation, and evaluation of health promotion programs in schools, work sites, nursing centers, and other community settings. Financial support for such programs can be sought from a variety of public and private sources. The health problems of today are best addressed by many sectors coming together in partnerships to improve social and environmental conditions that compromise health. Partnerships offer a way to communicate, collaborate, and empower to achieve solutions not attainable by single groups or organizations. Particularly exciting is the opportunity for schools of nursing to join with other health professions' schools, health care provider groups, and communities to build health partnerships. These partnerships, designed in a community-sensitive, culturally appropriate manner, will improve prevention and health promotion services provided to diverse populations.

Summary

Health promotion services should be offered in multiple settings to reach diverse populations. Development and maintenance of healthy lifestyles and healthy environments must be a central goal. Programs that involve the community and are tailored to its members' needs enhance cultural appropriateness and likelihood of success. Formation of community partnerships creates a network of community residents and health care providers to offer quality health promotion and prevention services.

Learning Activities

1. Identify a community-based health promotion program in your community and assess its effectiveness by interviewing two citizens who live in the community (e.g., the Red Dress Campaign to recognize heart disease as the major killer of women in the United States).
2. Investigate the level of interagency collaboration in a program to promote health or prevent disease in your community. What agencies are

represented? What agencies should be involved that are not represented?

3. Describe the steps you would take to work with an impoverished community to improve access to immunizations for children.

4. Identify a work site program in your community. Assess its strengths and limitations from the perspective of the employer, employee, and community.

Selected Web Sites

South Carolina Children and Family Healthcare Center
http://www.sc.edu/nursing/practice/chfc.html
The South Carolina Children and Family Healthcare Center is an example of a successful nurse-managed health care center.

The Community Guide (U.S. Centers for Disease Control and Prevention)
http://thecommunityguide.org/
The Community Guide provides evidence-based recommendation of what is known about effectiveness, economic efficiency, and feasibility of interventions to prevent disease and promote health for a variety of public health concerns.

The Community Tool Box
http://ctb.ku.edu/en/
The Community Tool Box is the world's largest resource for free information on essential skills for building healthy communities.

Cochrane Collaboration
http://www.cochrane.org/
The Cochrane Collaboration reviews standards for health care interventions and appropriate treatments.

Health Resources and Services Administration, Primary Health Care: The Health Center Program
http://bphc.hrsa.gov/
This Health Resources and Services Administration Web site offers information on developing centers to increase access to health care in the nation's most needy communities.

Centers for Disease Control and Prevention Workplace Safety & Health
http://www.cdc.gov/workplace/
The CDC Workplace Safety & Health Agency works with partners throughout the nation to monitor health in the workplace.

The Youth Risk Behavior Surveillance System
http://www.cdc.gov/healthyyouth/yrbs
The Youth Risk Behavior Surveillance System monitors priority health risk behaviors and the prevalence of obesity and asthma among youth and young adults.

Turning Information into Health Behavioral Risk Factor Surveillance System
http://cdc.gov/brfss/index.htm
The Behavioral Risk Factor Surveillance System is a state-based system of health surveys that collects information on health risk behaviors, preventive health practices, and health care access.

Healthy People in Healthy Communities
http://www.healthypeople.gov/Publications /HealthyCommunities2001/default.htm
Health People in Healthy Communities is a guide for building coalitions, measuring outcomes, and creating partnerships dedicated to improving the health of the community.

PEP—A Personal Empowerment Plan
http://www.cdc/needphp/dnpa/pep.htm
PEP is a strategy for work sites to promote employee physical activity and healthy eating. Visit this Web site to access basic tools for work site health promotion planning.

References

Abood, D. A., Black, D. R., & Coster, D. C. (2008). Evaluation of a school-based teen obesity prevention program. *Journal of Nutrition Education and Behavior, 40*(3), 168–174.

Aldana, S. G., Merrill, R. M., Price, K., Hardy, A., & Hager R. (2005). Financial impact of a comprehensive multisite workplace health promotion program. *Preventive Medicine, 40*(2), 131–137.

Beets, M. W., Beighle, A., Erwin, H. E., & Huberty, J. L. (2009). After-school program impact on physical activity and fitness: A meta-analysis. *American Journal of Preventive Medicine, 36*(6), 527–537.

Christensen, P. (2004). The health-promoting family: A conceptual framework for future research. *Social Science & Medicine, 59*(2), 377–387.

Currie, M., King, G., Rosenbaum, P., Law, M., Kertoy, M., & Specht, J. (2005). A model of impacts of research partnerships in health and social services. *Evaluation and Program Planning, 28*(4), 400–412.

Eime, R. M., Payne, W. R., & Harvey, J. T. (2008). Making sports clubs healthy and welcoming environments: A strategy to increase participation. *Journal of Science and Medicine in Sport, 11*, 146–154.

Jenerette, C. M., Funk, M., Ruff, C., Grey, M., Adderley-Kelly, B., & McCorkle, R. (2008) Models of inter-institutional collaboration to build research capacity for reducing health disparities. *Nursing Outlook, 56*(1), 16–24.

Jordan, K. C., Erikson, E. D., Cox, R., Carlson, E. C., Heap, E., Friedrichs, M., et al. (2008). Evaluation of the Gold Medal schools program. *Journal of the American Dietetic Association, 108*, 1916–1920.

King, E. S. (2008). A 10-year review of four academic nurse-managed centers: Challenges and survival strategies. *Journal of Professional Nursing, 24*, 14–20.

Kushto-Reese, K., Maguire, M. C., Silbert-Flagg, J. A., Immelt, S., & Shaefer, S. J. M. (2007). Developing community partnerships in nursing education for children's health. *Nursing Outlook, 55*(2), 85–94.

Lerner, R. M., & Thompson, L. S. (2002). Promoting healthy adolescent behavior and development: Issues in the design and evaluation of effective youth programs. *Journal of Pediatric Nursing, 17*(5), 338–344.

Lubans, D. R., & Sylva, K. (2009). Mediators of change following a senior school physical activity intervention. *Journal of Science and Medicine in Sport, 12*, 134–140.

McCullum-Gomez, C., Barroso, C. S., Hoelscher, D. M., Ward, J. L., & Kelder, S. H. (2006). Factors influencing implementation of the Coordinated Approach to Child Health (CATCH) eat smart school nutrition program in Texas. *Journal of the American Dietetic Association, 106*, 2039–2044.

Minkler, M. (2004). *Community organizing and community building for health* (2nd ed., pp. 20–29). New Brunswick, NJ: Rutgers University Press.

Mobley, A. R., Lawyer, H., Faith, J., & Mobley, S. L. (2007). Motivational influences for participating in a worksite wellness program. *Journal of the American Dietetic Association, 107*(8) (Suppl 1), A104.

Naughton G. A., Carlson, J., & Greene, D. A. (2006). A challenge to fitness testing in primary schools. *Journal of Science and Medicine in Sport, 9*(1–2), 40–55.

Ockene, J. K., Edgerton, E. A., Teutsch, S. M., Marion, L. N., Miller, T., Genevro, J., et al. (2007). Integrating evidence-based clinical and community strategies to improve health. *American Journal of Preventive Medicine, 32*(3), 244–252.

Ohta, M., Takigami, C., & Ikeda, M. (2007). Effect of lifestyle modification on workers' job satisfaction through the collaborative utilization of community-based health promotion program. *International Congress Series, 1294*, 123–126.

Östlin, P., Eckermann, E., Shankar Mishra, U., Knowane, M., & Wallstam, E. (2006). Gender and health promotion: A multisectoral policy approach. *Health Promotion International, 21*(Suppl 1), 25–35.

Parks, K. M., & Steelman, L. A. (2008). Organizational wellness programs: A meta-analysis. *Journal of Occupational Health Psychology, 13*(1), 58–68.

Patton, G., Bond, L., Butler, H., & Glover, S. (2003). Changing schools, changing health? Design and implementation of the gatehouse project. *Journal of Adolescent Health, 33*, 231–239.

Potvin, L., Cargo, M., McComber, A. M., Delormier, T., & Macaulay, A. C. (2003). Implementing participatory intervention and research in communities: Lessons from the Kahnawake schools diabetes prevention project in Canada. *Social Science & Medicine, 56*, 1295–1305.

Powell, D. L., & Gilliss, C. L. (2005). Building capacity and competency in conducting health disparities research. *Nursing Outlook, 53*(3), 107–108.

Powell, D. R., & Peet, S. H. (2008). Development and outcomes of a community-based intervention to improve parents' use of inquiry in informal learning contexts. *Journal of Applied Developmental Psychology, 29*(4), 259–273.

Reed, K. E., Warburton, D., MacDonald, H. M., Naylor, P. J., & McKay, H. A. (2008). Action Schools! BC: A school based physical activity intervention designed to decrease cardiovascular disease risk factors in children. *Preventive Medicine, 46*, 525–531.

Ridgers, N., Stratton, G., Clark, E., Fairclough, S. J., & Richardson, D. J. (2006a). Day-to-day and seasonal variability of physical activity during school recess. *Preventive Medicine, 42*, 372–374.

Ridgers, N., Stratton, G., Fairclough, S. J., & Twisk, J. W. R. (2006b). Long-term effects of a playground markings and physical structures on children's recess physical activity levels. *Preventive Medicine, 44*(5), 393–397.

Stoler, F. D., Touger-Decker, R., O'Sullivan-Maillet, J., & Debchoudhary, I. (2006). Wellness in the workplace: A 12 week group and individual program. *Journal of the American Dietetic Association, 106*(8) (Suppl 1), A9.

Straub, D. M., Deeds, B. G., Willard, N., Castor, J., Peralta, L., Francisco, V. T., et al. (2007). Partnership selection and formation: A case study of developing adolescent health community–researcher partnerships in fifteen U.S. communities: Adolescent Trials Network for HIV/AIDS Interventions. *Journal of Adolescent Health, 40*(6), 489–498

Tandon S. D., Marshall, B., Templeman, A. J., & Sonenstein, F. L. (2008). Health access and status of adolescents and young adults using youth employment and training programs in an urban environment. *Journal of Adolescent Health, 43*(1), 30–37.

Taymoon, P., & Lubans, D. R. (2008). Mediators of behavior change in two tailored physical activity interventions for adolescent girls. *Psychology of Sport and Exercise, 9*, 605–619.

Turner, L. M., & Stanhope, M. (2008). The Good Samaritan nursing center: A commonwealth collaborative. *Nursing Clinics of North America, 43*, 341–356.

Tyler, D., & Horner, S. D. (2008). Family-centered collaborative negotiation: A model for facilitating behavior change in primary care. *Journal of the American Academy of Nurse Practitioners, 20*(4), 194–203.

Vargas, R. B., Jones, L., Terry, C., Nicholas, S. B., Kopple, J., Forge, N., et al. (2008). Community-partnered approaches to enhance chronic kidney disease awareness, prevention, and early intervention: Building Bridges to Optimum Health World Kidney Day Los Angeles 2007 Collaborative. *Advances in Chronic Kidney Disease, 15*(2), 153–161.

Wakefield, S., & Poland, B. (2005). Family, friend or foe? Critical reflections on the relevance and role of social capital in health promotion and community development. *Social Science & Medicine, 60*(12), 2819–2832.

Webber, L. S., Catellier, D. J., Lytle, L. A., Murray, D. M., Pratt, C. A., Young, D. R., et al. (2008). Promoting physical activity in middle school girls: Trial of Activity for Adolescent Girls. *American Journal of Preventive Medicine, 34*(3), 173–184.

Williams, C. L., Carter, B. J., Kibbe, D. J., & Dennison, D. (2009). Increasing physical activity in preschool: A pilot study to evaluate Animal Trackers. *Journal of Nutrition Education and Behavior, 41*, 47–52.

CHAPTER 14

Promoting Health Through Social and Environmental Change

OBJECTIVES

1. Justify the rationale for describing health as a social goal.
2. List common health-damaging factors in the environment and their etiology.
3. Discuss two opposing approaches to behavior change and the pros and cons of each approach.
4. Describe the role of financial incentives in behavior change.

Outline

Recognition that health is influenced by the social and physical environments in which people live has resulted in new approaches to achieve behavior change. As mentioned in previous chapters, large-scale change is best accomplished by focusing on altering social and environmental structures that influence health, in addition to individual and group behaviors. Effective health promotion must take into consideration the dynamic relationships between individuals and families and their social and environmental contexts. Health and social policies that fail to directly address inequitable living conditions, such as poverty, abuse, violence, hunger, and unemployment; environmental threats, such as pollution in work sites and communities; and disparities in access and care will not change the health of individuals and communities. Individual and family efforts to adopt healthy behaviors are also likely to be ineffective in the presence of environmental constraints and policies that do not promote healthy living. Strategies for health promotion that focus only on individual behavior change will fail without simultaneous efforts to alter the physical and social environment and the collective behavior of the community.

HEALTH AS A SOCIAL GOAL

Health must be identified as a social goal as well as an individual one, as the health of societies, communities, families, and individuals are integrated and inseparable. Publication of the social determinants of health by the World Health Organization (WHO) was a significant milestone, as it documents the social, cultural, economic, and political factors, as well as biological and psychological factors that influence health (WHO, 2008). Health promotion efforts involve working with communities and policy makers to ameliorate conditions that contribute to poor health, such as inadequate housing, an unsafe water supply, poor nutrition or insufficient food supply, chemical toxins, poor recreational facilities, inadequate access to care, and lack of economic opportunity. Globally, governments acknowledge that behavior-change strategies must be directed beyond the individual to include community and policy-level factors.

Health as a social goal requires the integration of theories that address community change (Chapter 3) with theories that address individual behavior change (Chapter 2) and family change (family stress theory, family development theory, family systems theory). The three theoretical perspectives are complementary. When nurses think only in terms of one-to-one relationships, the range and success of intervention possibilities are severely limited.

Health behavior change is more likely to be successful when the social context in which the individual lives is also targeted. For example, smoking cessation programs must not only target the individual addictive properties of smoking; the social context in which smoking occurs must also be addressed, including the advertising and sale of cigarettes, the influence of the tobacco industry on certain sectors of the population, and the role of public policy in changing smoking behaviors. Tobacco public policy interventions have been successful in changing smoking behaviors through laws that reduce exposure to secondhand smoke in public facilities, excise taxes that increase the costs of cigarettes, and regulations to limit advertising and promotion of tobacco products. In 2009, the Family Smoking Prevention and Tobacco Control Act was signed. This historic legislation grants authority to the U.S. Food and Drug administration (FDA) to regulate tobacco products (U.S. FDA,

2009). The FDA is responsible for protecting the public health, so major public policy changes are likely to occur as the result of this legislation.

Similar strategies and legislation that target the obesity problem in the United States are needed. Environmental changes for obesity, such as modifying how food is marketed and priced, establishing standards for foods served in cafeterias and vending machines on government property, increasing availability of healthy foods at lower costs, increasing mass media campaigns to promote healthy eating and physical activity, designing green spaces in communities, and changing school food and activity policies will help counter obesity. Increasing individual health choices, although effective for some people, will not be effective unless the health-damaging environmental factors are eliminated and healthy options are accessible (Walls, Peeters, Loff, & Crammond, 2009). Individuals, communities, and government must have a sustained commitment to stop the increasing trend in obesity in children and adults. Enduring, large-scale behavior change is best achieved by changing the standards of acceptable behavior in a community instead of attempting to change the behavior of individuals against overwhelming social odds.

The pursuit of health as a social goal requires that people of a community engage in the process of change to accommodate various social, political, and economic developments. Central concepts in community-building models include participation, empowerment, critical consciousness, community competence, and issue selection (Minkler, Wallerstein, & Wilson, 2008). *Empowerment* is a social action process through which individuals and communities gain control over their lives and their environment to improve their health and quality of life. *Community competence*, a closely related concept, focuses on problem-solving ability as a central goal of the community. Competent communities can identify their problems and needs, achieve a working consensus on goals and priorities, agree on ways to implement goals, and collaborate effectively in actions that need to be taken (Minkler et al., 2008). Health care professionals can assist in the development of community competence by identifying natural community leaders who will undertake community assessments and actions necessary to strengthen the community. Leadership development is a critical component in developing community competence. Community leaders can stimulate people in the community to identify problems and solutions and act as facilitators to build group effectiveness. As a community gains competence in negotiating for resources to address a particular problem, the community becomes empowered. This empowerment enhances problem-solving ability and capacity to cope with other problems that may arise. In addition, community members gain a sense of ownership and empowerment by initiating and promoting change.

Ecological models focus on changing the environmental context, including regulatory changes to support healthy behaviors (see Chapter 3). The Healthy People 2020 objectives emphasize an ecological approach to health promotion to create health-enhancing social and physical environments (U.S. Department of Health and Human Services [USDHHS], 2009). Social ecological models focus on the social context to produce large-scale social change. Social change is generally followed by changes in the normative structures, or the shared rules and expectations (rules of conduct) that govern everyday life.

Social change may occur either through a functionalist view or a conflict view (Anderson, Scrimshaw, Fullilove, & Fielding, 2003). In the *functionalist* view, change is a gradual adaptive process oriented toward community reform and is based on cooperation and consensus. As the community changes, social norms change and new rules of conduct arise for the changed community. Social change focuses on the community's strengths and how these strengths can be used to foster continuing development of community competence. In the *conflict* view, the system changes by coercive means or social control. Those who control important parts of the community attempt to change social norms. A functionalist perspective is consistent with an expansive view of health. The two perspectives are contrasted in Figure 14–1. Social ecological models hold promise for successful health promotion, as individuals and their social environments are considered in behavior change. More research is needed on the effectiveness of changing environments on health behavior.

In summary, when health is considered a social goal as well as an individual one, the focus for health promotion includes the community as well as the individual. Individuals can govern their own behavior and should do so. Government formulates broad policies and allocates funding. However, priority decisions and strategies for social change for more complex lifestyle issues can best be made collectively by members of the community. This strategy ensures that programs are relevant and appropriate for these involved and encourages greater buy-in and participation in the planning and implementation process.

HEALTH IN A CHANGING SOCIAL ENVIRONMENT

Health reform continues to proceed at a rapid rate in the United States with antici-pated comprehensive reform in 2010. The U.S. health care system is considered one of the most extravagant and wasteful in the Western world (Editorial, 2009). Excess

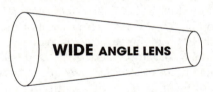

Models for Intervention

Social change	*Social control*
Social analysis	Epidemiologic and demographic analysis
Focus on strengths	Focus on weaknesses
Goal is health outcome and increased community competence	Goal is health outcome
Organized around human categories	Organized around disease categories
Asks what people's motives are	Asks how can we motivate people

FIGURE 14–1 Comparison of Social Change with Social Control Models *Source:* Eng, E., Salmon, M. E., & Mullen, F., 1992, "Community Empowerment: The Critical Base for Primary Care," *Family Community Health, 15*(1), 1–2. Used with permission.

administrative costs, excess profits, and excess costs of prescription drugs has been estimated to exceed the costs of providing health care to all uninsured Americans (Dalen & Alpert, 2008). Factors responsible for the priority to pass reform measures in the United States include rising health care costs for consumers (higher premiums, rising deductibles, higher co-payments, and escalating out-of-pocket expenses) and lack of access to care for those who are unable to purchase health insurance (Halle & Seshamani, 2009). Health reform must address health care costs, prevention and wellness, safety, and quality, and ensure affordable, high-quality health coverage for all Americans. Every community should be able to provide services and monitor the health status of its members and assist its members in accessing health care services.

In addition to health reform, information and communication technology (ICT) has transformed our society to an information- and knowledge-based one in which we are connected globally (Abbott & Coenen, 2008). ICT has the potential to contribute to reducing health inequities through the delivery of education and access to new therapies, techniques, and knowledge resources to improve health care. Poverty and illiteracy in developing countries, cost, resistance, and lack of standards in the United States are all challenges to the application of ICT.

One form of ICT, cellular telephony, has rapidly expanded into health education and health care. Short messaging service, or text messaging, is being used to educate and answer questions about sexual health for teens, send reminders to take medications, enter health data, and deliver health alerts. This technology opens the door to new methods to enhance empowerment through the delivery of health information and care in developed as well as developing nations.

Comprehensive, computerized health assessments can be used to tailor health promotion programs to the knowledge, beliefs, motivations, and prior health behavior histories of diverse individuals and families. Health promotion activities are taking advantage of computer-based technologies such as CD-ROM and the Internet to target audiences, tailor health promotion messages, and promote interactive ongoing exchanges about health. Personal computers in the home offer informational resources to answer questions and provide access to support and discussion groups.

Clients and their health care professionals can link electronically as well. Client data has become standardized and easily communicated with the electronic personal health record (PHR) (see Chapter 4). An electronic PHR enables clients to have access to their personal data, act as stewards of their information, and take an active role in their own health (Halamka, Mandl, & Tang, 2008). In contrast, an electronic health record (EHR) is managed by health care professionals or institutions. The PHR is a tool to help maintain health and wellness through access to credible information and data, as well as a means to help manage an illness (Tang, Ash, Bates, Overhage, & Sands, 2006). Technological challenges, organizational barriers, economic and market forces, and individual obstacles have limited the nationwide adoption of both the EHR and PHR. However, all levels of government as well as the private sector have encouraged adoption and made it a national priority.

The information era has also brought about changes to empower families. Interactive computer technology enables parents to work at home as well as obtain health information without visiting a health care provider. The Internet revolution is reshaping health education, as individuals conduct health information searches, share information with their families, and ask informed questions of their health care providers. Computer-assisted health education is also being successfully implemented with the Internet (see Chapters 9 and 11).

The information revolution continues to challenge health professionals to think creatively about the delivery of health promotion, new ways to educate health professionals, and the potential consequences of this technology on society. Application of these technologies must be critically evaluated so that the nurse stays at the forefront in helping clients enhance their health amid conditions of rapid social and environmental change.

PROMOTING HEALTH THROUGH PUBLIC POLICY

The importance of shaping health policies in the public and private sectors to improve health for populations is widely advocated. Policies set goals and limits and define choices. Public policy shapes the quality of social determinants of health (Raphael, 2007). Personal, social, and political factors all influence the development and implementation of health policy. For example, at the personal level, changes in public sentiment have influenced the development of health policy related to smoking in public places in the United States. At the political level, lobbyists have been successful in maintaining the economic interests of the drug industries to prevent lower drug costs. On a more positive note, public policy has resulted in removal of cigarette commercials from television.

The idea of developing policies for healthier communities is not new. Historically, local governments provided environmental safeguards against infectious diseases. However, healthy communities include social and economic factors as well as environmental ones. An underlying assumption of developing healthy communities is that local government plays a significant role through the development and implementation of policies to improve health, whereas community members actively participate in the decision-making process. Thus, policy formulation to promote health begins at the local level, through identification of problems and development of local ordinances to implement change.

The role of the U.S. government in regulating health behavior remains nebulous. State and federal policies regulate a range of health behaviors, including alcohol, tobacco, seat belt use, food safety, and drug use. In addition, state and federal governments play a major role in the payment of health care services. In many cases, a uniform health policy is missing. This is due in part to the continued attention to racial and ethnic health differences and individual behavioral risk factors rather than addressing the social determinants and accompanying economic, political, and social resources needed (Raphael, 2007).

The Healthy People 2020 initiative's overarching goals are to achieve health equity and eliminate health disparities, and to create social and physical environments that promote good health for all. These goals challenge local, state, and federal governments, as well as policy-makers, to make policy changes that affect entire populations to address social determinants at all levels. For example, local governments can limit youth access to tobacco in local markets and vending machines. Local and state policies can also be developed to target economic development in communities with high unemployment or promote safe housing in poor neighborhoods. Long-term changes occur as a result of modifying the conditions under which people live. Healthy People 2020 emphasizes changing the physical and social environments to improve health behaviors.

Although policy making is usually thought to occur at the national and international level, local and regional policy making can be just as fruitful in health promotion efforts. Local and regional policy making can occur through social service agencies, local transportation authorities, public safety commissions, economic development zones, and professional organizations. An advantage of beginning at the local level for policy making is that the trickle-down time is eliminated: Policy will have an influence in the community almost immediately. Community and political leaders, along with the local and state health departments, can advise and advocate large-scale changes to promote health.

Policy making is driven by stakeholder interests and uses both science-based and non-science-based information (Metcalfe & Higgins, 2009). Policy making is value driven, dynamic, often chaotic, and is about social influence, as it involves persuasion, attitude change, decision making, and compromise. Facts, or science-based information, are usually used in the early phases of policy development to identify problems and solutions, including the economic costs. However, non-science-based, or less verifiable, information presented by stakeholders who offer their informed judgments and personal experiences is also used to promote the legitimacy of a proposed policy. Both types of knowledge are needed to gain support for successful policy making. Although scientific knowledge is critical, stakeholders also need other information such as the political costs as well as the resources necessary to implement the policies. This additional information assists in the development of consensus to achieve policy development.

Barriers to public health policy formulation are numerous (Metcalfe & Higgins, 2009). First, policy-makers may not be committed to maintaining the health change. Second, a research policy practice gap may exist, in which the research has not been translated in a user-friendly language. Third, the dominance of a strong commercial market, such as the food industry, may also hinder the success of a policy formulation Fourth, policy-makers need timely information that is relevant to the problem area, continued and personal communication, and clear and simple explanations of findings and implications for policy (Ensor, Clapham, & Prasai, 2009). This points to an important component to health policy formation: a political champion or knowledge broker. This person is a respected and articulate proponent of a particular policy and recognizes how best to work with policy-makers to develop policy.

An example of a prime area for health policy formulation and implementation is physical activity. The evidence is clear that physical inactivity has negative health consequences across the life span (Haskell, Blair, & Hill 2009). Evidence also indicates that physical activity plays a role in health promotion and disease prevention. Despite the growing body of evidence, the majority of youth and adults in this country remain inactive. Local and state health departments are positioned to serve as catalysts for the institutional and community changes needed to promote physical activity (Simon, Gonzales, Ginsburg, Abrams, & Fielding, 2009). Local departments usually have connections with other community organizations, and state agencies can facilitate communication and partnerships across regions. Health policies are also needed to support the development and financing of physical activity programs in schools, communities, and work sites, and the creation of activity-friendly community environments. Health policies are needed that encourage individuals and communities to place a higher value on health and provide the resources necessary to make healthy changes. Collaborative partnership models to develop health policy must be implemented and tested to increase access to information and resources. Individuals, communities, local and state governments, and the national government are all active partners in this effort.

PROMOTING HEALTH THROUGH ENVIRONMENTAL CHANGE

The quality of the physical environment in which people live is critical to the health of populations. Traditionally, environmental health practices have focused on controlling factors that are beyond the power of most people. However, individuals and communities have control over many external factors. The goal is to help people change these factors to promote healthy environments. Not only should health-damaging features of the environment be eliminated, but health-enhancing features should be augmented and actively used to promote health and well-being.

Eliminating Health-Damaging Features of the Environment

The harmful effects of toxic substances in the environment have been vividly illustrated. Although there has been a dramatic reduction in the number of children with elevated lead levels, lead paint hazards in older houses still remains a major childhood environmental disease in the United States (Jacobs & Nevin, 2006). The major source of lead is contaminated lead dust that settles on floors and window sills and is ingested through normal hand-to-mouth contact. Exposure to high levels of lead can be fatal, but even low exposures can be toxic to the central nervous system, resulting in delayed learning, impaired hearing, and growth deficits. Children under age 6 years are especially vulnerable because their nervous systems are still developing. Regulatory changes, namely the Residential Lead Hazard Reduction Act in 1992, resulted in a decline in childhood lead poisoning in the 1990s. Research forecasting data suggest that window replacement in pre-1975 housing has resulted in lead poisoning prevention. A lead-safe window replacement initiative would be a major step toward lead poisoning prevention in children (Jacobs & Nevin, 2006).

Leading indoor air hazards to which many thousands of people are exposed each year are tobacco smoke and radon. Environmental tobacco smoke causes lung cancer in nonsmokers. Children of parents who smoke are more likely to develop lower respiratory tract infections and middle ear infections than are children of parents who do not smoke. Asthma and other respiratory diseases are triggered or worsened by tobacco smoke and other substances in the air. Other indoor hazards include tight building syndrome, which is attributed to recycled air in buildings that may breed fungi and bacteria.

The second leading cause of lung cancer, after smoking, is exposure to radon, a natural by-product of the breakdown of uranium. It is a heavy gas and has a tendency to collect in basements or other low places in homes, offices, and schools (U.S. Environmental Protection Agency, 2009). Radon can also dissolve in water and is found in homes that have their own well. Radon is inhaled and deposited in the lungs, so it is potentially damaging to surrounding lung tissues. The best way to assess radon is to measure its concentration in the air in buildings. Do-it-yourself kits are available in retail stores, or the test can be done by a licensed contractor.

Outdoor air quality continues to be a widespread environmental problem nationally and internationally. The effects are noted in premature deaths, cancer, respiratory, and cardiovascular diseases. Motor vehicles account for one-fourth of emissions that produce ground-level ozone, the largest problem in air pollution. Although emission controls that were implemented in Europe and North America have decreased ozone precursors to a small degree, concerns remain due to the increased emission of these precursors in the rapidly developing areas of the world such as South and East Asia (Cape, 2008). Employers are now encouraging and rewarding individuals to walk or use public transportation rather than drive their cars. Local and regional governments can devise public transportation systems that are amenable to communities and design streets that facilitate bicyclists and pedestrians. The increasing popularity of hybrid automobiles, which use alternative fuels, is a positive development. Nationally, support must be increased for the development and use of alternative fuels such as ethanol by commercial and private vehicles.

Water quality remains a concern because of protozoa and chemical contaminants. Industry and agricultural runoff may contaminate water. For example, the development of intensive animal feeding operations has resulted in the discharge of improperly treated animal wastes into recreational and drinking water. Mercury has been found in breast milk of mothers who live near gold-mining areas and consume fish from contaminated runoff water from the mines (Bose-O'Reilly, Lettmeier, Roider, Siebert, & Drasch, 2008). Mercury is used to extract the gold from the ore. Mercury is neurotoxic and a hazard to infant health development. The development of new molecular technologies to detect and monitor water contamination has eliminated the inability to detect parasitic contamination. These new technologies will greatly improve water monitoring and surveillance techniques.

The environment has three functions important to health promotion. First, the environment is one of a complex group of factors that lead to healthy and unhealthy behaviors. Second, the environment moderates the effects of health promotion efforts. Last, the environment can be changed to achieve health promotion goals. Changing the environment requires targeting policy-makers in private industry as well as in government.

Risk assessment is the means by which currently available information about environmental public health problems can be organized and understood. Four major steps are involved in the risk assessment process:

1. Hazard identification
2. Dose–response assessment
3. Exposure assessment
4. Risk characterization

In hazard identification, the ranges of toxic effects for a substance are identified from the literature. The second step, dose–response assessment, is used to describe as accurately as possible the relationship between magnitude, duration, frequency, and timing of exposure to the hazard and the frequency of manifestation of the hazard's adverse effects. Human exposure assessment identifies the range of exposures experienced by the target population of concern. In the fourth step, the particular risks that are likely to be experienced by the population of interest under actual expected exposure conditions are described. This four-step assessment framework can be applied to many types of health threats that arise in the environment. Comprehensive risk assessment directs attention to the sources of risk that, if reduced, will yield the greatest public health benefits.

Health professionals should note that the tolerance for risks on the part of individuals and families is based on the characteristics of the risk itself.

1. Voluntarily assumed risks are tolerated better than those imposed by others.
2. Risks over which scientists debate and are uncertain are more feared than those in which scientific consensus endorses a risk.
3. Risks of natural origin are considered to be less threatening than those created by humans.

Responses differ according to the characteristics of the risk being considered, alternating from undue alarm to apathy. Individuals should be encouraged to consider objective information about the nature and extent of various environmental risks, rather than relying on feelings and emotions. Further, some societies base risk reduction priorities on the relative ease with which risk reduction can be achieved. Ease of resolution sometimes has a poor correspondence with the public health importance of the risks being attacked. Environmental risk reduction objectives should be based on the best available scientific knowledge about the relative risks of various pollutants to health rather than on what is emotionally appealing or politically attractive at a particular point in time.

Many major environmental risks require intensive, multifaceted, and often long-term interventions to change attitudes and reallocate resources for their control. Nurses and other health professionals need to play a proactive role in promoting health by focusing on environmental change in the local community and its work sites, such as methods to reduce environmental pollutants; safe waste disposal; monitoring and surveillance to ensure good quality water; and worker protection from toxic substances.

Augmenting Health-Promoting Features of the Environment

Major advances in public health have occurred through improvements in the built environments, such as sanitary reforms. Evidence continues to link the built environment with health outcomes. The *built environment*, defined as the way in which communities and neighborhoods are designed, includes buildings, spaces, transportation systems, homes, schools, workplaces, parks, and recreation facilities (Sallis, 2009). Physical activity and obesity have been linked to the physical attributes of neighborhoods (Sallis et al., 2009). Living in walkable neighborhoods has been found to be associated with greater physical activity and lower overweight and obesity. Policies are needed to enhance existing neighborhoods by creating green spaces and walking trails, as research also shows that older people who live in environments that support walking have better health (Sugiyama & Thompson, 2007).

Where people live makes a difference in their health. Health is related to the built environment and social capital. The neighborhood should be considered a setting in which health is enhanced. Numerous factors determine the health and wellness, as shown in health map in Figure 14–2. These factors range from individual lifestyle behaviors to the global ecosystem (Rao, Prasad, Adshead, & Tissera, 2007).

Collective efficacy, the perception of mutual trust and willingness to help each other, is a measure of neighborhood social capital that has been associated with healthy neighborhoods (Cohen, Inagami, & Finch, 2008). *Neighborhood cohesion,*

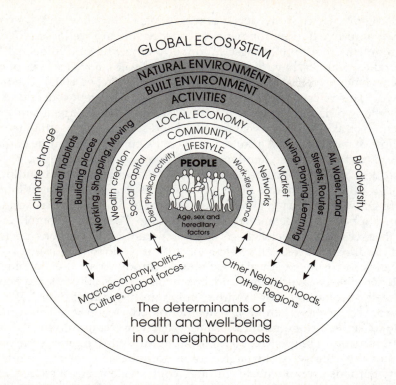

FIGURE 14–2 Health Map for Healthy Communities   *Source:* Reprinted from *The Lancet*, Volume 370, M. Rao, S. Prasad, F. Adshead and H. Tissera, "The Built Environment and Health," pages 1111–1113, Copyright 2007, with permission from Elsevier. http://www.sciencedirect.com/

another measure of social capital, refers to neighborhood's residents' sense of shared norms, values, and feelings of belonging within their local area. Perceived levels of safety can result from neighborhood social capital. Neighborhood cohesion and safety have also been shown to be associated with differences in neighborhood health (Baum, Ziersch, Zhang, & Osborne, 2009) Community-participatory interventions, along with local government involvement to create policy changes and provide resources, can change communities to become health enhancing for all of its members.

Latinos are the most physically inactive racial/ethnic group in the United States (Macera et al., 2005). The consequences are seen in the high rates of obesity and diabetes. Many Latinos live in places that are overcrowded, have high crime rates, have excessive traffic, and lack access to parks and other recreational facilities. Low-income Hispanic children are more likely to live in unsafe neighborhoods with poor street environments and greater dangers from traffic and crime (Zhu & Lee, 2008). In California, Latino communities have begun to play an active role in changing their environments by working with civic officials and school districts to address the lack of open space. Community capacity building has resulted in the "browning of the green movement," which reflects the emerging power base of the Latinos to push for transformation of their neighborhoods (Latino Coalition for a Healthy California, 2006).

Continued community capacity development along with policy and system changes are needed to improve the environments to foster health and wellness.

Environments that promote restoration, or a renewing of diminished functional resources and capabilities, have beneficial effects on health. Four features of restorative environments have been identified (Herzog, Maguire, & Nebel, 2003). The first feature is being away. This refers to settings that call on mental content that is different from normal; in other words, getting away from it all. The second feature of a restorative setting is extent. Extent refers to sufficient content and structure of a setting to occupy the mind to allow rest to occur. An example of such a setting is a Japanese garden. Third, fascination refers to effortless attention. Fascination is restorative when it is characterized by effortless attention and aesthetic beauty in the setting. Natural settings serve as an example of offering moderate fascination. The last feature is compatibility. A compatible setting is when there is a good fit between the individual's purpose and the type of activities supported or demanded by the setting. These four components can be measured to assess the beneficial effects of environments. Interventions can then be implemented to address the restorative elements that are lacking to improve well-being.

Strategies to foster health and well-being through health-enhancing environments in inner cities, at work sites, and in school settings are important for prevention and health promotion. For example, community gardens have been shown to facilitate social connections, strengthen neighborhoods, increase leisure-time physical activity, build skills, bridge ethnically and age diverse communities, and improve community nutrition (Teig et al., 2009). Community gardens have the potential to promote healthy lifestyles through community-based environmental change. Community gardens promote health through collective efficacy, a shared willingness to intervene for the good of the community. Other areas of the environment, including housing, water quality, waste disposal, and air quality; all need attention to promote the health of its citizens.

Nurses play a pivotal role in promoting community interventions to promote health. Assisting communities to define health goals, engaging sectors in the community to support safe living conditions, providing health education, teaching family health promotion skills, promoting culturally appropriate preventive services, working with schools to develop health promotion curriculum and facilitate physical activity, and promoting health in the workplace are few of the many areas in which nurses and other health care professionals can contribute.

VOLUNTARY CHANGE VERSUS LEGISLATIVE POLICY

In a democratic society, it is widely assumed that matters of risk critical to survival and security are subject to regulatory decisions, whereas risks not clearly vital to general health and welfare are issues for personal decision and action. In a democracy, even vital risks may be left to individual decision, providing that they do not infringe on the rights of others. The role of government continues to be questioned in relation to legislating environmental and behavioral changes that promote good health and increase longevity. On one hand, if the government uses the means at its disposal to regulate changes in behavior, it may be faced with problems of an ethical nature. On the other hand, voluntary, individual approaches may fall short of achieving widespread change in self-damaging behaviors.

How far policy should go in terms of individual behavior continues to be debated. Public health policy plays a major role in the regulation of advertising and taxation of harmful products as well as communicable disease control, such as quarantine and surveillance. For example, pandemic influenza preparedness requires health policy. Public policy and laws may make the task of policy-makers easier for large-scale health threats. However, the balance between public good and individual rights is a difficult dilemma (Martin, 2007). If the state has a moral obligation to protect the right of its citizens, can health measures that benefit the population as a whole be subverted by minority beliefs? The appropriate balance between public good and individual rights is a challenging one and must be continually examined.

Government involvement in lifestyle reform is to some extent supported by the long-standing role of the federal government as a health care provider. Although federal regulations might be cost-effective, many individuals may consider health promotion legislation to be unethical or place undue intrusion on their individual freedom. Ethical issues, including individual autonomy, must be thoughtfully considered in matters of health.

Two philosophical views of the role of government have been labeled individualism and paternalism (Ribisl & Humphries, 1998). *Individualism* is the American ideal, in which individuals are given maximum freedom in the area of health promotion. Health habits are considered personal, so outside interventions by governmental policy are not warranted. Poor health is attributed to individuals; thus, society's responsibility is minimized. *Paternalism*, the counterpoint, holds that experts (professionals and policy-makers) have a moral responsibility to solve health problems because individuals lack the ability to do so. Therefore, interventions, such as laws and public policies, are justified for the health of society. The role of individuals in this model is to adhere to policies. Individuals are not blamed for their problems, as they are viewed as victims of circumstance. Both views have strengths. In the individualism model, control is in the hands of the individuals, promoting a sense of efficacy and empowerment. Second, diversity of opinions is respected in the individualistic view. The strength of the paternalistic view is that it has the potential to reduce health inequities. Health policies are socially responsible as they apply to all segments of the population. In addition, problems over which individuals have no control, such as environmental issues, are recognized and addressed.

Both approaches have limitations as well. As stated throughout the book, an emphasis on individualism or personal responsibility for health may promote victim blaming, which becomes problematic, as social and environmental factors are also major determinants of health. However, overemphasis on paternalism or social responsibility may discount individual and group differences in human responses as well as the contributions of individuals to lifestyle change. Both approaches are needed to promote health in individuals and communities. Collaborative models of health promotion will promote community empowerment, embrace diversity, address environmental issues, and incorporate civic leaders and policy-makers to eliminate health inequities.

Deciding whether social changes to enhance health should be voluntary or mandatory presents a complex dilemma. Is coercion ever appropriate? If so, how, and to what extent? Is it coercive to increase cigarette taxes to help defray the cost of smoking-induced disease? Should highly refined sugar products and high-cholesterol foods also be taxed more heavily to pay for the cost of health problems due to obesity and atherosclerosis? Should taxes on large, high-speed automobiles be proportionately higher than taxes on smaller cars with limited speed and greater fuel economy? Which lifestyle, organizational, and social changes should be voluntary and which should be mandated through legislation? A balance of voluntary and mandatory action is needed, while continuing to pay close attention to the ethical dimensions of such health-related decisions.

Economic Incentives for Disease Prevention and Health Promotion

The dependence of the American people on diagnosis and treatment of disease to improve health and increase longevity is economically and socially rooted in our culture. Until recently, Americans were willing to spend escalating proportions of both personal and public dollars on an increasing array of medical services, hoping for "magic bullets" to cure all ills. However, the availability of health care technology and medical interventions exceeds society's ability to afford them. In addition, medical care is considered to account for only 10–15% of the declines in premature death in the twentieth century; factors that help to prevent illness have been responsible for the remaining decline. Health care systems are now undergoing restructuring, and new health care policies are being implemented to attempt to achieve a balance among prevention, health promotion, and disease treatment services.

Health promotion programs continue to be at a competitive disadvantage for time and money, in spite of mounting evidence that health promotion and prevention efforts reduce morbidity and mortality. Those allocating resources require evidence of cost savings, and health promotion changes may not be immediately evident. It is important for lawmakers as well as the public to understand the difference between screening for disease and prevention, as well as the difference between health promotion and disease prevention. Health promotion focuses on lifestyle changes to promote wellness. Primary prevention focuses on promoting good health practices to avoid disease. Both promote a healthy lifestyle. Goetzel (2009) states that we should ask what the most cost-effective way to improve population health is, not whether prevention saves money. With scarce resources, promoting healthy lifestyles—such as eating a healthy diet, being physically active, maintaining a normal weight, not smoking, drinking in moderation, managing stress, and surrounding oneself with family and friends—do not require costly medical treatment and have been documented to prevent and/or reduce chronic diseases such as cardiovascular disease and diabetes.

Cost-effective analysis (CEA), cost–benefit analysis, and other economic evaluations discussed in Chapter 10 have assumed an important role in research and health care policy decisions. These methods, particularly CEA, are useful for evaluating and comparing different health promotion strategies and providing health care professionals with important information related to patient preferences and priorities for prevention and health promotion. However, the results of these analyses may also be controversial if the social implications are not taken into account.

Positive effects from any health promotion program require a chain of events: (1) a structured program, (2) sustained participation, and (3) health enhancement or reduction of risk (measured by specified outcome criteria). Health-promotion program costs are incurred as the program is implemented, although benefits may not be seen until some future time. An extended time period between costs and benefits can be reconciled with cost-analysis procedures. However, consumers may not be willing to spend to protect themselves from a health problem with 20-year latency when they feel well. Emphasizing both short- and long-term benefits may enhance consumer acceptance of interventions that require individual behavioral and environmental change.

High demands for medical services result in high rates of use of resource-intensive services and less emphasis on self-care, preventive, and health promotion services. Traditional insurance coverage has offered little in the way of incentives to increase motivation for engaging in prevention and health promotion activities. Individuals and families who have insurance rarely have coverage for health promotion services, because such services cannot be related to a specific diagnosis or medical complaint. The working poor, defined as working adults who live in poverty, are less likely to use preventive care (including breast and prostate cancer screening and cholesterol screening) than nonpoor working adults (Ross, Bernheim, Bradley, Teng, & Gallo, 2007). Employers are well-positioned to play a role in promoting the health of poor and nonpoor working adults. Offering insurance coverage and work site screening programs for blood pressure, cholesterol, and influenza and other vaccinations, and educational programs that promote health are some of the strategies that can be implemented in the workplace to increase participation in prevention and health promotion. Insurance coverage for both primary and secondary prevention decreases the insurance costs spent on medical treatments, making it cost-effective for insurers (Ellis & Manning, 2007).

The current fee-for-service and per-patient models of reimbursement encourage volume-driven care rather than value-driven care. The PROMETHEUS payment model is currently being tested by the Robert Wood Johnson Foundation (Robert Wood Johnson Foundation, 2009). In this model, payment centers on paying for a comprehensive episode of care based on clinical guidelines or expert opinion for best treating the condition from beginning to end. The costs are calculated based on an evidenced-informed case rate, which creates a budget for the entire episode of care. In addition, bonuses are earned through a quality scorecard that is tied to the reduction of potentially avoidable complications (PACs). This is based on PROMETHEUS team evidence that up to 40% of every dollar spent on chronic conditions and 15–20% of every dollar spent on acute hospitalizations and procedures are attributable to PACs. This new model has potential to offer a blueprint for a new health care payment system that promotes and rewards high-quality, efficient, patient-centered care. Although the pilot program covers acute, chronic, and inpatient procedures, this model has potential for coverage of health promotion and primary prevention activities as well.

All evidence to date indicates that if health reform is not enacted to make health insurance more accessible and affordable, the United States will continue to face accelerating costs for individuals, employers, and government (Holahan, Garrett, Headen, & Lucas, 2009). The rate of health care costs will continue to increase along with the numbers of uninsured. Health reform will change who bears the burden of financing the health care system and how the burden is shared. Although health reform will be very difficult and expensive, it is projected to ultimately improve both the health and financial security of Americans.

OPPORTUNITIES FOR RESEARCH IN SOCIAL AND ENVIRONMENTAL CHANGE

Social and environmental change approaches to promote health offer many opportunities for nursing research. Suggested directions for nursing and interdisciplinary research efforts include the following:

1. Test the effects of both family and community health promotion interventions on positively altering health-related social norms among children and adolescents.
2. Develop and test environmental change strategies to reduce health threats.

3. Analyze the cost-effectiveness of financial incentives in health care plans that focus on health promotion and disease prevention services.
4. Test the effectiveness of policy changes that eliminate environmental barriers to healthy food choices and active lifestyles to treat and prevent obesity.

The study of interactive effects of human and environmental factors in health and disease is complex and requires interdisciplinary research collaboration to address the many gaps in knowledge that exist.

CONSIDERATIONS FOR PRACTICE TO PROMOTE SOCIAL AND ENVIRONMENTAL CHANGE

Health promotion and prevention interventions can no longer focus exclusively on the individual to achieve large-scale behavior change. The comprehensive view of health promotion emphasizes the need for collaboration between health care professionals, health care organizations, and policy-makers at the local, state, and national levels. Nurses will need to help build healthy communities by implementing interventions that focus on developing community competence and empowerment. Skills are needed to work with communities to identify resources, problems, and opportunities. The nurse also must learn how to implement strategies to involve community members and be able to teach leadership skills neeeded to play an active role in the change process.

Because of the multiple factors involved in behavior change that go beyond the individual, nurses also must become active in the promotion of health policy to decrease social and environmental risks present in many communities. This can be accomplished by working with local health departments and state legislatures to make change as well as participating in lobbying efforts to increase funds and services. Health promotion in the 21st century brings many challenges due to the rapid, ongoing changes in the population, workforce, technology, and health care environment. However, these challenges bring new opportunities for nurses, who, with other members of an interdisciplinary team, can create innovative plans to improve health.

Summary

This chapter focuses on society as a collective and the impact of public policy and social and physical environments on the health status of individuals, families, and communities. Attempts to promote healthy lifestyles without changes in the environments in which people live will result in frustration and failure of health promotion efforts. A balanced approach to disease prevention and health promotion requires attention to (1) quality of the social and physical environments, (2) inequities in health-promoting options available for all, and (3) changes in health policy to create healthier communities. Because health is no longer viewed as an aim in itself, but as a resource for personal and social development as well as a product of social conditions, changes in public policies should become part of any effort to promote health.

Learning Activities

1. Conduct a home or work site assessment to identify a health-damaging environmental factor. Describe the history of the problem, its effects on the health of the family or workers, barriers to solving the problem, resources needed to solve the problem, and resources available to solve the problem.
2. Develop at least three community strategies to solve the problem identified in Activity 1, and outline an evaluation plan of your possible solutions.
3. Write a letter to your state legislatures voicing your concerns about the environmental problem identified in Activity 1 and suggest how they might help solve the problem.

Selected Web Sites

Clearinghouse for Occupational Safety and Health Information
http://www.cdc.gov/niosh/homepage.html

Drug Policy Information Clearinghouse
http://whitehousedrugpolicy.gov

Food and Drug Administration
www.fda.gov

Health Resources and Services Administration
http://www.hrsa.gov

Indoor Air Quality Information Clearing House
http://www.epa.gov/iaq

National Lead Information Center
http://www.epa.gov/lead/nlic.htm

Office on Smoking and Health
www.cdc.gov/tobacco

Kaisernetwork Health Policy as it Happens
http://www.kaisernetwork.org

National Academy for State Health Policy
http://www.nashp.org

References

Abbott, P. A., & Coenen, A. (2008). Globalization and advances in information and communication technologies: The impact of nursing and health. *Nursing, Outlook, 56*, 238–246.

Anderson, L. M., Scrimshaw, S. C., Fullilove, M. T., & Fielding, J. E. (2003). The community guide's model for linking the social environment to health. *American Journal of Preventive Medicine, 24*(3S) 12–20.

Baum, F. E., Ziersch, A. M., Zhang, G., & Osborne, K. (2009). Do perceived neighborhood cohesion and safety contribute to neighborhood differences in health? *Health & Place, 15*(4), 925–934.

Bose-O'Reilly, Lettmeier, B., Roider, G., Siebert, U., & Drash, G. (2008). Mercury in breast milk: A hazard for infants in gold mining areas? *International Journal of. Hygiene and Environmental Health, 211*, 615–623.

Cape, J. N. (2008). Surface ozone concentrations and ecosystem health: Past trends and a guide to future projections. *Science of the Total Environment, 400*, 257–269.

Cohen, D. A., Inagami, S., & Finch, B. (2008). The built environment and collective efficacy. *Health & Place, 14*, 198–208.

Dalen, J. E., & Alpert, J. S. (2008). National health insurance: Could it work in the U.S.? *The American Journal of Medicine, 121*, 553–554.

Editorial. (2009, 5 March). What price health? *Nature, 458*(7234), 7 (published online 4 March 2009). Retrieved from http://www.nature.com/nature/journal/v458/n7234/pdf/458007a.pdf

Ellis, R. P., & Manning, W. G. (2007). Optimal health insurance for prevention and treatment. *Journal of Health Economics, 26*, 1128–1150.

Ensor, T., Clapham, S., & Prasai, P. (2009). What drives health policy formulation? Insights from the Nepal maternity incentive scheme. *Health Policy, 90,* 247–253.

Goetzel, R. Z. (2009). Do prevention or treatment services save money? The wrong debate. *Health Affairs, 28,* 37–41.

Halamka, J. D., Mandl, K. D., & Tang, P. C. (2008). Early experiences with the personal health record. *Journal of the American Medical Informatics Association, 15,* 1–7.

Halle, M., & Seshamani, M. (2009). Hidden costs of health care. Retrieved from http://www .healthreform.gov

Haskell, W. L., Blair, S. N., & Hill, J. O. (2009). Physical activity: Health outcomes and importance for public health policy. *Preventive Medicine, 49*(4), 280–282.

Herzog, T. R., Maguire, C. P., & Nebel, M. B. (2003). Assessing the restorative components of environments. *Journal of Environmental Psychology, 23,* 159–170.

Holahan, J., Garrett, B., Headen, I., & Lucas, A. (2009). *Health reform: The cost of failure.* Princeton, NJ: RWJ Urban Institute.

Jacobs, D. E. & Nevin, R. (2006). Validation of a 20-year forecast of U.S. childhood lead poisoning: Updated prospects for 2010. *Environmental Research, 102,* 352–364.

Latino Coalition for a Healthy California. (2006). Retrieved from http://www.lchc.org /documents/obesity/LatinosLCHV.pdf

Macera, C. A., Ham, S. A., Yore, M. M., Jones D. A., Ainsworth B. E., Kimsey C. D., et al. (2005, April). Prevalence of physical activity in the United States: Behavioral Risk Factor Surveillance System, 2001. *Prevention of Chronic Disease* [serial online]. Retrieved from http://www.cdc.gov/pcd/issues/2005

Martin, R. (2007). Law as a tool in promoting and protecting public health: Always in our best interests? *Public Health, 121,* 846–853.

Metcalfe, G., & Higgins, C. (2009). Health public policy: Is health impact assessment the cornerstone? *Public Health, 123,* 296–310.

Minkler, M., Wallerstein, N., & Wilson, N. (2008). Improving health through community organization and community building. In K. Glanz, B. K. Rimer, & K. Viswanath (Eds.), *Health behavior and health education* (4th ed.,

pp. 287–309). San Francisco: Jossey-Bass Publishers.

Rao, M., Prasad, S., Adshead, F., & Tissera, H. (2007). The built environment and health. *The Lancet, 370,* 1111–1113.

Raphael, D. (2007). Public policies and the problematic USA populations' health profile. *Health Policy, 84,* 101–111.

Ribisl, K. M., & Humphries, K. (1998). Collaboration between professionals and mediating structures in the community: Towards a "Third Way" in health promotion. In S. A. Shumaker, E. B. Schron, J. K. Ockene & W. L. McBee, (Eds.), *The handbook of health behavior change* (2nd ed., pp. 535–554). New York: Springer.

Robert Wood Johnson Foundation. (2009). What is PROMETHEUS payment? An evidence-informed model for payment reform. Retrieved from http://www .PrometheusPayment.org

Ross, J. S., Bernheim, S. M., Bradley, E. H., Teng, H., & Gallo, W. T. (2007). Use of preventive care by the working poor in the United States. *Preventive Medicine, 44,* 254–259.

Sallis, J. F. (2009). Measuring physical activity environments. A brief history. *American Journal of Preventive Medicine, 36*(4S), S86–S92.

Sallis, J. F., Saelens, B. E., Frank, L. D., Conway, T. L., Slymen, D. J., Cain, K. L., et al. (2009). Neighborhood built environment and income: Examining multiple health outcomes. *Social Science & Medicine, 68,* 1285–1293.

Simon, P., Gonzales, E., Ginsburg, D., Abrams, J., & Fielding, J. (2009). Physical activity promotion: A local and state health department perspective. *Preventive Medicine, 49*(4), 297–298.

Sugiyama, T., & Thompson, C. W. (2007). Older people's health, outdoor activity and supportiveness of neighborhood environments. *Landscape and Urban Planning, 83,* 168–175.

Tang, P. C., Ash, J. S., Bates, D. W., Overhage, J. M., & Sands, D. Z. (2006). Personal health records: Definitions, benefits, and strategies for overcoming barriers to adoption. *Journal of the American Medical Informatics Association, 13,* 121–126.

Teig, E., Amulya, J., Bardwell, L., Buchenau, M., Marshall, J. A., & Litt, J. S. (2009). Collective efficacy in Denver, Colorado: Strengthening neighborhoods and health through community gardens. *Health & Place, 15*(4), 1115–1122.

U.S. Department of Health and Human Services. (2009). Healthy People 2020. Retrieved from http://www.healthypeople2020.gov

U.S. Environmental Protection Agency. (2009). *Radon*, Retrieved July 10, 2009, from http://www.epa.gov/radiatoin/radionuclides/radon.htm

U.S. FDA. (2009). *FDA & tobacco regulation.* Retrieved July 10, 2009 from http://www.fda.gov/NewsEvents/PublicHealthFocus/ucm168412.htm

Walls, H. L., Peeters, A., Loff, B., & Crammond, B. R. (2009). Why education and choice won't solve the obesity problem. *American Journal of Public Health, 99,* 590–592.

World Health Organization. (2008). *Closing the gap in a generation.* Geneva, Switzerland: WHO. Retrieved from http://who.int/social determinants/the commission/final report/en/index.htm

Zhu, X., & Lee, C. (2008). Walkability and safety around elementary schools: Economic and ethnic disparities. *American Journal of Preventive Medicine, 34*(4), 282–290.

INDEX

Stress management approaches
  stress-inducing situation frequency minimization, 201–3
  stress resistance increasing, 203–6
Stressors, 196
Stress resistance, increasing
  assertiveness increasing in, 205
  coping resources building in, 205–6
  exercise promotion in, 203–4
  physical/pscyhologic, 203
  realistic goal setting in, 205
  self-efficacy enhancement in, 204–5
  self-esteem enhancement in, 204
SWEAT2. *See* Sedentary Exercise Adherence Trial
Systems theory, 70–71

T

Tannahill, A., 28
Technology advances influence, on global health promotion, 2–3
Theory of planned behavior (TPB), 40, 41–42
Theory of reasoned action (TRA), 40–41
Throughput, 71
TPB. *See* Theory of planned behavior
TRA. *See* Theory of reasoned action
Transtheoretical model, 51–53
True-false statements assessment, 108
Trunk flexion, 98

U

United States (U.S.). *See also specific U.S. topics*
  health care system/reform, 324–25, 334–35
  health policy, 326
  health promotion national progress, 3–5
University of South Carolina Children and Family Healthcare Center, 311
Uplifts, 101–3
Upstream interventions, 248
U.S. Department of Agriculture Food Guide, 171
U.S. Department of Health and Human Services, 3, 89
U.S. Department of Health and Human Services (USDHHS), 141–42, 171
U.S. Preventive Services Task Force (USPSTF), 122
U.S. Task Force on Community Interventions, 151
U.S. Task Force on Preventive Services *Community Guide*, 184, 185
USDHHS. *See* U.S. Department of Health and Human Services
USDHHS Physical Activity Guidelines Advisory Committee, 141–42
USPSTF. *See* U.S. Preventive Services Task Force

V

Virtual communities, and social support, 225–26
Vision, 313
Vulnerable populations, 287
Vulnerable populations health
  disparities, 287–89
  racial/ethnic, 288
  socioeconomic status and, 288
Vulnerable populations health promotion, 286
  characteristics to assess, 293–94
  considerations for practice, 299
  culturally appropriate intervention strategies, 297–98
  culturally relevant intervention strategies, 294, 295–96
  designing culturally competent programs for, 293–97
  health care professionals/cultural competence and, 291–93
  of health equity, 289–91
  research opportunities, 298–99

W

Ware, J. E., 29
Water quality, 329
Ways of Coping Questionnaire, 103, 206
Web-based behavior change interventions, 59
Weight
  gain and physical activity, 141
  healthy/unhealthy guidelines, 102
  maintenance strategies for recommended, 186
  reduction program initiation strategies, 186–88
Well-being, and individual health definition, 20–22
Wellness
  high-level, 20
  individual health definition as, 20, 21
WHO. *See* World Health Organization
Whole community interventions, 157–58
Women: Stay healthy at any age (AHRQ), 122
Work, and stress/health, 200–201
Work site
  adult physical activity promotion in, 156–57, 309–10
  health promotion, 308–10
Worksite Opportunities for Wellness (WOW), 157
World Health Organization (WHO), 1–2, 322
  Global Burden of Disease Survey, 196
  health definition, 17, 196
WOW. *See* Worksite Opportunities for Wellness
Wu, R., 22

Y

Youth Risk Behavioral Surveillance System (YRBSS), 4